T0259054

Sports Neurology

Guest Editor

CORY TOTH, MD, FRCPC

PHYSICAL MEDICINE AND REHABILITATION CLINICS OF NORTH AMERICA

www.pmr.theclinics.com

Consulting Editor
GEORGE H. KRAFT, MD, MS

February 2009 • Volume 20 • Number 1

SAUNDERS an imprint of ELSEVIER, Inc.

W.B. SAUNDERS COMPANY
A Division of Elsevier Inc.

1600 John F. Kennedy Boulevard • Suite 1800 • Philadelphia, Pennsylvania 19103

http://www.theclinics.com

PHYSICAL MEDICINE AND REHABILITATION CLINICS OF NORTH AMERICA Volume 20, Number 1
February 2009 ISSN 1047-9651, ISBN-10: 1-4377-0743-2, ISBN-13: 978-1-4377-0743-4

Editor: Debora Dellapena

Reprints. For copies of 100 or more of articles in this publication, please contact the Commercial Reprints Department, Elsevier Inc., 360 Park Avenue South, New York, NY 10010-1710. Tel.: 212-633-3812; Fax: 212-462-1935; E-mail: reprints@elsevier.com.

Physical Medicine and Rehabilitation Clinics of North America (ISSN 1047-9651) is published quarterly by Elsevier Inc., 360 Park Avenue South, New York, NY 10010-1710. Months of publication are February, May, August, and November. Business and Editorial Offices: 1600 John F. Kennedy Blvd., Suite 1800, Philadelphia, PA 19103-2899. Customer Service Office: 11830 Westline Industrial Drive, St. Louis, MO 63146. Periodicals postage paid at New York, NY and additional mailing offices. Subscription price per year is $213.00 (US individuals), $339.00 (US institutions), $107.00 (US students), $259.00 (Canadian individuals), $443.00 (Canadian institutions), $155.00 (Canadian students), $319.00 (foreign individuals), $443.00 (foreign institutions), and $155.00 (foreign students). Foreign air speed delivery is included in all *Clinics* subscription prices. All prices are subject to change without notice. **POSTMASTER:** Send address changes to *Physical Medicine and Rehabilitation Clinics of North America*, Elsevier Periodicals Customer Service, 11830 Westline Industrial Drive, St. Louis, MO 63146. **Customer Service: 1-800-654-2452 (US). From outside of the United States, call 314-453-7041. Fax: 314-453-5170. E-mail: JournalsCustomerService-usa@elsevier.com (for print support); JournalsOnlineSupport-usa@elsevier.com (for online support).**

Physical Medicine and Rehabilitation Clinics of North America is indexed in *Excerpta Medica, MEDLINE/ PubMed (Index Medicus), Cinahl,* and *Cumulative Index to Nursing and Allied Health Literature.*

Printed and bound by CPI Group (UK) Ltd, Croydon, CR0 4YY

Transferred to Digital Print 2011

Contributors

CONSULTING EDITOR

GEORGE H. KRAFT, MD, MS
Alvord Professor of Multiple Sclerosis Research; Professor, Rehabilitation Medicine; and Adjunct Professor, Neurology, University of Washington School of Medicine, Seattle, Washington

GUEST EDITOR

CORY TOTH, MD, FRCPC
Assistant Professor of Neurology, Department of Clinical Neurosciences, University of Calgary, Calgary, Alberta, Canada

AUTHORS

BARRY P. BODEN, MD
Adjunct Associate Professor in Surgery, The Uniformed Services University of the Health Sciences, Bethesda; and Orthopedic Surgeon, The Orthopaedic Center, Rockville, Maryland

FRANCESCO BOTRÈ
Professor, Laboratorio Antidoping, Federazione Medico Sportiva Italiana; and Dipartimento per le Tecnologie, le Risorse e lo Sviluppo, "Sapienza" Università di Roma, Rome, Italy

KEVIN BUSCHE, BSc, MD, FRCPC NEUROLOGY
Clinical Assistant Professor, Division of Neurology, Department of Clinical Neurosciences, Faculty of Medicine, University of Calgary Health Sciences Center; Division of Neurology, Calgary Health Region, Rockyview General Hospital, Calgary, Alberta, Canada

PETER A. CAMERON, MBBS, MD, FACEM
Professor, Department of Epidemiology and Preventive Medicine, Monash University, The Alfred Hospital, Melbourne, Victoria, Australia

IRA R. CASSON, MD
Mild Traumatic Brain Injury Committee, National Football League, New York; Department of Neurology, Long Island Jewish Medical Center, Albert Einstein College of Medicine, New Hyde Park, Bronx, New York

BRIAN CHAZE, BA
Section of Neurosurgery, University of Manitoba, Winnipeg, Manitoba, Canada

HOWARD B. COHEN, DDS, MA, PhD
Faculty of Dentistry, University of Toronto; Dufferin Rogers Dental, Toronto, Ontario, Canada

CRAIG A. CUMMINS, MD
Lake Cook Orthopedic Associates, Barrington, Illinois

MICHAELA C. DEVRIES, BSc, MSc
Pediatrics and Medicine, Division of Neurology, McMaster University, McMaster University Medical Center, Hamilton, Ontario, Canada

OLIVIER GIRARD, PhD
Lecturer, Motor Efficiency and Deficiency Laboratory, Faculty of Sport Sciences, University of Montpellier, Montpellier, France

JODI HAWES, MD, PT
Resident, Department of Neurology, Duke University Medical Center, Durham, North Carolina

CHRISTOPHER G. JARVIS, MD
Chief, Soldier Health Services, Family and Sports Medicine, Fort Campbell, Kentucky

JAMES KENNEDY, MD, PhD
Resident, Division of Plastic Surgery, Department of Surgery, Faculty of Medicine, University of Calgary; Foothills Hospital, Calgary, Alberta, Canada

MICHAEL L. LEVY, MD, PhD
Associate Professor of Surgery, Division of Neurological Surgery, University of California, San Diego Medical Center; Chief, Department of Pediatric Neurosurgery, Rady Children's Hospital, San Diego, California

MARK LOVELL, PhD
Director, Sports Medicine Concussion Program, Department of Orthopaedic Surgery, University of Pittsburgh Medical Center; Associate Professor, University of Pittsburgh, Pittsburgh, Pennsylvania

E. WAYNE MASSEY, MD, FAAN, FACP
Professor of Medicine, Department of Neurology, Duke University Medical Center, Durham, North Carolina

KELLY A. McKEAN, MSc
Nike Sports Research Laboratory, Beaverton, Oregon

PAUL R. McCRORY, MBBS, PhD, FRACP, FACSP, FASMF, FACSM, FRSM, GradDipEpidStats
Associate Professor, Centre for Health, Exercise, and Sports Medicine and the Brain Research Institute, University of Melbourne, Carlton, Melbourne, Victoria, Australia

PATRICK McDONALD, MD, MHSc, FRCSC
Assistant Professor, Section of Neurosurgery, University of Manitoba; Director, Pediatric Neurosurgery, Winnipeg Children's Hospital, Winnipeg, Manitoba, Canada

GRÉGOIRE P. MILLET, PhD
Senior Physiologist, ASPIRE Academy for Sports Excellence, Doha, Qatar

ANTONIO PAVAN, MD
Professor, Servizio di Immunoematologia e Medicina Trasfusionale, II Facoltà di Medicina e Chirurgia, Azienda Ospedaliera Sant'Andrea, "Sapienza" Università di Roma, Via di Grottarossa, Rome, Italy

MIN S. PARK, MD
Resident-Physician, Division of Neurological Surgery, University of California, San Diego Medical Center, San Diego, California

ELLIOT J. PELLMAN, MD
Mild Traumatic Brain Injury Committee, National Football League, New York; ProHEALTH Care Associates, LLP, Lake Success; Department of Medicine, Mount Sinai School of Medicine; Department of Orthopaedics, Mount Sinai School of Medicine, New York, New York

CHARLES SAMUELS MD, CCFP, DABSM
Medical Director, Centre for Sleep and Human Performance; Associate Adjunct Professor, Department of Family Medicine, Faculty of Medicine, University of Calgary, Calgary, Alberta, Canada; Principle Investigator, Calgary Police Service Health and Human Performance Research Initiative; Co-investigator, Canadian Sports Centre Sleep and Human Performance Research Project, Calgary, Alberta, Canada

DAVID S. SCHNEIDER, DO
Lake Cook Orthopedic Associates, Barrington, Illinois

MARK A. TARNOPOLSKY, MD, PhD, FRCPC
Pediatrics and Medicine, Division of Neurology, McMaster University, McMaster University Medical Center; and Neurometabolic, Neuromuscular Clinic, McMaster University, Hamilton, Ontario, Canada

CHARLES H. TATOR, MD, PhD, FACS, FRCSC
Professor of Neurosurgery, University of Toronto, Toronto; Toronto Western Hospital, Toronto, Ontario, Canada

CORY TOTH, MD, FRCPC
Assistant Professor of Neurology, Department of Clinical Neurosciences, University of Calgary, Alberta, Canada

DAVID C. VIANO, Dr. med., PhD
Mild Traumatic Brain Injury Committee, National Football League, New York, New York; ProBiomechanics LLC, Bloomfield Hills, Michigan

STEPHANIE R. WALKER, MA, MLS
Associate Librarian for Information Services, Brooklyn College of the City University of New York, Brooklyn, New York

RICHARD A. WENNBERG, MD, MSc, FRCPC
Associate Professor, Faculty of Medicine (Neurology), Division of Neurology, Toronto Western Hospital, University of Toronto, Toronto, Ontario, Canada

TSHARNI R. ZAZRYN, BAppSci (Human Movement)
Department of Health Science, Monash University, Frankston, Melbourne, Victoria, Australia

Contents

Sports and recreational activities are associated with a variety of injuries. Although many of these injuries are musculoskeletal in nature, both the peripheral nervous system and the central nervous system are at risk for injury as well. This article examines the incidence of nervous system injuries in particular sports. The association between particular forms of injuries and the sports in which they are likely to be incurred are also investigated. Further assessment of preventative measures is provided when possible.

With the increased conditioning, size, and speed of professional athletes and the increase in individuals engaging in sports and recreational activities, there is potential for rising numbers of traumatic brain injuries in sports. Fortunately, parallel strides in basic research technology and improvements in computer and video technology have created a new era of discovery in the study of the biomechanical aspects of sports-related head injuries. Although prevention will always be the most important factor in reducing the incidence of sports-related traumatic brain injuries, ongoing studies will lead to the development of newer protective equipment, improved recognition and management of concussions on the field of play, and modification of rules and guidelines to make these activities safer and more enjoyable.

This article provides a review of contemporary standards for the management of athletes who have sustained a sports-related head injury. Recent research regarding concussion management is reviewed with specific reference to clinical care. The use of neuropsychologic testing in sports also is reviewed, and a systematic protocol for the management of sports-related concussion is presented.

Athletic competition has long been a known source of spinal injuries. Approximately 8.7% of all new cases of spinal cord injuries in the United States are related to sports activities. The sports activities that have the highest risk of catastrophic spinal injuries are football, ice hockey, wrestling, diving, skiing, snowboarding, rugby, and cheerleading. Axial compression forces to the top of the head can lead to cervical fracture and quadriplegia in any sport. It is critical for any medical personnel responsible for athletes in team sports to have a plan for stabilization and transfer of an athlete who sustains a cervical spine injury.

Spinal injuries and spinal cord injuries in sports and recreation represent frequent and important causes of injury and disability. These injuries are virtually all preventable through strict adherence to the codes of conduct of the rules and regulations for sports and recreation and through an attitude of respect for one's own welfare and the welfare of the opponents or other participants. Adherence to guidelines for return to sport after injury can help to prevent worsening of deficits and the onset of new deficits.

Many different sports and recreational activities are associated with injuries to the peripheral nervous system (PNS). Although some of those injuries are specific to an individual sport, other peripheral nerve injuries occur ubiquitously within many sporting activities. This review of sport-specific PNS injuries should assist in the understanding of morbidity associated with particular sporting activities, professional or amateur. Proper recognition of these syndromes can prevent unnecessary diagnostic testing and delays in proper diagnosis. The sports most commonly associated with peripheral nerve injuries are likely football, hockey, and baseball, but many other sports have unique associations with peripheral nerve injury. This article should be of assistance for the neurologist, neurosurgeon, orthopedic surgeon, physiatrist, sports medicine doctor, and general physician in contact with athletes at risk for neurologic injuries.

The relative contribution and source of the fuels used during endurance exercise is dependent on the intensity and the duration of the exercise. Much work has been done to investigate the potential performance-enhancing effect of manipulating training and dietary interventions in athletes, as well as the influence of gender. Studies show that even patients with metabolic myopathies may derive benefits that counter the age-associated loss of muscle mass and strength. This article gives an overview of these different impacts on endurance exercise, concluding with an examination of the metabolic myopathies that impair substrate metabolism in skeletal muscle and result in exercise intolerance.

Section 3 – Variables in Sport

This article considers the health risks associated with the abuse of performance-enhancing drugs (PEDs) in sport. After an overview on the evolution of doping substances and methods and on the current international organization of the antidoping tests, the potential risks correlated with abuse of PEDs are presented. Specific problems of drug associations, designer steroids, and nutritional supplements also are discussed. Data from randomized clinical trials may not be sufficient to identify the complete range of adverse effects possible with abuse of PEDs; more specific studies are necessary to assess their actual toxic potential.

The relationship of sleep to post-exercise recovery (PER) and athletic performance is a topic of great interest because of the growing body of scientific evidence confirming a link between critical sleep factors, cognitive processes, and metabolic function. Sleep restriction (sleep deprivation), sleep disturbance (poor sleep quality), and circadian rhythm disturbance (jet lag) are the key sleep factors that affect the overall restorative quality of the sleep state. This article discusses these theoretic concepts, presents relevant clinical cases, and reviews pilot data exploring the prevalence of sleep disturbance in two groups of high-performance athletes.

This article describes the physiologic and neural mechanisms that cause neuromuscular fatigue in racquet sports: table tennis, tennis, squash, and badminton. In these intermittent and dual activities, performance may be limited as a match progresses because of a reduced central activation, linked to changes in neurotransmitter concentration or in response to afferent sensory feedback. Alternatively, modulation of spinal loop properties may occur because of changes in metabolic or mechanical properties within the muscle. Finally, increased fatigue manifested by mistimed strokes, lower speed, and altered on-court movements may be caused by ionic disturbances and impairments in excitation-contraction coupling properties. These alterations in neuromuscular function contribute to decrease in racquet sports performance observed under fatigue.

regions of the body can be used for contact, they are similar in competitor exposure time. Their acute injury rates are similar; thus their injuries can appropriately be considered together. Injuries of all types occur in combat sports, with injuries in between one fifth to one half of all fights in boxing, karate, and tae kwon do. Most boxing injuries are to the head and neck region. In other combat sports, the head and neck region are the second (after the lower limbs) or the first most common injury site.

Cycling is often considered a leisurely activity with minimal potential for severe or chronic injury. Acute head and spinal trauma can be devastating and can predominantly contribute to all-cause mortality in injuries attributed to cycling. Chronic overuse injuries primarily affecting the ulnar, median, and pudendal nerves are also a cause of significant morbidity for the cyclist.

Neurologic running injuries account for a small number of running injuries. This may be caused by misdiagnosis or underdiagnosis. Nerve injuries that have been reported in runners include injuries to the interdigital nerves and the tibial, peroneal, and sural nerves. In this article, the etiology, symptoms, diagnosis, and treatment of these injuries are reviewed. Differences between nerve injury and more common musculoskeletal injury have been presented to aid in differential diagnosis.

Interest in scuba (self-contained underwater breathing apparatus) diving increased in the 1970s, and undersea diving continues to be a popular sport early in the 21st century, with approximately 3 million certified divers in the United States. The Divers Alert Network (DAN), an institution created in 1981 by the Commerce Department, National Oceanic and Atmospheric Administration, has collected diving injury data for US and Canadian divers since 1987 that can be studied to suggest the epidemiologic characteristics of diving. This article examines neurologic injuries resulting from scuba diving.

Weight lifting and other forms of strength training are becoming more common because of an increased awareness of the need to maintain individual physical fitness. Emergency room data indicate that injuries caused by weight training have become more universal over time, likely because of increased participation rates. Neurologic injuries can result from weight lifting and related practices. Although predominantly peripheral nervous system injuries have been described, central nervous system disease

THE CLINICS ARE NOW AVAILABLE ONLINE!

Access your subscription at:
www.theclinics.com

Foreword

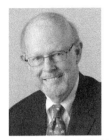

George H. Kraft, MD, MS
Consulting Editor

As I have mentioned in several previous forewords in *Physical Medicine and Rehabilitation Clinics,* sports medicine has become a popular part of our specialty. In many physical medicine and rehabilitation residency training programs, well over half of the graduates take sports and spine/musculoskeletal medicine fellowships. This is becoming a very important part of our field and we want to increase the frequency of *Clinics* issues dealing with such topics. For example, the most recent issue on sports was in May of 2008; and here, February, 2009, is another.

But this issue is different. In fact, it is unique in the entire history of this series. This issue was made possible because of a policy now being implemented by Saunders/Elsevier to allow "cross publishing" of appropriate issues. This issue on sports neurology was initially published as the February, 2008 (Volume 26, Number 1) issue of Saunders' *Neurologic Clinics*. It is now being made available to readers of the *Physical Medicine and Rehabilitation Clinics*.

This issue represents a logical inclusion to our intermittent series on sports medicine. A very important component of managing sports injuries is attending to the accompanying neurological injury—whether it be of the peripheral nerve, plexus, nerve root, spinal cord, or brain. That is the focus of this issue.

This issue draws upon an eclectic mix of physicians and scientists from various specialties: neurology, neurosurgery, orthopedics, preventive medicine, dentistry, pediatrics, plastic surgery, family medicine, and physiatry. These specialists hail from academia, trauma hospitals, military services, the National Football League, industry (Nike), and library science. It is a large issue, full of important information about the neurological sequelle of sports injuries, and will complement all of our previous publications on sports medicine.

I am indebted to the Guest Editor, Cory Toth, MD, FRCPC, of the Department of Clinical Neurosciences at the University of Calgary, in Calgary, Alberta, who initially brought together these experts and organized their contributions into a wide-ranging *tour de force*. Readers will benefit from his and the authors' efforts. Thanks also to Randolph W. Evans, MD, the Consulting Editor of the *Neurologic Clinics* for his concurrence in this project and to Deb Dellapena, Elsevier's in-house editor with whom I have happily worked for many years.

Phys Med Rehabil Clin N Am 20 (2009) xv–xvi
doi:10.1016/j.pmr.2008.11.001
1047-9651/08/$ – see front matter

Hopefully, the readers of the *Physical Medicine and Rehabilitation Clinics of North America*—especially those involved in sports medicine—will agree that this is a valuable issue for their collection. Please let us know if you agree. Here is to good reading, good patient care, and to eclecticism!

George H. Kraft, MD, MS
Alvord Professor of Multiple Scelerosis Research
Adjunct Professor, Neurology
Professor, Rehabilitation Medicine
University of Washington
1959 NE Pacific Street, Box 356490
Seattle, WA 98195-6490, USA

E-mail address:
ghkraft@u.washington.edu (G.H. Kraft)

Preface

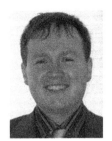

Cory Toth, MD, FRCPC
Guest Editor

The study of sporting biomechanics has been unmistakable for numerous civilizations and epochs. Beginning with the early works of Aristotle detailing human anatomy, Leonardo da Vinci's studies of anatomy concentrating upon muscles and tendons, and Etienne Jules Marey's examination of the heart beat, respiration, muscles, and movement of the body, assessment of the human body's abilities and activity has evolved over millenia. Since those early years, sports medicine has developed and grown with the emergence of new sports, new levels of competition, and new applications of biomechanics within human sporting activities. Special recognition of sport-specific problems has developed over time, such as with concussion from hockey and football, spinal cord problems from winter sports, and excessive pediatric injury associated with trampoline usage. The distinctiveness of many sports-related neurologic injuries has led to new interest in their prevalence, recognition, and prevention. This knowledge is important for diagnosis, immediate therapy, and rehabilitation following sports injuries.

This issue of *Physical Medicine and Rehabilitation Clinics* contains 19 articles examining aspects of sports-related injuries with emphasis on their impact to the nervous system. In addition to articles devoted to recognition and management of concussion and spinal cord injury, articles are also dedicated to the biomechanics of such injuries. Specialized articles have also been included to examine the importance of sleep deprivation, utilization of drugs of abuse, and the significance of fatigue to the athlete's well being and physiological functioning. The next section examines injuries related to the individual sports such as running and cycling, and team sports such as hockey and football. Topics both well-known and not so well-known to the physiatrist and other clinicians have been included. We have also designed this *Physical Medicine and Rehabilitation Clinics* issue to be of interest to the athlete, fan of athletic competitions, and the lay person as well. The issue may also be of interest to other physicians such as sports medicine specialists, neurosurgeons, neurologists, occupational medicine specialists, orthopedic surgeons, emergency medicine specialists, neuropsychologists, and general practitioners. We also hope that kinesiologists, physical therapists, sports trainers, and occupational therapists will be interested in many aspects of this issue.

Phys Med Rehabil Clin N Am 20 (2009) xvii–xviii
doi:10.1016/j.pmr.2008.11.002
1047-9651/08/$ – see front matter

I am very grateful to all of the outstanding contributors. I also appreciate the incentive by Randolph W. Evans to edit this collection, and all of the feedback provided by Deb Dellapena and her colleagues at Elsevier.

This is a great collection of important and timely articles that was composed with the contributors' visions, and I am pleased to assist in presenting this knowledge to the medical community and beyond. I hope that this collection is integral to the greater understanding of sports-related injuries in the rehabilitation community.

Cory Toth, MD, FRCPC
Department of Clinical Neurosciences
University of Calgary
3330 Hospital Drive NW
Rm 155, Heritage Medical Research Bldg
Calgary Alberta T2N 4N1, Canada

E-mail address:
corytoth@shaw.ca (C. Toth)

Section 1

Epidemiology

The Epidemiology of Injuries to the Nervous System Resulting from Sport and Recreation

Cory Toth, MD, FRCPC

KEYWORDS

- Epidemiology • Nerve entrapment • Concussion
- Spinal cord injury • Sport • Recreation

Sports-associated biomechanics have been observed and studied since the time of Aristotle, who studied human and animal gait. Leonardo da Vinci made observations regarding human motion and considered the importance of grade locomotion and the effects of running into the wind, centers of gravity, and standing and stepping. In recent years, sports medicine has grown with the appearance of new sports, new levels of competition, and new applications of biomechanics. Greater reporting of injury within sports has led to new levels of understanding of sports-related injuries. Recognition of excessive injury rates within particular sports has developed, such as concussion in hockey and football, spinal cord problems in winter sports, and excessive pediatric injury associated with trampoline use, and this knowledge has led to changes in prophylaxis and recommendations regarding methods of playing sports. Position statements regarding the avoidance of activities, such as children's use of trampolines, have arisen as a result of improved reporting.

Depending on the sporting activity, age of the participants, and level of competition, rates of injury to the nervous system and the types of nervous system injury vary. One of the unique qualities regarding sporting-related neurologic injuries is the uniform nature of injuries identified within particular individual sports. For example, injuries in racquet sports and volleyball are almost exclusively injuries to the peripheral nervous system around the dominant arm. The physician may be confronted with symptoms and signs reflecting injury to a number of neurologic levels, which may include the peripheral nerve, spinal roots, brachial plexus, spinal cord, or cerebrum. Recognition of the specific injury and its relationship to a specific sporting activity may help the physician make a prompt diagnosis and sound decisions regarding possible therapies.

This article originally appeared in *Neurologic Clinics*, volume 26, issue 1.
Department of Clinical Neurosciences, University of Calgary, Room 155, Heritage Medical Research Bldg., 3330 Hospital Drive NW, Calgary, Alberta T2N 4N1, Canada
E-mail address: corytoth@shaw.ca

This article reviews the epidemiology of injury, and particularly nervous system injury, for sports-related injuries reported in the scientific literature. Further information is given regarding specific aspects of the injury as related to the individual sport, whenever possible. In most cases, central nervous system (CNS) injuries are highlighted, because there is little epidemiology regarding the more infrequent injuries to the peripheral nervous system. Overall injury rates are provided as possible to place the impact of nervous system injuries into context (**Table 1**).

AUTOMOBILE RACING

A retrospective study over six seasons at the Indianapolis Raceway Park identified neurologic injuries in drivers during 61 open-wheel racing events. Four drivers required hospital admission, and two of these required admission to the ICU for head injuries.[1] Head trauma comprises 29% of all injuries in professional automobile racing, and open head injuries occur in 5% of these cases.[2,3] Closed head injuries rarely include intracranial hemorrhages, resulting instead in diffuse axonal injury.[2] Although exposure to emissions of carbon monoxide and vehicle fires certainly occurs in race car drivers (in one race an increased carboxyhemoglobin concentration was found in all race car drivers), no correlation has been demonstrated between carbon monoxide level and driver symptomatology.[4] Heat stroke has been reported rarely in automobile racing drivers.[5] Spinal injuries comprise 20% of sports-related injuries in professional automobile drivers and occur most often during a vehicular rollover; cervical spine or spinal cord injury seems to be the most common spinal injury.[3] One innovation that may improve the safety of race car drivers or racing motorcyclists is the introduction of additional chicanes, or turns placed in the fastest part of the racetrack. Their use on one racetrack decreased the risk of severe injury from 0.1% to 0.03%.[6]

BASEBALL AND SOFTBALL
Epidemiology

Acute injuries are more common than chronic injuries in baseball. Overall, however, baseball has one of the lower rates of injury among major sports. In children aged 7 to 13 years, the acute injury rate per 100 athlete exposures (AEs) was 1.7 for baseball and 1.0 for softball. Contusions were the most frequent type of injury; concussion comprised about 1% of all injuries.[7] The frequency of injury per team per season was 3.0 for baseball and 2.0 for softball, with more injuries occurring in games than in practices.[7] In high school student athletes, the overall injury rates per 100 player-seasons were 0.46 for softball and 0.23 for baseball.[8] At the collegiate level, baseball and softball injuries remain low.[9] Collegiate women's softball is subject to higher rates of preseason practice injuries than regular-season practice injuries (3.65/1000 AEs versus 1.68/1000 AEs). In games, collegiate women softball injury rates rise to 4.3 per 1000 AEs.[10] College male baseball players have higher rates of game-time injuries (5.78/1000 AEs) but similar rates of practice injuries (1.85/1000 AEs). Ten percent of all game injuries occurred from impact with a batted ball, an injury rate of 0.56 injuries per 1000 game AEs.[11] At an Olympian level, 29 injuries per 1000 player-matches occur in baseball, and neurologic injuries are extremely rare.[12] Of 10 different sports studied during a 3-year study period identifying mild traumatic brain injuries (MTBIs), softball accounted for only 2.1% and baseball accounted for only 1.2% of MTBIs.[8] These incidence rates are considerably lower than those for other major childhood sports such as football and hockey.

The incidence of MBTI is low among high school baseball players, with an injury rate of 0.23 per 100 player-seasons, 15 times less than that of football.[8] In Little League baseball players aged 7 to 18 years, the overall injury rate was 0.057 injuries per 100 player-hours, and the severe injury rate was 0.008 injuries per 100 player-hours; 46% of injuries were ball related, and 27% were collision related.[13] The most frequent mechanism of injury in Little League players is being hit by the ball (62% of acute injuries),[13] with the baseball usually striking the head.[14] Catastrophic injury rates in baseball are 0.37 per 100,000 high school player-games and 1.7 per 100,000 college player-games.[15] Fatality rates in baseball players are 0.067 per 100,000 high school athletes and 0.86 per 100,000 college baseball players.[15]

For collegiate baseball players, concussion comprises about 5% of all injuries.[16] One nonrandomized study found that an intervention leading to a relative reduction in injury without adverse effect on player performance or player acceptability was the use of a face guard on the batter's helmet.[17] Serious intracranial injuries affecting baseball players (eg, epidural hematoma secondary to a baseball bat striking the head or fatalities resulting from head injury) are rare.[15,18]

BASKETBALL

Injury rates generally are lower in basketball than in other popular team sports. For high school basketball players in an observational cohort study, injury rates per 100 high school player-seasons were 1.04 for girls' basketball and 0.75 for boys' basketball.[8] The incidence of MTBIs in high school basketball players is lower than in other organized sports, such as football, wrestling, and soccer. In a United States national survey, basketball injuries leading to ambulatory clinic visits were more common in male participants (5.7/1000) than in female participants (0.9/1000),[19] with neurologic injuries occurring rarely. In collegiate women basketball players, injury rates during a game (7.68/1000 AEs) are double those in practice (3.99/1000 AEs).[20] Likewise, male collegiate basketball players have more injuries in games (9.9/1000 AEs) than during practice (4.3/1000 AEs).[11] In Olympian basketball players, male injuries occur at a rate of 64 per 1000 athlete-matches, and female injuries occur at a rate of 67 per 1000 athlete-matches[12] with no indication of the rate of neurologic injuries in either group. In professional basketball players, the injury rates are 24.9 per 1000 AEs for women and 19.3 per 1000 AEs for men.[21]

Most basketball injuries are musculoskeletal injuries affecting the lower extremity. Concussion rates are estimated to be 0.3 to 0.5 per 1000 AEs.[11,20] Multiple studies have found that women collegiate basketball players are more subject to concussion, which represents 9% of all injuries in women compared with only 5% in male collegiate basketball players.[11,14,20] In one study in trauma center hospitals, basketball injuries capable of causing head injuries in 10- to 19-year-olds usually were related to striking the basketball pole or rim or being struck by a falling pole or backboard.[16]

BICYCLING

Although the incidence of injuries caused by bicycling accidents is largely unknown, some studies have provided estimates. In Norway, all bicycle injuries and fatalities are expected to be recorded but probably remain underreported (eg, single-bicycle accidents seem to be almost completely unreported in Norway, whereas in Canadian reports isolated crashes are the most common mode of injury).[22,23] Among Canadian recreational bicyclists, collision with vehicles accounts for 64% of bicycle-related deaths.[22] Although anecdotally suggested, there is no evidence that bicycle accidents are more common with bicycle motocross (BMX) style bikes than with non-BMX bikes.[24] In fact, it remains unclear which forms of bicycling may be more injury prone, and BMX bicycle riders have a lower proportion of serious injuries than bicycle racers,

Table 1
Rates of injury in major sports

Sport	Acute Injury Rate per 100 Athlete-Exposures	Acute Injury Rate per 100 Athlete-Seasons	Frequency of Injury per Team per Season	Incidence of Mild Traumatic Brain Injury per 100 Player-Seasons	Incidence of Mild Traumatic Brain Injury per 1000 Athlete-Exposures
Baseball	—	—	—	—	—
Age 7–13 y	1.7	—	3.0	—	—
Age 7–18 y	—	—	—	0.2	0.2
Age 13–17 y	—	0.2	—	—	—
Age 17–23 y	0.2	—	—	0.2	0.2
Badminton	5.0	—	—	—	—
Basketball	—	—	—	—	—
Age 13–18 y (male)	—	0.8	—	—	—
Age 13–18 y	—	1.0	—	—	—
Age 18–23 y (male)	1.0	—	—	—	0.3
Age 22–39 y (female)	0.4	—	—	—	0.5
Age 22–39 y (male)	1.9–6.4	1.0	—	—	—
Age 22–39 y (female)	2.5–6.7	1.0	—	—	—
Boxing	—	—	—	—	—
Amateur (male)	14–20	—	—	—	11–77
Professional (male)	21–45	—	—	—	186–251
Cheerleading	—	—	—	—	—
Age 6–11 y	0.1	—	—	—	<0.1
Age 12–17 y	0.8	—	—	—	<0.1
Cricket	<0.1	—	—	—	<0.1
Field hockey	—	0.5	—	—	—
Age 17–23 y (female)	7.9	—	—	—	0.5–0.7
Age 17–23 y (male)	12.6	—	—	—	1.1

Football	—	—	—	—	—
Age 7–13 y	—	—	—	—	—
Age 15–18 y	1.2	3.7	14.0	—	1.3
Age 18–23 y	1.5–4.0	—	—	6.1	2.3–6.1
Golf	1.5–4.0	—	—	6.1	2.3–6.1
Gymnastics	—	—	—	—	—
Age 18–23 y (female)	1.5	—	—	—	—
Hockey	—	—	—	—	—
Age 14–18 y (male)	0.9	75	—	3.7	3.7
Age 14–18 y (female)	0.8	—	—	—	—
Age 18–23 y (male)	0.5	—	—	4.2	1.5–4.2
Age 18–23 y (female)	1.3	—	—	—	2.7
Age 20–36 y (male)	11.9	—	—	6.6	6.6
Luge	—	39	—	—	—
Martial arts	—	—	—	—	—
Amateur	2.4	—	—	—	—
Professional	0.7–2.8	—	—	—	—
Age 7–14 y	0.6	—	—	—	—
Taekwandoe	6.3	—	—	—	—
Mountain climbing	0.2	—	—	—	—
Rodeo riding	3.2	—	—	—	—
Roller hockey	13.9	—	—	—	—
Skiing	0.2	—	—	—	2.1
Skiing, cross country	0.1	—	—	—	—
Ski Jumping	0.1–0.4	9.4	—	—	—
Snowboarding	0.4	—	—	—	6.1
Soccer	—	—	—	—	—
Age 14–18 y (male)	—	0.9	—	—	—

(continued on next page)

Table 1
(continued)

Sport	Acute Injury Rate per 100 Athlete-Exposures	Acute Injury Rate per 100 Athlete-Seasons	Frequency of Injury per Team per Season	Incidence of Mild Traumatic Brain Injury per 100 Player-Seasons	Incidence of Mild Traumatic Brain Injury per 1000 Athlete-Exposures
Age 14–18 y (female)	—	1.1	—	—	—
Age 18–23 y (female)	16.4	—	—	—	1.4
Age 18–23 y (male)	18.8	—	3.0	—	1.1
Age 22–35 y (female)	109	—	—	—	—
Age 22–35 y (male)	105	2.3	—	—	—
Softball					
Age 7–13 y (female)	1.0	—	2.0	—	—
Age 13–17 y (female)	—	0.5	—	—	—
Age 17–23 y (female)	0.4	—	2.0	—	0.3
Surfing	5.7	—	—	—	—
Volleyball	4.6	0.1	—	—	0.1–0.2
Wrestling					
Age 12–17 y (male)	2.3	1.6	—	—	—
Age 17–23 y (male)	7.3	—	—	—	1.3

including fewer head injuries.[24] Most accidents occurring in BMX riders are related to performing stunts or to poor cycling technique.[24] Approximately 7% of the injuries caused by BMX riding are concussions.[25] Although most injuries occurring in off-road bicycle racing are musculoskeletal in nature, a small incidence of concussion (< 1%) occurs, about 40% less than in other forms of cycling.[26,27] This low incidence may relate to a significantly higher rate of helmet use in bikers going off road.[27] Women seemed to be much more likely than men to sustain an serious injury while off-road biking,[28] although males have higher numbers of injuries, including cervical spinal cord injuries,[29] because of their more frequent participation.[30]

Children are subject to bicycling injuries, but it is unclear as to whether they suffer more injuries than older riders. Among pediatric admissions to a trauma center, 6% of injuries were related to bicycling.[31] Sixty-four percent of cycling-related injuries presenting to a pediatric emergency department were head and neck injuries.[32] Potentially avoidable head injuries resulting from bicycling accidents in which the participants were not wearing helmets have received media and political attention. In Canada, helmet use was associated with less likelihood of hospital admission following injury, a lower incidence of head and facial injury, and a lower incidence of concussion.[33] In the United States, the use of bicycle safety helmets for children led to a 88% risk reduction in intracranial injury and prevented skull fractures and possibly death caused by head injuries, end results possible in helmet-less children.[34]

BOXING

Boxing is perhaps the most controversial sport for physicians because of the degree of neurologic injury, questions about long-term sequelae, and the occurrence of death during a competition that is intended to injure the opponent. Both the American Medical Association and the American Academy of Pediatrics have stated opposition to both amateur and professional boxing. A major problem with determining the rates of injury in boxing is the regulatory policy–induced minimization of injuries. Nonetheless, the incidence of serious acute head injury in amateur boxing and noncompetitive boxing is believed to be lower than in the professional ranks, perhaps because of the greater degrees of regulation and reporting of injuries at the amateur level. In one study of instructional boxing in the United States Marine Corps, only one serious head injury occurred per 60,000 participants, only 0.3% of all boxing-related injuries during the study period.[35] Amateur boxing participants suffered a severe concussion or multiple knockouts in 0.58% of competitions.[36] Again, these studies may be subject to underreporting. In professional boxers, most early studies examining the sport in New York State demonstrated knockout rates of 3% per participant in the 1950s, and about three head injuries per 10 boxers in the 1980s.[37,38] A more recent study of professional boxing from Nevada has documented an overall injury rate of of 17.1 per 100 boxer-matches.[39] Male professional boxers are more likely to be injured than are female professional boxers.[39] Boxers who lose by knockout have twice the risk of injury as those boxers who do not.[39] Although the incidence of intracranial hemorrhage in boxers is unknown, acute subdural hematomas are the major cause of boxing-related mortality.[40] Despite these deaths related to acute injury, there is no evidence that boxers had a shorter life span than participants in other sports when data from the late nineteenth century and early to mid-twentieth century were assessed.[41] Assessment of neurologic injuries caused by boxing must be categorized to illuminate two important points. First, acute neurologic injuries must be distinguished from chronic brain injuries. Second, the level of competitive boxing, amateur versus professional, must be considered because of different regulations and protective gear. Obviously, acute neurologic injuries such as concussion, postconcussion syndrome, and intracranial hemorrhage are more easily identified than chronic neurologic injuries because of their immediate impact and obvious relationship to recently inflicted trauma. Serious acute intracranial injuries caused by boxing are recognized but are said by some to be rare.[40] In the case of a knockout, the boxer has sustained a concussion, which is easily recognizable.

Amateur boxing differs from professional boxing in the duration of fights, the nature of rules and regulatory policies, the degree of medical evaluation, and the use of protective devices (ie, headgear). The incidence of serious acute head injury in amateur boxing and noncompetitive boxing is thought to be lower than in the professional ranks, perhaps because of more regulation and greater reporting of injuries.[42] In amateur boxing, studies have reported the incidence of concussion or other head injury to be between 6.5% and 51.6% of all injuries.[43–46] For professional boxers, concussion and head injury rates may be higher, estimated to be between 16% and 70% of all injuries.[37,38,47] Concussion rates for both amateur and professional boxing are substantially higher than in other sports, ranging between 14 and 45 per 100 AEs.[37,38,46–48]

Chronic neurologic injuries from boxing are insidious in onset and often do not present until after the boxing career has ended.[49] Among former professional boxers who had participated in the sport for at least 3 years, 17% were found to have clinical evidence of CNS deficit considered to be attributable to boxing.[50] Measures of more chronic effects of boxing and neuropsychologic and cognitive effects have been studied many times with varying results. In fact, a systematic review has determined that there is no strong evidence associating chronic traumatic brain injury with participation in amateur boxing, although much of the available evidence is of poor quality.[51] The most severe abnormalities of neurologic functioning can be identified in the most severe cases of retired boxers who have post-boxing encephalopathy; these abnormalities, which include cerebellar, extrapyramidal, and intellectual impairments, have been termed "dementia pugilistica."[50] Other clinical features in patients who have dementia pugilistica can include tremor, dysarthria, and psychiatric changes such as explosive behavior and paranoid and jealous delusions.[52] Risk factors for a persistent CNS deficit have been varied and remain controversial. Some of the more consistent risk factors include a long boxing career with many bouts and the presence of the apolipoprotein E4 phenotype, a risk factor for other causes of neurodegeneration, including Alzheimer's disease.[46,50,53–58]

Neuropathologic abnormalities reported in former professional boxers include scarring of cerebellar folia with loss of cerebellar Purkinje cells, degeneration of the substantia nigra, the presence of neurofibrillary tangles in limbic gray matter, and the presence of cavum septum pellucidum.[59,60] Neurofibrillary tangles in dementia pugilistica brains are concentrated in the superficial neocortical layers, in contrast to Alzheimer's disease, where they predominate in deep layers.[61] As well, tau pathology in patients who have chronic traumatic injury, including boxers who have dementia pugilistica, possess the same tau epitopes found in filamentous tau inclusions in Alzheimer's disease brains, suggesting that pathologic mechanisms similar to those in Alzheimer's disease may be present.[62] Serum glial protein S-100B, postulated to have a relationship to cognitive deficits, increases immediately after boxing matches and correlates significantly with the number and severity of head blows.[63] These are all nonspecific markers of dysfunction, but their co-presence is strongly suggestive of boxing-induced encephalopathic changes.

CHEERLEADING

Cheerleading involves many high-risk maneuvers, including high team throws and daring aerial drills, frequently leading to accidents, particularly during pyramid building.[64]

Severe head injuries including skull fractures, hematomas, or cerebral edema have occurred. Mortality at the time of or within days of a head injury has occurred in two cheerleaders.[64] The number of injuries caused by cheerleading per 1000 participants per year ranges from 8.1 for 12- to 17-year-olds to 1.2 for 6- to 11-year-olds.[65] Concussion comprises 7% of all injuries (9.36/100,000 AEs) in high school cheerleaders, but catastrophic head injuries have not been reported.[66,67] In one study of concussion rates in high school athletes, cheerleading was the only sport for which the concussion rate was greater for practices than for games.[67]

CRICKET

Mean match injury incidences are quite low in cricket, ranging from 48.7 per 10,000 player-hours in test matches to 40.6 per 10,000 player-hours in 1-day international cricket, with injury prevalences of 11.3% and 8.1%, respectively. In domestic cricket matches, the incidence rates of match injury are 13.9 per 10,000 player-hours for first-class cricket, and 25.4 per 10,000 player-hours in 1-day domestic competitions.[68] Batsmen and fast bowlers are most likely to be injured.[69] Neurologic injuries seem to be very rare.

DIVING

The most common mechanism of injury associated with water activities is diving, with ervical spinal cord injury comprising 4.9% of all water-related accidents in children.[70] Cervical spinal cord injury is so common in divers that one large, retrospective study reported all spinal cord injuries associated with diving were at the cervical level[71] and led almost uniformly to quadriplegia. No further epidemiologic studies have been attempted to determine the prevalence of diving-related injuries, however.

EQUESTRIAN SPORTS

Surprisingly, injuries in equestrian sports are very common, perhaps 20 times more common than in motorcycling.[72] Closed head injuries are a common cause of injury in riders because of falls. Sixty percent of equestrian-related injuries are caused by falls from the horse;[73] 40% result from being kicked by a horse.[73] More females than males are injured in equestrian events because of the female predominance in this activity.[74] Helmet use reduces the risk and severity of head injuries,[75] but most riders are helmetless; only about 9% of riders involved in equestrian trauma were wearing helmets.[73,76,77]

FIELD HOCKEY AND LACROSSE

Despite the use of a hard ball and sticks by aggressive players, injury rates in lacrosse and field hockey tend to be much lower than other major sports. Neurologic injuries are extremely rare.[12] Field hockey was the least likely sport of 10 sports studied to cause head injury (1.1% of all MTBIs).[8] Most head injuries in field hockey are caused by ball contact.[78] The rate of concussion has increased during the last decade (0.5/1000 AEs); again, concussion rates are much higher during competition than during practice.[79,80]

In Olympian field hockey players, injury rates of 55 and 8 per 1000 player-matches occur in males and females, respectively. For collegiate women field hockey players the injury rate during games is twice that during practice (7.9 versus 3.7 injuries/1000 AEs).[79] The most common mechanisms for injury affecting female field hockey players were falls while ball handling or contact with a stick while ball handling.[80] Ankle sprains are most common injuries in both female and male field hockey players.[81]

Lacrosse-related trauma is more common among male players (81% of all cases in a male-dominated sport) and is most common among teenaged players (mean age, 16.9 years).[78] Male lacrosse players at the collegiate level also are much more likely to sustain injuries in games than during practice (12.6 versus 3.2 injuries/1000 AEs).

Of all major women's collegiate sports, lacrosse seems to have the highest percentage of injuries as concussions (14%), higher than in male lacrosse players (10%).[16] Females are more likely to suffer head or face injury (30%, versus 18% in males), perhaps because female lacrosse players are less likely to wear helmets,[78] although concussion rates seem to be slightly higher in male players.[81] One case of epidural intracranial hematoma was reported after the player was hit by a lacrosse stick.[82] Closed head injuries comprise 6% of all lacrosse-related injuries. These statistics have led to recommendations for the use of protective head/face gear.[78]

FOOTBALL
Epidemiology

Most studies report football as the sport most likely to be associated with serious injury as well as neurologic injury. Rates of injury per 1000 AEs in male high school football players are higher during games (12.0) than during practices (2.6).[8,83] The rates of injury per 1000 AEs in collegiate football players are even higher, with 40.2 injuries per 1000 AEs in games and 5.8 injuries per 1000 AEs in practice.[7,83] As would be expected, contact with another player is the most frequent method of injury in football.[7] Of all injuries reported, 14% are considered serious (fracture, dislocation, or concussion). In professional players, the overall frequency of injuries per professional team per season is 14, more than three times greater than in other team sports.[7]

Concussions are a frequent injury complication of football, with an estimated rate of 6.1 per athlete-season in one study,[84] more than twice the incidence in other team sports. High school football players self-reported a 47% incidence of concussion of over one season, with 35% of all players reporting multiple concussions.[85] Another study of both high school and college football players reported that 5% of players sustained only one concussion, whereas 15% of players sustained a second concussion during the same season.[86] The most common specific diagnosis among Canadian varsity football players was concussion.[87] A study of Canadian Football League professional players suggested a one-season concussion incidence rate of 45%, with a 70% incidence of multiple concussions in players reporting at least one concussion.[88]

Collegiate male football players have the highest injury rates of all collegiate athletes for both practices and games, with 9.6 to 36 injuries per 1000 AEs and 35.9 injuries per 1000 AEs, respectively.[9,89,90] In college football players, the incidence of concussion is distributed approximately equally between games and practice;[90,91] this distribution is unique for this sport and injury type, because the incidence of most sports-related injuries is higher during competition. A slightly increased incidence of concussion was noted among offensive and defensive lineman[91] and in special teams players.[92] It has been suggested that blocking may lead to more concussions than tackling.[92]

The incidence of cervical spine injury in football has fallen over time. From 1971 to 1975, the National Football Head and Neck Injury Registry suggested a rate of 4.14 per 100,000 AEs for cervical fractures and dislocations and 1.58 per 100,000 AEs for quadriplegia.[93] In all likelihood, the introduction of modern helmets led to further increases in spinal injuries. Over time, increased protection and rules preventing head-first contact have reduced the incidence of spinal injuries. From 1976 to 1987, the rate of cervical injuries fell by 70% from 7.72 per100,000 to 2.31 per 100,000 at the high school level.[94] Traumatic quadriplegia also decreased by 82% during the same period. Most recent data indicate a plateau in the incidence of traumatic quadriplegia. In 2002, the incidence of this traumatic quadriplegia was 0.33 per 100,000 in high school football and 1.33 per 100,000 in college football, according to a report by the National Center for Catastrophic Sport Injury Research in 2003. The incidence of catastrophic cervical spine injuries is 1.10 per 100,000 participants per year for high school football players and 4.72 injuries per 100,000 participants for college players.[95] Quadriplegia caused by cervical spinal cord injury occurs in 0.50 per 100,000 high school football players and 0.82 per 100,000 college football players.[95]

Brachial plexus injury is one of the most common football-associated peripheral nerve injuries. In Canadian varsity football players, brachial plexus injuries were the third most common specific diagnosis in football injuries,[78] whereas the incidence at two University centers was 49% of all peripheral nervous system injuries.[96] The incidence of plexus injury has been reported to be as high as 2.2 cases per 100 players.[84] Initially called "pinched nerve syndrome," this phenomenon now is colloquially termed a "stinger" or "burner." The stinger comprises approximately 36% of all neurologic upper extremity injuries related to football.[97]

More severe brain injuries are less commonly reported in the football literature. The presence of chronic traumatic brain injury, as seen in boxing, has been postulated in football, but without significant evidence.[98] Intracranial hemorrhage, particularly subdural hematoma, has been reported rarely in football.[8] Persistent cerebral traumatic injury caused by football has been documented in 66 players over the past 3 decades.[99] Players who tackle with the head down and use the head as a battering ram may be at increased risk for more severe forms of injuries to the head and neck.[99]

GOLF

Most golf injuries that occur independently of a golf cart–related accident result from the golf swing. The 1-year incidence rate of golf injury is 0.36 to 0.60 injuries per 1000 participant-hours, although neurologic injuries are distinctly uncommon.[100] Nearly all golf-related injuries affecting the head and spine are related to golf cart accidents, often involving inebriated passengers and drivers.

GYMNASTICS

In some studies the prevalence of injuries to the cervical spine among gymnasts is next to that in football and wrestling, with most of the spinal cord lesions occurring at the mid-cervical levels.[101,102] For collegiate female gymnasts, the rate of injury in competition (15.2/1000 AEs) is double that in practice (6.1 /1000 AEs).[103] High school and college gymnasts are also at greater risk of death than are participants in other sports.[104]

In recent years the trampoline has been identified as a common cause of injury and of spinal cord injuries in particular. Trampolines have been held responsible for more than 6500 pediatric cervical spine injuries in 1998 in the United States, a fivefold increase in reported injuries compared with the previous 10 years.[105,106] Trampoline-related injuries occur equally in females and males, with a median age of 7 years.[106]

HOCKEY

Ice hockey is associated with high rates of injury in both amateur and professional leagues, although good epidemiologic studies of hockey-related injuries have been completed only recently. In children aged 9 to 16 years, overall injury rates are 30 injuries per 100 players per season or 4.13 injuries per 1000 player-hours,[107] with injury rates rising with increasing age in general. For high school hockey players, total injury rates of 75 cases per 100 players, or 5 injuries per 1000 player-hours, have been reported.[108] Of these injuries, 12% were concussions experienced by 9% of the players. In collegiate female hockey players, the rate of injury in games (12.6/1000 AEs) is more than five times higher than the rate in practice (2.5/1000 AEs).[109] Unlike male hockey players, concussions are the most common injury for female hockey players both in games (21.6%) and in practices (13.2%).[109] In collegiate men's hockey the injury rate is more than eight times higher in games (16.3/1000 AEs) than in practice (2.0/000 AEs).[110,111] A Danish study of adult hockey players found an equally high injury rate, 90 cases per 100 players per season, or 4.7 injuries per 1000 exposure-hours.[112] Female and male hockey players have similar overall injury rates (9.19/1000 AEs for males versus 7.77/1000 AEs for females), even though intentional body checking is not allowed in women's hockey.[113] Injury rates in ice hockey are much higher in males under the age of 18 years (9:1), however.[114]

Most hockey injuries affect the head and neck. Peak accelerations inside the helmet, which probably contribute to the risk of head injury, are significantly higher for hockey players than for football players.[115] Body checking remains the most common cause of injury in hockey, because children and teenaged players in contact leagues are four times more likely to be injured and are 12 times more likely to receive a fracture than players of the same age in noncontact leagues.[116] Some of the other risk factors for injury in ice hockey are distinct from those in other sports: more experienced players are significantly more likely to sustain injury;[108] the older, taller, and heavier a player is, the greater is the risk of injury as well.[108] Particular events associated with injury include forechecking and breakout plays (head injury) and backchecking.[108] Illegal activities such as elbowing and high sticking were responsible for 26% of hockey injuries.[108]

Concussion rates are high at every level of hockey play. Every season, 10% to 12% of minor league hockey players 9 years to 17 years old suffer a head injury, usually concussive in nature.[117] The rate of concussion has a positive correlation with the age of the player: youth players aged 5 to 17 years suffer 2.8 concussions per 1000 player-hours; college hockey players have a rate of 4.2 per 1000 player-hours; and elite amateur players have a rate of 6.6 per 1000 player-hours.[118] This positive association with increasing age is probably related to higher rates of body checking. At the professional level, concussion rates are even higher, 20 to 30 concussions per 1000 player-hours[119] or 3.7 per athlete-season.[84] Of even greater concern is the continuing rise in the concussion rates in professional ice hockey players in recent seasons.[119] Again in contrast to other sports, the incidence of concussion increases with higher levels of play and greater player experience.[118] Although this increase may reflect greater rates of recognition and reporting, other factors, such as larger and faster players, harder boards, and the presence of glass over the boards may contribute also.[119]

Since 1981, hockey-related spinal injuries have been on the rise, although reporting bias, increasing numbers of hockey players, and better diagnostic and reporting skills may contribute to the increase.[120] An average of 17 major spinal injuries occurs annually in Canada,[121] and there have been six deaths in Canada caused by spinal injury during this period.[120] Most of the athletes suffering major spinal injuries were males aged 16 to 20 years.[121] A Canadian registry of hockey-related spinal injuries has been created to capture spinal injury cases from 1966 to 1996.[120]

IN-LINE AND ROLLER-SKATING

Although less common than ice hockey, professional roller hockey, also called "in-line hockey," may have higher overall injury rates than ice hockey, perhaps because of differences in playing surfaces or difficulty in stopping while in-line skating.[122] One study found similar total injury rates between roller hockey (139/1000 AEs) and ice hockey (119/1000 AEs) but noted that more games were lost because of injuries in ice hockey (8.3 games per season) than in in-line hockey (6.5 games per season).[123] Roller hockey may have a lower incidence of head and neck injuries than ice hockey.[123] In children involved in ice skating, roller skating, and in-line skating, ice skating leads to a higher proportion of head injuries (13%) including concussions (4%), probably because of the greater likelihood of loss of balance and the higher impact with the ice surface.[124]

Recreational in-line skating most frequently leads to injuries in boys (61%) with a mean age of 12 years.[125,126] Head injuries resulting from in-line skating (34%) are significantly less common than with skateboarding (51%),[126,127] however, and the severity of injury is significantly less than with skateboarding.[127] Helmet use has been advocated in all three sports.[126]

JUDO, KARATE, KICKBOXING, AND RELATED SPORTS

The incidence of injuries occurring among the martial arts disciplines is roughly similar, at least between karate, taekwondo, and Muay Thai kickboxing.[128] Next to contusion, concussion was the most common form of head injury in both sexes.[129,130] As expected, the most common mechanism of head injury was a direct blow to the head.[130] Male adult full-contact taekwondo competitors suffer slightly higher rates of head injury (7.04/1000 AEs) than child athletes, but the dominant injury mechanism remains a blow to the head (6.46/1000 AEs).[129]

MOTOR BIKING

Injuries to motorcycle racers are quite common and often are associated with mortality (9% of all injuries).[131] Because racing motorcycles can reach speeds greater than 306 km/h, neurologic injuries would be expected.[131] The vulnerability of being on a motorcycle, however, does not lead to injury rates higher than those in automobile racers overall.[132] Of all injuries, only 10% to 30% are head injuries; 25% of these head injuries are severe with associated intracranial hemorrhage or mortality.[131,133] Spinal fractures are uncommon, representing 4% of all injuries.[133]

MOUNTAIN CLIMBING/HIKING

Injury rates among mountain climbers are low, estimated at 2 cases per 1000 climbers.[134] There are few data regarding the incidence of specific injuries, however. A unique form of sports-related neurologic dysfunction is cerebral edema. Headache, perhaps caused by cerebral edema, is a prominent feature of acute mountain sickness,[135] which also leads to dyspnea, weakness, asthenia, and nausea. Headache may be caused by intracranial vascular dilatation secondary to hypercapnia before the development of hyperventilation caused by hypoxia.[135] Cerebral edema usually occurs only above 12,000 feet and generally requires about 2 to 3 days to develop.[136] The incidence of cerebral edema in all climbers above 12,000 feet may be as high as 1.8%, and it can occur even in experienced climbers.[136] Vasogenic edema probably predominates early, with cytotoxic edema developing later; the development of cerebral edema is often fatal.[136] High-altitude cerebral edema has documented MRI changes with reversible white matter edema, having a predilection for the splenium of the corpus callosum.[137]

RODEO

Rodeo injury rates vary by event but are the highest in bull-riding, bareback riding, and saddle bronc events.[138] The incidence of rodeo-related injury is high, reported as 32.2 injuries per 1000 AEs,[138,139] although the overall injury rate is 2.3 per 100 AEs, lower than in most contact sports.[138] Concussions account for 9% of all reported rodeo injuries,[138] second only to knee injuries. Head and neck injuries in rodeo occur most commonly during dismount because of the violent motions of the animal.[140] Concussions typically occur from violent dismounts or from sustaining a blow from the animal.[140,141] In contrast to other sporting events, inexperienced rough-stock rodeo competitors have a lower overall rate of injury and severe injury than experienced competitors.[142]

RUGBY AND AUSTRALIAN RULES FOOTBALL

The overall incidence of injuries in professional rugby players is 55.4 injuries per 1000 player-hours during games, with 4.3 injuries per 1000 player-hours in practice.[143] Rugby and Australian rules football are both highly subject to cerebral concussion, the largest neurologic concern within both of these sports.[144] As with ice hockey, concussion rates seem to be rising within Australian rules football.[145] A statistic that is cause for concern is that junior Australian rules football players have higher concussion rates than senior players.[146,147]

The majority of rugby-related injuries are to the head and neck. Overall, the rate of head, neck, and orofacial injuries in Australian football is 2.6 injuries/1000 participation-hours.[148] The average annual incidence of acute spinal cord injuries in Australian football and rugby players is between 1.5 and 3.2 per 100,000 players.[149] The incidence of spinal injuries in professional rugby players is 10.9 per 1000 player match-hours and is lower during practice (0.37/1000 player training-hours).[150] The most common mechanism of injury seems to be cervical spine hyperflexion, often during scrimmaging or tackling, producing fracture dislocations of C4-C5 or C5-C6.[151] The number of serious spinal injuries has increased during the past decade despite changes in rules to prevent injury.[152] The phenomenon of transient quadriparesis, most common in American football, has been reported in rugby as well.[152] Overall, 39% of injured players became permanently wheelchair-dependent.[153]

A study of childhood and teenage rugby players has reported that currently used headgear does not protect against concussion.[154] Although helmet use in rugby players has not been validated, headgear performance may improve with incorporated thickened polyethylene foam.[155]

SKIING, SNOWBOARDING, SNOWBLADING, SLEDDING, SKATING, AND SKI JUMPING

Although most winter sport–related injuries are orthopedic in nature, neurologic injuries may occur. Cross-country skiers are subject to an injury rate of 0.72 injuries per 1000 skier-days, with more injuries occurring in inexperienced skiers.[156] The incidence of downhill skiing injuries is 2.05 per 1000 skier-days,[157] and the mortality rate is 1.6 per 1,000,000 skier-days. Older skiers have the highest skiing-related injury rates: 29.0 per 1000 participants for skiers between 55 and 64 years old and 21.7 per 1000 participants for skiers age 65 years or older, followed by 15.5 per 1000 participants in skiers between 45 and 54 years old.[158] Head and spinal injuries are most common. In

Germany, 25% of sports-related spinal cord injuries resulted from downhill skiing accidents.[71] Most spinal injuries (70%) caused by downhill skiing result from a simple fall; the next most common cause is striking a tree.[159,160]

In contrast to the greater propensity for injury in older skiers, snowboarding-related injuries are most common in the 10- to 13-year-old age group (15.9/1000 participants), followed by the 14- to 17-year-old age group (15.0/1000 participants) and the 18- to 24-year-old age group (13.5/1000 participants).[158] Intermediate or expert snowboarders are more likely to be injured than beginners, usually because of jumping.[160,161] Intentional jumping is a cause of injury in 77% of snowboarders, compared with 20% of skiers.[162]

Head injuries, although not as widely publicized as spinal injury, are common in downhill skiing.[163] Traumatic brain injury rates in skiers are highest among older skiers (2.15/1000 participants in skiers 55–64 years old) and very young skiers (1.69/1000 participants in skiers 10–13 years old).[158] Snowboarders seem to have even higher rates of head injury, up to three times higher than in skiers.[164,165] Competitive snowboarders have an injury incidence rate of 4.0 ± 0.7 injuries per 1000 AEs.[166]

Although ski jumping would be expected to have high injury rates, the injury rates for non–World Cup and for World Cup competitions are low, estimated at 4.3 and 1.2 injuries per 1000 skier-days, respectively, roughly equivalent to injury rates of alpine skiing.[167]

The risk of sustaining an injury in luge, a winter sport in which either an individual or a team rides a sled down a winding ice track, is 0.39 per person per year. Most injuries are musculoskeletal in nature.[168] In luge, crashes can lead to concussions, which comprise 2% of all injuries.[168]

In contrast to the level of spinal injury in other sports and recreational activities, most skiing-related spinal traumas occur in the thoracolumbar region (47%), followed by the cervical region (39%).[172] Serious injuries to the spinal canal in snowboarding-related injuries occur mostly at the cervical level.[160,169]

Snowblading is a relatively new sport that uses short, maneuverable skis. Head injury, including concussion, composes 11% of all injuries in snowbladers.[170]

Injury in short-track speed skating is uncommon, but 6% of elite level speed skaters suffer concussion because of accidents in competition. Likewise, junior figure skaters can be subject to head injuries, which are much more common in pairs skaters (10% of injuries) than in single figure skaters.[171]

Recreational sledding has similar degrees of overall injury as skiing, but the incidence of head injuries is significantly greater,[172] as high as 34%, and in children 3% of injuries affect the spinal column.[173] Sledding injuries are most common in boys 5 to 14 years of age.[174]

SNOWMOBILING, ALL-TERRAIN-VEHICLE RIDING

Brachial plexus injuries occur in 4.8% of snowmobile accident victims.[175] A complete brachial plexopathy is seen in 67% of snowmobile accidents, often in conjunction with orthopedic shoulder injury.[176] Participants injured using snowmobiles are typically male (85%–90%) and have an average age of 25 to 29 years.[177,178] Helmets are used sparingly (35%), and alcohol intake is present in 44% of cases.[177] Serious head injuries comprise 34% of all injuries, and spinal injuries comprise 18%.[177]

Injuries caused by the use of popular all-terrain vehicles (ATVs) have become more common, especially in pediatric populations, which comprise 65% of injured riders.[173] The most common ATV-related injuries include skull fracture, closed head injury, intracranial hemorrhage, and spinal fractures.[179] The most common mechanisms of injury are falling off the ATV to the ground, striking a tree, or flipping backward.[180] Next to orthopedic injuries, closed head injuries are the most commonly reported injury.[181] Cranial injuries comprise 64% of the number of the neurologic injuries, and spinal injuries comprise 36%.[180]

SOCCER

Most soccer-related injuries are musculoskeletal in nature and usually affect the lower extremities, but head and neck injuries can occur. Injury rates in collegiate-level soccer players are estimated at 2.1 per 100 AEs during total events (games plus practices), with 1% of all injuries considered serious.[7] The frequency of injuries per team per season for soccer is three for total events, much less than for football.[7] Of all injuries over a 3-year period, mild traumatic brain injuries accounted for 6.2% of injuries in both boys' and girls' soccer at the childhood and high school levels.[8] At the high school level, injury rates per 100 player-seasons were 1.14 for girls' soccer and 0.92 for boys' soccer.[8] In collegiate female soccer players, rates of injury are more than three times higher in games than during practice (16.4/1000 AEs versus 5.2/1000 AEs).[182] Even though heading is a major part of the sport, concussions are relatively uncommon in female soccer players (1.4/1000 AEs).[182] Statistics for male collegiate soccer players are similar, with injury rates four times higher during games than in practices (18.8/1000 AEs versus 4.3/1000 AEs).[183] Concussions are less common among male collegiate soccer players, however (1.1/1000 AEs).[183] In Olympian soccer players, rates of injury are 109 and 105 injuries per 1000 player-matches for male and female players, respectively, with neurologic injuries occurring extremely rarely.[12] Professional male soccer players from the 2006 Fédération Internationale de Football Association World Cup had overall injury rates of 69 per 1000 match-hours, or 2.3 injuries per match.[184] In professional female soccer players, injury rates are considerably higher in defenders (9.4/1000 hours) and strikers (8.4/1000 hours) than goalkeepers (4.8/1000 hours) and midfielders (4.6/1000 hours).[185] Overall, female soccer players have injury rates of 67.4 injuries per 1000 player-hours or approximately 2.2 injuries per match, comparable to those in their male counterparts.[186]

Despite controversy regarding the use of artificial turf, there are no major differences in the incidence, severity, or type of injuries sustained on new-generation artificial turf and grass by either male or female soccer players.[187,188]

Most soccer injuries seem to be caused by unintentional collisions with other players or goal posts or by mishaps in attempting to strike or head the ball. When heading the ball is measured with a triaxial accelerometer, peak accelerations are significantly higher (160%–180%) than in impacts occurring in football or hockey.[115] Although heading the ball leads to most reported concussions, injuries resulting from striking the goal posts have been reported as well.[189] As a result, head injuries account for 4% to 22% of soccer injuries.[189,190] As in other sports, the recognition of concussions is limited: 63% of Canadian University soccer players self-reported having symptoms of a concussion during the previous year, but only 20% of these soccer players realized that they had suffered a concussion.[88] Of the soccer players experiencing concussion, 82% experienced multiple concussions; this finding may suggest that particular players are more susceptible to head injury.[88] A recognized risk factor for concussion is female sex;[88] next to lacrosse, women's soccer has the highest percentage of injuries occurring as concussion (11%), a higher percentage than seen for male soccer players (7%).[16] Of all soccer positions, goalies were the players most commonly affected by concussion, even though they rarely head the ball.[91]

Although the force and repetitive nature of heading the soccer ball and collisions with other players might suggest the development of long-term neuropsychologic dysfunction, this association is unclear. In other studies, neither participation in soccer nor a history of soccer-related concussions was found to be associated with impaired performance of neurocognitive function in high-level soccer players or teenage players.[86,190] Another study compared neuropsychologic functioning in soccer players and collegiate athletes engaged in sports in which head injuries would be unusual. It failed to demonstrate any difference in neurocognitive function or scholastic aptitude even in players who had an average of more than 15 seasons of soccer.[191] Therefore, it is unlikely that the subconcussive impact of purposeful heading is responsible for neurocognitive changes.

SURFING

Surfing has an injury rate of 5.7 per 1000 AEs, or 13 per 1000 hours of competitive surfing. The risk of injury increase when surfing in waves overhead or when surfing over a rock or reef bottom.[192]

TENNIS AND OTHER RACQUET SPORTS

Although the epidemiology of racquet sport–related injuries is largely unknown, badminton has an overall incidence rate of 5.04 injuries per 1000 player-hours. Essentially all injuries are musculoskeletal in nature.[193]

VOLLEYBALL

Overall, volleyball is one of the safest competitive and recreational sports played by high school and collegiate athletes. In high school volleyball players, the injury rate is only 0.14 per 100 player-seasons, the lowest of 10 high school sporting activities examined in one study.[8] In female collegiate volleyball players, the rate of injury in a game (4.6/1000 AEs) is similar to that in practice (4.11000 AEs).[185] The rate of concussion in female collegiate volleyball players is exceptionally low (0.2/1000 AEs),[194] with concussion comprising only about 4% of all injuries in collegiate-level female volleyball players.[16]

Although injuries are uncommon in volleyball, peripheral nerve injuries caused by volleyball are unique, related to the overhand motion of serving. The most frequently reported form of mononeuropathy is an isolated entrapment of the suprascapular nerve at the spinoglenoid notch of the patient's serving arm; this injury presents with painless weakness of dominant arm external rotation with infraspinatus atrophy identifiable on examination.[195,196] The overall prevalence of suprascapular neuropathy in international-level volleyball players ranges from 33% to 45%, based on clinical and electrophysiologic examination.[197,198] Up to 12% of volleyball players also may have subclinical suprascapular neuropathy.[195,196] This susceptibility may be caused by an increased range of motion of the shoulder joint[199] or impingement of the nerve by the medial tendinous margin between the infraspinatus and supraspinatus muscles.[200] Isolated mononeuropathies of the axillary nerve and long thoracic nerve also have been reported in younger volleyball players, perhaps related to a quadrilateral space syndrome in the case of axillary mononeuropathy.[201,202] Also, asymptomatic ulnar neuropathy at the elbow is more common among volleyball players than among healthy control subjects.[203]

WAKEBOARDING

Wakeboarding is a relatively new water sport that is similar to snowboarding except that the rider is pulled behind a boat. Head injuries represent most injuries (29%) for wakeboarders; in contrast, head injuries represent the smallest percentage of injuries (4%) in water skiers.[204]

WRESTLING

Amateur wrestling is an aggressive sport with an injury rate among high school competitors of 1.58 per 100 player-seasons, second only to football.[8] Wrestling also accounts for the second-highest rate (10.5%) of MTBIs in collegiate athletes (after football).[8] The rate of concussion in wrestling has been estimated at 2.5 per athlete-season, composing about 6% of all injuries in collegiate male wrestlers.[16,84] High school wrestlers have an injury rate of 2.33 injuries per 1000 AEs, but collegiate wrestlers have higher injury rates (7.25/1000 AEs) and moderate rates of concussion (1.3/1000 AEs).[205]

Most severe head injuries result from head-to-head collision during takedown attempts, but slams to the mat also can result in head injury.[206] Severe injuries in amateur wrestlers have included cervical spinal fractures (77%), spinal cord contusions with transient quadriparesis (12%), severe closed head injury (8%), and acute lumbar disc herniation (3%), sometimes resulting in quadriplegia (33%), residual neurologic deficits (20%), paraplegia (3%), and death caused by head injury (3%).[206]

Although professional wrestlers clearly are subjected to repetitive trauma leading to traumatic brain injuries and spinal injuries, there is very little literature examining the prevalence of injuries in this sports population. Female professional wrestlers, particularly those with long careers, are subject to head trauma and recurrent retrograde amnesia.[207]

SUMMARY

Although many sports have unique forms of injury, such as the atypical mononeuropathies occurring in volleyball players and thoracolumbar spinal injuries occurring in skiers, most sports such as football and hockey are dominated by nonspecific injuries such as brachial plexopathy, concussion, and spinal injuries. It is clear that nervous system injury can occur with almost any competitive sport. Even apparently benign sporting activities such as cheerleading, golf, and dancing have been associated with nervous system injuries. Epidemiologic reviews have identified certain sports, such as football and hockey, as being associated with very high injury rates. True injury rates probably are much higher in sports that are not evaluated formally because of probable underreporting. It is hoped that this article will help the health care professional in the recognizing sport-specific injuries and in determining prognosis.

REFERENCES

1. Steele AG. Emergency medical care for open wheel racing events at Indianapolis Raceway Park. Ann Emerg Med 1994;24:264–8.
2. Gennarelli TA. Cerebral concussions and diffuse brain injuries. In: Cooper PR, editor. Head injury. 2nd edition. Baltimore (MD): Wilkins and Wilkins; 1987. p. 108–24.
3. Trammell TR, Olivary SE. Crash and injury statistics from Indy-car racing 1985–1989. In: Proceedings of the 34th Annual Conference, Association for Advancement of Automotive Medicine. Scottsdale (AZ); 1991. p. 329–35.

4. Holley JE, Butler JW, Mahoney JM. Carbon monoxide poisoning in racing car drivers. J Sports Med Phys Fitness 1999;39:20–3.
5. Jareno A, de la Serna JL, Cercas A, et al. Heat stroke in motor car racing drivers. Br J Sports Med 1987;21:48.
6. Leonard L, Lim A, Chesser TJ, et al. Does changing the configuration of a motor racing circuit make it safer? Br J Sports Med 2005;39:159–61.
7. Radelet MA, Lephart SM, Rubinstein EN, et al. Survey of the injury rate for children in community sports. Pediatrics 2002;110:E28.
8. Powell JW, Barber-Foss KD. Traumatic brain injury in high school athletes. JAMA 1999;282:958–63.
9. Hootman JM, Dick R, Agel J. Epidemiology of collegiate injuries for 15 sports: summary and recommendations for injury prevention initiatives. J Athl Train 2007;42:311–9.
10. Marshall SW, Hamstra-Wright KL, Dick R, et al. Descriptive epidemiology of collegiate women's softball injuries: National Collegiate Athletic Association Injury Surveillance System, 1988–1989 through 2003–2004. J Athl Train 2007;42:286–94.
11. Dick R, Sauers EL, Agel J, et al. Descriptive epidemiology of collegiate men's baseball injuries: National Collegiate Athletic Association Injury Surveillance System, 1988–1989 through 2003–2004. J Athl Train 2007;42:183–93.
12. Junge A, Langevoort G, Pipe A, et al. Injuries in team sport tournaments during the 2004 Olympic Games. Am J Sports Med 2006;34:565–76.
13. Pasternack JS, Veenema KR, Callahan CM. Baseball injuries: a Little League survey. Pediatrics 1996;98:445–8.
14. Cheng TL, Fields CB, Brenner RA, et al. Sports injuries: an important cause of morbidity in urban youth. District of Columbia Child/Adolescent Injury Research Network. Pediatrics 2000;105:E32.
15. Boden BP, Tacchetti R, Mueller FO. Catastrophic injuries in high school and college baseball players. Am J Sports Med 2004;32:1189–96.
16. Covassin T, Swanik CB, Sachs ML. Epidemiological considerations of concussions among intercollegiate athletes. Appl Neuropsychol 2003;10:12–22.
17. Danis RP, Hu K, Bell M. Acceptability of baseball face guards and reduction of oculofacial injury in receptive youth league players. Inj Prev 2000;6:232–4.
18. Rice JO, Walters C, Olson RE, et al. Epidural hematoma after minor oral trauma. J Oral Surg 1976;34:639–41.
19. Hammig BJ, Yang H, Bensema B. Epidemiology of basketball injuries among adults presenting to ambulatory care settings in the United States. Clin J Sport Med 2007;17:446–51.
20. Agel J, Olson DE, Dick R, et al. Descriptive epidemiology of collegiate women's basketball injuries: National Collegiate Athletic Association Injury Surveillance System, 1988–1989 through 2003–2004. J Athl Train 2007;42:202–10.
21. Deitch JR, Starkey C, Walters SL, et al. Injury risk in professional basketball players: a comparison of Women's National Basketball Association and National Basketball Association athletes. Am J Sports Med 2006;34:1077–83.
22. Konkin DE, Garraway N, Hameed SM, et al. Population-based analysis of severe injuries from nonmotorized wheeled vehicles. Am J Surg 2006;191:615–8.
23. Veisten K, Saelensminde K, Alvaer K, et al. Total costs of bicycle injuries in Norway: correcting injury figures and indicating data needs. Accid Anal Prev 2007;39:1162–9.
24. Worrell J. BMX bicycles: accident comparison with other models. Arch Emerg Med 1985;2:209–13.

25. Illingworth CM. BMX compared with ordinary bicycle accidents. Arch Dis Child 1985;60:461–4.
26. Kronisch RL, Chow TK, Simon LM, et al. Acute injuries in off-road bicycle racing. Am J Sports Med 1996;24:88–93.
27. Rivara FP, Thompson DC, Thompson RS, et al. Injuries involving off-road cycling. J Fam Pract 1997;44:481–5.
28. Kronisch RL, Pfeiffer RP, Chow TK, et al. Gender differences in acute mountain bike racing injuries. Clin J Sport Med 2002;12:158–64.
29. Apsingi S, Dussa CU, Soni BM. Acute cervical spine injuries in mountain biking: a report of 3 cases. Am J Sports Med 2006;34:487–9.
30. Kim PT, Jangra D, Ritchie AH, et al. Mountain biking injuries requiring trauma center admission: a 10-year regional trauma system experience. J Trauma 2006;60:312–8.
31. Mezhir JJ, Glynn L, Liu DC, et al. Handlebar injuries in children: should we raise the bar of suspicion? Am Surg 2007;73:807–10.
32. Pedal-cycle injuries among children aged <6 years–Wisconsin, 2002–2004. MMWR Morb Mortal Wkly Rep 2006;55:1345–8.
33. Linn S, Smith D, Sheps S. Epidemiology of bicycle injury, head injury, and helmet use among children in British Columbia: a five year descriptive study. Canadian Hospitals Injury, Reporting and Prevention Program (CHIRPP). Inj Prev 1998;4:122–5.
34. Shafi S, Gilbert JC, Loghmanee F, et al. Impact of bicycle helmet safety legislation on children admitted to a regional pediatric trauma center. J Pediatr Surg 1998;33:317–21.
35. Ross RT, Ochsner MG Jr. Acute intracranial boxing-related injuries in U.S. Marine Corps recruits: report of two cases. Mil Med 1999;164:68–70.
36. Blonstein JL, Clarke E. Further observations on the medical aspects of amateur boxing. Br Med J 1957;1:362–4.
37. McCown IA. Boxing injuries. Am J Surg 1959;98:509–16.
38. Jordan BD, Campbell E. Acute boxing injuries among professional boxers in New York State. Physical Sports Medicine 1988;12:53–67.
39. Bledsoe GH, Li G, Levy F. Injury risk in professional boxing. South Med J 2005;98:994–8.
40. Unterharnscheidt F. About boxing: review of historical and medical aspects. Tex Rep Biol Med 1970;28:421–95.
41. Bianco M, Fabbricatore C, Sanna N, et al. Elite athletes: is survival shortened in boxers? Int J Sports Med 2007;28:697–702.
42. Unterharnscheidt F. A neurologist's reflections on boxing. V. Concluding remarks. Rev Neurol 1995;23:1027–32.
43. Estwanik J, Boitano M, Ari N. Amateur boxing injuries at the 1981 and 1982 USA/ABF national championships. Phys Sportsmed 1984;12:123–8.
44. Larsson LE, Melin KA, Nordstrom-Ohrberg G, et al. Acute head injuries in boxers; clinical and electroencephalographic studies. Acta Psychiatr Neurol Scand Suppl 1954;95:2–42.
45. Jordan B, Voy R, Stone J. Amateur boxing injuries at the US Olympic Training Center. Phys Sportsmed 1990;18:81–90.
46. Porter M, O'Brien M. Incidence and severity of injuries resulting from amateur boxing in Ireland. Clin J Sport Med 1996;6(2):97–101.
47. Zazryn TR, Finch CF, McCrory P. A 16 year study of injuries to professional boxers in the state of Victoria, Australia. Br J Sports Med 2003;37:321–4.
48. Welch M, Sitler M, Kroeten H. Boxing injuries from an instructional program. Phys Sportsmed 1986;14:81–9.

49. Jordan BD. Neurologic aspects of boxing. Arch Neurol 1987;44:453–9.
50. Roberts AH. Brain damage in boxers. London: Pittman Medical Scientific Publishing; 1969.
51. Loosemore M, Knowles CH, Whyte GP. Amateur boxing and risk of chronic traumatic brain injury: systematic review of observational studies. BMJ 2007;335:809.
52. Mendez MF. The neuropsychiatric aspects of boxing. Int J Psychiatry Med 1995; 25:249–62.
53. Jordan B, Relkin N, Ravdin L, et al. Apolipoprotein E e4 associated with chronic traumatic brain injury in boxing. JAMA 1997;278(2):136–40.
54. Casson I, Siegel O, Sham R, et al. Brain damage in modern boxers. JAMA 1984; 251(20):2663–7.
55. Haglund Y, Edman G, Murelius O, et al. Does Swedish amateur boxing lead to chronic brain damage? 1. A retrospective medical, neurological and personality trait study. Acta Neurol Scand 1990;82:245–52.
56. Jordan B. Boxing. In: Caine D, Caine C, Lindner K, editors. Epidemiology of sports injuries. Champaign, Illinois: Human Kinetics Publishers, Inc; 1996. p. 113–23.
57. Brooks N, Kupshik G, Wilson L, et al. A neuropsychological study of active amateur boxers. J Neurol Neurosurg Psychiatry 1987;50:997–1000.
58. Jordan B, Kanik A, Horwich M, et al. Apolipoprotein E e4 and fatal cerebral amyloid angiopathy associated with dementia pugilistica. Ann Neurol 1995;38(4): 698–9.
59. Bodensteiner JB, Schaefer GB. Dementia pugilistica and cavum septi pellucidi: born to box? Sports Med 1997;24:361–5.
60. Corsellis JA, Bruton CJ, Freeman-Browne D. The aftermath of boxing. Psychol Med 1973;3:270–303.
61. Hof PR, Bouras C, Buee L, et al. Differential distribution of neurofibrillary tangles in the cerebral cortex of dementia pugilistica and Alzheimer's disease cases. Acta Neuropathol 1992;85:23–30.
62. Schmidt ML, Zhukareva V, Newell KL, et al. Tau isoform profile and phosphorylation state in dementia pugilistica recapitulate Alzheimer's disease. Acta Neuropathol 2001;101:518–24.
63. Otto M, Holthusen S, Bahn E, et al. Boxing and running lead to a rise in serum levels of S-100B protein. Int J Sports Med 2000;21:551–5.
64. Boden BP, Tacchetti R, Mueller FO. Catastrophic cheerleading injuries. Am J Sports Med 2003;31:881–8.
65. Shields BJ, Smith GA. Cheerleading-related injuries to children 5 to 18 years of age: United States, 1990–2002. Pediatrics 2006;117:122–9.
66. Schulz MR, Marshall SW, Yang J, et al. A prospective cohort study of injury incidence and risk factors in North Carolina high school competitive cheerleaders. Am J Sports Med 2004;32:396–405.
67. Schulz MR, Marshall SW, Mueller FO, et al. Incidence and risk factors for concussion in high school athletes, North Carolina, 1996–1999. Am J Epidemiol 2004;160:937–44.
68. Mansingh A, Harper L, Headley S, et al. Injuries in West Indies cricket 2003–2004. Br J Sports Med 2006;40:119–23.
69. Orchard JW, James T, Portus MR. Injuries to elite male cricketers in Australia over a 10-year period. J Sci Med Sport 2006;9:459–67.
70. Hwang V, Shofer FS, Durbin DR, et al. Prevalence of traumatic injuries in drowning and near drowning in children and adolescents. Arch Pediatr Adolesc Med 2003;157:50–3.

71. Schmitt H, Gerner HJ. Paralysis from sport and diving accidents. Clin J Sport Med 2001;11:17–22.
72. Gierup J, Larsson M, Lennquist S. Incidence and nature of horse-riding injuries. A one-year prospective study. Acta Chir Scand 1976;142:57–61.
73. Kriss TC, Kriss VM. Equine-related neurosurgical trauma: a prospective series of 30 patients. J Trauma 1997;43:97–9.
74. Bixby-Hammett DM, Brooks WH. Common injuries in horseback riding. A review. Sports Med 1990;9:36–47.
75. Fleming PR, Crompton JL, Simpson DA. Neuro-ophthalmological sequelae of horse-related accidents. Clin Experiment Ophthalmol 2001;29:208–12.
76. Bond GR, Christoph RA, Rodgers BM. Pediatric equestrian injuries: assessing the impact of helmet use. Pediatrics 1995;95:487–9.
77. Ball CG, Ball JE, Kirkpatrick AW, et al. Equestrian injuries: incidence, injury patterns, and risk factors for 10 years of major traumatic injuries. Am J Surg 2007; 193:636–40.
78. Diamond PT, Gale SD. Head injuries in men's and women's lacrosse: a 10 year analysis of the NEISS database. National Electronic Injury Surveillance System. Brain Inj 2001;15:537–44.
79. Dick R, Hootman JM, Agel J, et al. Descriptive epidemiology of collegiate women's field hockey injuries: National Collegiate Athletic Association Injury Surveillance System, 1988–1989 through 2002–2003. J Athl Train 2007;42:211–20.
80. Dick R, Lincoln AE, Agel J, et al. Descriptive epidemiology of collegiate women's lacrosse injuries: National Collegiate Athletic Association Injury Surveillance System, 1988–1989 through 2003–2004. J Athl Train 2007;42:262–9.
81. Dick R, Romani WA, Agel J, et al. Descriptive epidemiology of collegiate men's lacrosse injuries: National Collegiate Athletic Association Injury Surveillance System, 1988–1989 through 2003–2004. J Athl Train 2007;42:255–61.
82. Rimel RW, Nelson WE, Persing JA, et al. Epidural hematoma in lacrosse. Physical Sports Medicine 1983;11:140–4.
83. Shankar PR, Fields SK, Collins CL, et al. Epidemiology of high school and collegiate football injuries in the United States, 2005–2006. Am J Sports Med 2007; 35:1295–303.
84. Clarke KS. Prevention: an epidemiologic view. In: Torg JS, editor. Athletic injuries in the head, neck and face. Philadelphia: Lea and Febiger; 1982. p. 15–26.
85. Langburt W, Cohen B, Akhthar N, et al. Incidence of concussion in high school football players of Ohio and Pennsylvania. J Child Neurol 2001;16:83–5.
86. Guskiewicz KM, Weaver NL, Padua DA, et al. Epidemiology of concussion in collegiate and high school football players. Am J Sports Med 2000;28:643–50.
87. Meeuwisse WH, Hagel BE, Mohtadi NG, et al. The distribution of injuries in men's Canada West university football. A 5-year analysis. Am J Sports Med 2000;28: 516–23.
88. Delaney JS, Lacroix VJ, Leclerc S, et al. Concussions during the 1997 Canadian Football League season. Clin J Sport Med 2000;10:9–14.
89. Knowles SB, Marshall SW, Bowling JM, et al. A prospective study of injury incidence among North Carolina high school athletes. Am J Epidemiol 2006;164: 1209–21.
90. Dick R, Ferrara MS, Agel J, et al. Descriptive epidemiology of collegiate men's football injuries: National Collegiate Athletic Association Injury Surveillance System, 1988–1989 through 2003–2004. J Athl Train 2007;42:221–33.
91. Delaney JS, Lacroix VJ, Leclerc S, et al. Concussions among university football and soccer players. Clin J Sport Med 2002;12:331–8.

92. Alves WM, Rimel RW, Nelson WE. University of Virginia prospective study of football-induced minor head injury: status report. Clin Sports Med 1987;6:211–8.
93. Torg JS, Quedenfeld TC, Burstein A, et al. National football head and neck injury registry: report on cervical quadriplegia, 1971 to 1975. Am J Sports Med 1979;7:127–32.
94. Torg JS, Vegso JJ, O'Neill MJ, et al. The epidemiologic, pathologic, biomechanical, and cinematographic analysis of football-induced cervical spine trauma. Am J Sports Med 1990;18:50–7.
95. Boden BP, Tacchetti RL, Cantu RC, et al. Catastrophic cervical spine injuries in high school and college football players. Am J Sports Med 2006;34:1223–32.
96. Clancy WG Jr, Brand RL, Bergfield JA. Upper trunk brachial plexus injuries in contact sports. Am J Sports Med 1977;5:209–16.
97. Krivickas LS, Wilbourn AJ. Peripheral nerve injuries in athletes: a case series of over 200 injuries. Semin Neurol 2000;20:225–32.
98. Rabadi MH, Jordan BD. The cumulative effect of repetitive concussion in sports. Clin J Sport Med 2001;11:194–8.
99. Cantu RC, Mueller FO. Catastrophic football injuries: 1977–1998. Neurosurgery 2000;47:673–5.
100. McHardy A, Pollard H, Luo K. One-year follow-up study on golf injuries in Australian amateur golfers. Am J Sports Med 2007;35:1354–60.
101. Noguchi T. A survey of spinal cord injuries resulting from sport. Paraplegia 1994;32:170–3.
102. Bailes JE, Hadley MN, Quigley MR, et al. Management of athletic injuries of the cervical spine and spinal cord. Neurosurgery 1991;29:491–7.
103. Marshall SW, Covassin T, Dick R, et al. Descriptive epidemiology of collegiate women's gymnastics injuries: National Collegiate Athletic Association Injury Surveillance System, 1988–1989 through 2003–2004. J Athl Train 2007;42:234–40.
104. Mueller FO, Cantu RC. Catastrophic injuries and fatalities in high school and college sports, fall 1982–spring 1988. Med Sci Sports Exerc 1990;22:737–41.
105. Brown PG, Lee M. Trampoline injuries of the cervical spine. Pediatr Neurosurg 2000;32:170–5.
106. Furnival RA, Street KA, Schunk JE. Too many pediatric trampoline injuries. Pediatrics 1999;103:E57.
107. Emery CA, Meeuwisse WH. Injury rates, risk factors, and mechanisms of injury in minor hockey. Am J Sports Med 2006;34(12):1960–9.
108. Gerberich SG, Finke R, Madden M, et al. An epidemiological study of high school ice hockey injuries. Childs Nerv Syst 1987;3:59–64.
109. Agel J, Dick R, Nelson B, et al. Descriptive epidemiology of collegiate women's ice hockey injuries: National Collegiate Athletic Association Injury Surveillance System, 2000–2001 through 2003–2004. J Athl Train 2007;42:249–54.
110. Agel J, Dompier TP, Dick R, et al. Descriptive epidemiology of collegiate men's ice hockey injuries: National Collegiate Athletic Association Injury Surveillance System, 1988–1989 through 2003–2004. J Athl Train 2007;42:241–8.
111. Flik K, Lyman S, Marx RG. American collegiate men's ice hockey: an analysis of injuries. Am J Sports Med 2005;33:183–7.
112. Jorgensen U, Schmidt-Olsen S. The epidemiology of ice hockey injuries. Br J Sports Med 1986;20:7–9.
113. Schick DM, Meeuwisse WH. Injury rates and profiles in female ice hockey players. Am J Sports Med 2003;31:47–52.
114. Hostetler SG, Xiang H, Smith GA. Characteristics of ice hockey-related injuries treated in US emergency departments, 2001–2002. Pediatrics 2004;114:E661–6.

115. Naunheim R, McGurren M, Standeven J, et al. Does the use of artificial turf contribute to head injuries? J Trauma 2002;53:691–4.
116. Juhn MS, Brolinson PG, Duffey T, et al. Position statement. Violence and injury in ice hockey. Clin J Sport Med 2002;12:46–51.
117. Biasca N, Wirth S, Tegner Y. The avoidability of head and neck injuries in ice hockey: an historical review. Br J Sports Med 2002;36:410–27.
118. Honey CR. Brain injury in ice hockey. Clin J Sport Med 1998;8:43–6.
119. Wennberg RA, Tator CH. National Hockey League reported concussions, 1986–87 to 2001–02. Can J Neurol Sci 2003;30:206–9.
120. Tator CH, Carson JD, Cushman R. Hockey injuries of the spine in Canada, 1966–1996. CMAJ 2000;162:787–8.
121. Tator CH, Carson JD, Edmonds VE. New spinal injuries in hockey. Clin J Sport Med 1997;7:17–21.
122. Varlotta GP, Lager SL, Nicholas S, et al. Professional roller hockey injuries. Clin J Sport Med 2000;10:29–33.
123. Hutchinson MR, Milhouse C, Gapski M. Comparison of injury patterns in elite hockey players using ice versus in-line skates. Med Sci Sports Exerc 1998; 30:1371–3.
124. Knox CL, Comstock RD, McGeehan J, et al. Differences in the risk associated with head injury for pediatric ice skaters, roller skaters, and in-line skaters. Pediatrics 2006;118:549–54.
125. Naunheim RS, Standeven J, Richter C, et al. Comparison of impact data in hockey, football, and soccer. J Trauma 2000;48:938–41.
126. Schieber RA, Branche-Dorsey CM, Ryan GW. Comparison of in-line skating injuries with rollerskating and skateboarding injuries. JAMA 1994;271:1856–8.
127. Osberg JS, Schneps SE, Di SC, et al. Skateboarding: more dangerous than roller skating or in-line skating. Arch Pediatr Adolesc Med 1998;152:985–91.
128. Gartland S, Malik MH, Lovell ME. Injury and injury rates in Muay Thai kick boxing. Br J Sports Med 2001;35:308–13.
129. Pieter W, Zemper ED. Incidence of reported cerebral concussion in adult taekwondo athletes. J R Soc Health 1998;118:272–9.
130. Pieter W, Zemper ED. Head and neck injuries in young taekwondo athletes. J Sports Med Phys Fitness 1999;39:147–53.
131. Varley GW, Spencer-Jones R, Thomas P, et al. Injury patterns in motorcycle road racers: experience on the Isle of Man 1989–1991. Injury 1993;24:443–6.
132. Chapman MA, Oni J. Motor racing accidents at Brands Hatch, 1988/9. Br J Sports Med 1991;25:121–3.
133. Horner CH, O'Brien AA. Motorcycle racing injuries on track and road circuits in Ireland. Br J Sports Med 1986;20:157–8.
134. Schusman LC, Lutz LJ. Mountaineering and rock climbing accidents. Physical Sports Medicine 1982;10:52–61.
135. Foulke GE. Altitude-related illness. Am J Emerg Med 1985;3:217–26.
136. Hackett PH. High altitude cerebral edema and acute mountain sickness. A pathophysiology update. Adv Exp Med Biol 1999;474:23–45.
137. Hackett PH, Yarnell PR, Hill R, et al. High-altitude cerebral edema evaluated with magnetic resonance imaging: clinical correlation and pathophysiology. JAMA 1998;280:1920–5.
138. Butterwick DJ, Hagel B, Nelson DS, et al. Epidemiologic analysis of injury in five years of Canadian professional rodeo. Am J Sports Med 2002;30:193–8.
139. Downey DJ. Rodeo injuries and prevention. Curr Sports Med Rep 2007;6:328–32.

140. Nebergall R. Rodeo. In: Calne PJ, Caine CG, Lindner KJ, editors. Epidemiology of sports injuries. Champaign, Ill: Human Kinetics; 1996. p. 350–6.

141. Butterwick DJ, Nelson DS, LaFave MR, et al. Epidemiological analysis of injury in one year of Canadian professional rodeo. Clin J Sport Med 1996;6:171–7.

142. Butterwick DJ, Meeuwisse WH. Effect of experience on rodeo injury. Clin J Sport Med 2002;12:30–5.

143. Holtzhausen LJ, Schwellnus MP, Jakoet I, et al. The incidence and nature of injuries in South African rugby players in the rugby Super 12 competition. S Afr Med J 2006;96:1260–5.

144. Orchard J, Wood T, Seward H, et al. Comparison of injuries in elite senior and junior Australian football. J Sci Med Sport 1998;1:83–8.

145. Orchard J. AFL 1996 injury report. Melbourne Australian Football League Medical Officers Association. Melbourne; 1995. p. 7–8.

146. Seward H, Orchard J, Hazard H, et al. Football injuries in Australia at the elite level. Med J Aust 1993;159:298–301.

147. Marshall SW, Spencer RJ. Concussion in rugby: the hidden epidemic. J Athl Train 2001;36:334–8.

148. Braham R, Finch CF, McCrory P. The incidence of head/neck/orofacial injuries in non-elite Australian football. J Sci Med Sport 2004;7:451–3.

149. Berry JG, Harrison JE, Yeo JD, et al. Cervical spinal cord injury in rugby union and rugby league: are incidence rates declining in NSW? Aust N Z J Public Health 2006;30:268–74.

150. Fuller CW, Brooks JH, Kemp SP. Spinal injuries in professional rugby union: a prospective cohort study. Clin J Sport Med 2007;17:10–6.

151. Quarrie KL, Cantu RC, Chalmers DJ. Rugby union injuries to the cervical spine and spinal cord. Sports Med 2002;32:633–53.

152. Scher AT. Rugby injuries to the cervical spine and spinal cord: a 10-year review. Clin Sports Med 1998;17:195–206.

153. Carmody DJ, Taylor TK, Parker DA, et al. Spinal cord injuries in Australian footballers 1997–2002. Med J Aust 2005;182:561–4.

154. McIntosh AS, McCrory P. Effectiveness of headgear in a pilot study of Under 15 Rugby Union football. Br J Sports Med 2001;35:167–9.

155. McIntosh A, McCrory P, Finch CF. Performance enhanced headgear: a scientific approach to the development of protective headgear. Br J Sports Med 2004;38: 46–9.

156. Boyle JJ, Johnson RJ, Pope MH, et al. Cross-country skiing injuries. In: Johnson RJ, Mote CD Jr, editors. Skiing trauma and safety. 5th International Symposium, ASTM STP 860. Philadelphia: American Society for Testing and Materials; 1985. p. 411–22.

157. Corra S, Conci A, Conforti G, et al. Skiing and snowboarding injuries and their impact on the emergency care system in South Tyrol: a retrospective analysis for the winter season 2001–2002. Inj Control Saf Promot 2004;11:281–5.

158. Xiang H, Kelleher K, Shields BJ, et al. Skiing- and snowboarding-related injuries treated in U.S. emergency departments, 2002. J Trauma 2005;58: 112–8.

159. Myles ST, Mohtadi NG, Schnittker J. Injuries to the nervous system and spine in downhill skiing. Can J Surg 1992;35:643–8.

160. Yamakawa H, Murase S, Sakai H, et al. Spinal injuries in snowboarders: risk of jumping as an integral part of snowboarding. J Trauma 2001;50:1101–5.

161. Wakahara K, Matsumoto K, Sumi H, et al. Traumatic spinal cord injuries from snowboarding. Am J Sports Med 2006;34:1670–4.

162. Tarazi F, Dvorak MF, Wing PC. Spinal injuries in skiers and snowboarders. Am J Sports Med 1999;27:177–80.

163. Nakaguchi H, Fujimaki T, Ueki K, et al. Snowboard head injury: prospective study in Chino, Nagano, for two seasons from 1995 to 1997. J Trauma 1999; 46:1066–9.

164. Hentschel S, Hader W, Boyd M. Head injuries in skiers and snowboarders in British Columbia. Can J Neurol Sci 2001;28:42–6.

165. Levy AS, Hawkes AP, Hemminger LM, et al. An analysis of head injuries among skiers and snowboarders. J Trauma 2002;53:695–704.

166. Torjussen J, Bahr R. Injuries among competitive snowboarders at the national elite level. Am J Sports Med 2005;33:370–7.

167. Wright JR Jr, Hixson EG, Rand JJ. Injury patterns in Nordic ski jumpers. A retrospective analysis of injuries occurring at the Intervale Ski Jump Complex from 1980 to 1985. Am J Sports Med 1986;14:393–7.

168. Cummings RS Jr, Shurland AT, Prodoehl JA, et al. Injuries in the sport of luge. Epidemiology and analysis. Am J Sports Med 1997;25:508–13.

169. Genelin A, Kathrein A, Daniaux A, et al. [Current status of spinal injuries in winter sports]. Schweiz Z Med Traumatol 1994;17–20 [in German].

170. Bridges EJ, Rouah F, Johnston KM. Snowblading injuries in Eastern Canada. Br J Sports Med 2003;37:511–5.

171. Dubravcic-Simunjak S, Pecina M, Kuipers H, et al. The incidence of injuries in elite junior figure skaters. Am J Sports Med 2003;31:511–7.

172. Federiuk CS, Schlueter JL, Adams AL. Skiing, snowboarding, and sledding injuries in a northwestern state. Wilderness Environ Med 2002;13:245–9.

173. Shorter NA, Mooney DP, Harmon BJ. Childhood sledding injuries. Am J Emerg Med 1999;17:32–4.

174. Skarbek-Borowska S, Amanullah S, Mello MJ, et al. Emergency department visits for sledding injuries in children in the United States in 2001/2002. Acad Emerg Med 2006;13:181–5.

175. Midha R. Epidemiology of brachial plexus injuries in a multitrauma population. Neurosurgery 1997;40:1182–8.

176. Braun BL, Meyers B, Dulebohn SC, et al. Severe brachial plexus injury as a result of snowmobiling: a case series. J Trauma 1998;44:726–30.

177. Beilman GJ, Brasel KJ, Dittrich K, et al. Risk factors and patterns of injury in snowmobile crashes. Wilderness Environ Med 1999;10:226–32.

178. Farley DR, Orchard TF, Bannon MP, et al. The care and cost of snowmobile-related injuries. Minn Med 1996;79:21–5.

179. Mangano FT, Menendez JA, Smyth MD, et al. Pediatric neurosurgical injuries associated with all-terrain vehicle accidents: a 10-year experience at St. Louis Children's Hospital. J Neurosurg 2006;105:2–5.

180. Russell A, Boop FA, Cherny WB, et al. Neurologic injuries associated with all-terrain vehicles and recommendations for protective measures for the pediatric population. Pediatr Emerg Care 1998;14:31–5.

181. Lister DG, Carl J III, Morgan JH III, et al. Pediatric all-terrain vehicle trauma: a 5-year statewide experience. J Pediatr Surg 1998;33:1081–3.

182. Dick R, Putukian M, Agel J, et al. Descriptive epidemiology of collegiate women's soccer injuries: National Collegiate Athletic Association Injury Surveillance System, 1988–1989 through 2002–2003. J Athl Train 2007;42:278–85.

183. Agel J, Evans TA, Dick R, et al. Descriptive epidemiology of collegiate men's soccer injuries: National Collegiate Athletic Association Injury Surveillance System, 1988–1989 through 2002–2003. J Athl Train 2007;42:270–7.

184. Dvorak J, Junge A, Grimm K, et al. Medical report from the 2006 FIFA World Cup Germany. Br J Sports Med 2007;41:578–81.
185. Faude O, Junge A, Kindermann W, et al. Risk factors for injuries in elite female soccer players. Br J Sports Med 2006;40:785–90.
186. Junge A, Dvorak J. Injuries in female football players in top-level international tournaments. Br J Sports Med 2007;41(Suppl 1):I3–7.
187. Fuller CW, Dick RW, Corlette J, et al. Comparison of the incidence, nature and cause of injuries sustained on grass and new generation artificial turf by male and female football players. Part 2: training injuries. Br J Sports Med 2007; 41(Suppl 1):I27–32.
188. Fuller CW, Dick RW, Corlette J, et al. Comparison of the incidence, nature and cause of injuries sustained on grass and new generation artificial turf by male and female football players. Part 1: match injuries. Br J Sports Med 2007; 41(Suppl 1):I20–6.
189. Tysvaer AT. Head and neck injuries in soccer. Impact of minor trauma. Sports Med 1992;14:200–13.
190. Janda DH, Bir CA, Cheney AL. An evaluation of the cumulative concussive effect of soccer heading in the youth population. Inj Control Saf Promot 2002; 9:25–31.
191. Collins MW, Grindel SH, Lovell MR, et al. Relationship between concussion and neuropsychological performance in college football players. JAMA 1999;282: 964–70.
192. Nathanson A, Bird S, Dao L, et al. Competitive surfing injuries: a prospective study of surfing-related injuries among contest surfers. Am J Sports Med 2007;35:113–7.
193. Yung PS, Chan RH, Wong FC, et al. Epidemiology of injuries in Hong Kong elite badminton athletes. Res Sports Med 2007;15:133–46.
194. Agel J, Palmieri-Smith RM, Dick R, et al. Descriptive epidemiology of collegiate women's volleyball injuries: National Collegiate Athletic Association Injury Surveillance System, 1988–1989 through 2003–2004. J Athl Train 2007;42:295–302.
195. Ferretti A, Cerullo G, Russo G. Suprascapular neuropathy in volleyball players. J Bone Joint Surg Am 1987;69:260–3.
196. Montagna P, Colonna S. Suprascapular neuropathy restricted to the infraspinatus muscle in volleyball players. Acta Neurol Scand 1993;87:248–50.
197. Eggert S, Holzgraefe M [Compression neuropathy of the suprascapular nerve in high performance volleyball players]. Sportverletz Sportschaden 1993;7:136–42 [in German].
198. Holzgraefe M, Kukowski B, Eggert S. Prevalence of latent and manifest suprascapular neuropathy in high-performance volleyball players. Br J Sports Med 1994;28:177–9.
199. Witvrouw E, Cools A, Lysens R, et al. Suprascapular neuropathy in volleyball players. Br J Sports Med 2000;34:174–80.
200. Sandow MJ, Ilic J. Suprascapular nerve rotator cuff compression syndrome in volleyball players. J Shoulder Elbow Surg 1998;7:516–21.
201. Distefano S. Neuropathy due to entrapment of the long thoracic nerve. A case report. Ital J Orthop Traumatol 1989;15:259–62.
202. Paladini D, Dellantonio R, Cinti A, et al. Axillary neuropathy in volleyball players: report of two cases and literature review. J Neurol Neurosurg Psychiatry 1996; 60:345–7.
203. Ozbek A, Bamac B, Budak F, et al. Nerve conduction study of ulnar nerve in volleyball players. Scand J Med Sci Sports 2006;16:197–200.

204. Hostetler SG, Hostetler TL, Smith GA, et al. Characteristics of water skiing-related and wakeboarding-related injuries treated in emergency departments in the United States, 2001–2003. Am J Sports Med 2005;33:1065–70.
205. Yard EE, Collins CL, Dick RW, et al. An epidemiologic comparison of high school and college wrestling injuries. Am J Sports Med 2007, epub ahead of print.
206. Snook G. A survey of wrestling injuries. Am J Sports Med 1980;8:450–3.
207. Nomoto J, Seiki Y, Nemoto M, et al. Head trauma in female professional wrestlers. Neurol Med Chir (Tokyo) 2007;47:147–51.

Section 2

Mechanisms of Injury and Activity

Biomechanical Aspects of Sports-Related Head Injuries

Min S. Park, MD[a],*, Michael L. Levy, MD, PhD[a,b]

KEYWORDS

• Head injury • Sports • Biomechanics

"Players live for it, fans love it, media celebrate it—and all bemoan its devastating consequences. The brutal collision of bodies is football's lifeblood, and the NFL's biggest concern".[1]

The dangers and long-term consequences of sports-related head injuries take center stage in the national media. In a cover story for the sports weekly, *Sports Illustrated*, Tim Layden explored the locker room culture of the professional football player and the seemingly insatiable appetite of the news media and the viewing and paying public for violent, and occasionally injurious, football collisions.[1]

A recent epidemiologic study detailed the increased risks of depression and cognitive impairment in retired professional football players who sustained concussions during their playing career.[2,3] Those athletes who had sustained one or two concussions were 1.5 times more likely to suffer from depression compared with athletes who had no significant concussion history, and those who had sustained three or more concussions were three times more likely to suffer from depression.[2] This latter group also experienced a higher prevalence of mild cognitive deficits and memory difficulties, as well as a tendency for an earlier onset of Alzheimer's disease, when compared with their colleagues who had no concussion history.[3] In an effort to better understand concussions in professional football, the National Football League (NFL) formed the Commission on Mild Traumatic Brain Injury in 1994 to examine the biomechanics of concussions sustained on the football field and to recommend policies to minimize injury to its players.[4–9]

This article originally appeared in *Neurologic Clinics*, Volume 26, Issue 1.

a Division of Neurological Surgery, University of California, San Diego Medical Center, 200 West Arbor Drive, MC 8893, San Diego, CA 92103–8893, USA

b Department of Pediatric Neurosurgery, Rady Children's Hospital, 8010 Frost Street, Suite 502, San Diego, CA 92123, USA

* Corresponding author.

E-mail address: minpark1@hotmail.com (M.S. Park).

Sports-related traumatic brain injuries (TBI) are not only limited to the professional athlete. The Centers for Disease Control and Prevention (CDC) recently estimated approximately 207,830 patient emergency department visits annually for sports and recreation-related non-fatal TBI over a recent 4-year interval in the United States.[10] When individuals not seeking medical care are included, there are an estimated 1.6 to 3.8 million sports-related TBI per year.[11]

Because of the large number of sports-related TBI sustained each year, it is important to have a more complete understanding of the biomechanical pathophysiology of this condition. This article examines recent information regarding sports-related TBI, beginning with a basic description of the critical biomechanical forces based on Newtonian or classical physics, and ending with a review of the literature as it relates more specifically to head injuries in sports.

INTRODUCTION TO BIOMECHANICAL FORCES

The general biomechanical forces involved in the description and understanding of head injuries rely heavily on the principles of Newtonian physics. The human head can be represented as a point particle, an idealized model without regard to its size, shape, or structure, characterized by its position in relative space, its mass, and its ability to be placed in motion by force application. Generally, a point particle is placed at the origin of an arbitrarily defined coordinate system. For a three-dimensional model, the point particle is placed at the intersection of the X, Y, and Z coordinate planes (**Fig. 1**). Any displacement of the point particle is then measured as a vector with a magnitude and direction of change of position along these three axes. In the international system of units, the position of a point particle is measured in meters and its mass is measured in kilograms. As the position of a point particle changes, the velocity of the object can be determined by its displacement in meters with respect to the time interval in seconds:

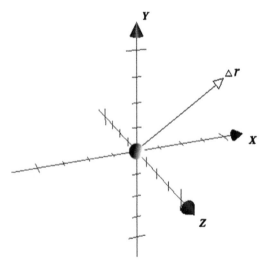

Fig. 1. X, Y, Z coordinate system demonstrating direction and magnitude of change in vector r. The vector is determined by the direction and length of the arrow.

$$v \ (m/s^2) = \Delta r \ (m) \ / \ \Delta t \ (s)$$

where v is the velocity, Δr is the change in position, and Δt is the change in time.

The acceleration of an object is determined by the change in its velocity with respect to time:

$$a \ (m/s^2) = \Delta v \ (m/s)/\Delta t \ (s)$$

where a is the acceleration and Δv is the change in velocity. Because displacements are measured as vectors, either a change in magnitude of the velocity or a change in the direction of velocity can result in the acceleration of an object. A deceleration of an object results from a decrease in the magnitude of the velocity.

Building upon these initial principles, Newton's second law of motion describes the relationship between the force and momentum of an object:

$$F \ (kg \cdot m/s^2) = \Delta[m(kg) \cdot v(m/s)]/\Delta t(s)$$

where F is the force applied to a point particle and m is the mass of the point particle. The numerator of the equation also represents an object's momentum. Assuming that the mass of an object does not change during its acceleration, the equation can be simplified to the following:

$$F \ (kg \ m/s^2) = m \ (kg) \cdot a \ (m/s^2)$$

Work is defined as the product of the force on a point particle and the resulting displacement of the particle:

$$W \ (kg \cdot m^2/s^2) = F \ (kg \cdot m/s^2) \ \Delta s(m)$$

where W is the work and Δs is the displacement of a point particle. The total amount of work done on a point particle is the sum of its applied forces. The kinetic energy is determined by the amount of work done on a particle to accelerate from a zero velocity to a given velocity:

$$E_k \ (kg \cdot m^2/s^2) = 1/2m \ (kg) \cdot v^2 \ (m^2/s^2)$$

where E_k is the kinetic energy.

In reality, the human head cannot simply be characterized as a point particle, but instead possesses a distinct shape and size. If the vector of force runs directly through its center of gravity, the head will accelerate in a linear fashion without rotation. If, however, the vector of force runs through a point other than the center of gravity, there will be both a linear and rotational component to the acceleration.[12] With this introduction to Newtonian physics in mind, we can more closely analyze the biomechanical forces applied to the head during an impact.

BIOMECHANICS OF HEAD INJURIES IN SPORTS

Head injuries in athletes often result from collisions sustained during the normal context of the particular sport. In football, for example, low- and high-impact collisions involving the head are relatively common during the course of a particular play. Soccer players routinely use their heads to strike the ball, and can inadvertently sustain injuries from direct head-to-head or head-to-body challenges with another individual. Boxers and other prize fighters, on the other hand, often sustain repeated blows to the head during a bout.

Head injuries involving athletes involve two types of biomechanical stresses. Acceleration-deceleration injuries result either from an athlete's head striking a stationary object and coming to an abrupt stop, or from a stationary head being struck by a moving object passing through the center of gravity of the head. These translational impacts impart linear, tensile, and compressive forces on the individual's brain.[13] Rotational or angular acceleration results because the brain is relatively fixed along the long axis of the spine. If the vector of force passes outside of the head's center of gravity, it will be subject to rotational acceleration.[12] Early studies by Holbourn in 1943[14] and later by Gennarelli and colleagues[15] demonstrated that angular kinematics were more likely to result in injury to the brain.

To measure the tolerance of the human head to blunt impacts, Gurdjian and colleagues[16,17] developed the Wayne State Tolerance Curve (WSTC) based upon their experimental work with cadaveric skulls. The WSTC was created to depict the relationship between the acceleration level and impulse duration necessary for a blunt impact to cause a skull fracture. High acceleration impacts require a shorter impulse duration than slow acceleration impacts to fracture the skull. The Gadd Severity Index (SI),[18] proposed in 1966, was created to place more emphasis on the acceleration component of the impact versus the time duration by raising the acceleration value by a power of 2.5.

$$SI = \int a^{2.5} \cdot dt$$

Ultimately, the Head Injury Criterion (HIC) was created in 1971 to focus on the relevant aspect of the impact that would most likely cause injury to the brain[12,19]

$$HIC = (t_2 - t_1)\left[1/(t_2 - t_1)\int_{t1}^{t2} a(t) \cdot dt\right]^{2.5}$$

where $(t_2 - t_1)$ represents the time interval and $a(t)$ is the resultant acceleration of the head. The HIC relies on linear acceleration to produce injury at the brainstem as well as concussion. Although the HIC is the most commonly used criterion for assessing the risk of traumatic brain injury from a non-penetrating impact, several other systems have been developed to account for the effects of angular kinematics, energy, or tissue stress in producing brain injury.[12,20]

FOOTBALL

With an estimated 1.5 million participants in the United States each year, American football is one of the most popular sports activities for young athletes. In the early history of football, injuries and fatalities were more prevalent and related to tackling drills and head injuries. Cantu and Mueller[21] analyzed 497 fatalities related to brain and spine injuries in football from 1945 to 1999, and reported that 69% of the fatalities were related to brain injuries and 16% were related to injuries to the cervical spine. The greatest numbers of fatal injuries, however, occurred during earlier time periods, from 1965 to 1969, with the lowest occurrences in the last 2 decades of their study.[21] A more recent study of severe head injuries in collegiate and high school football players also demonstrated an overall low rate of catastrophic head injuries with the advent of newer helmet designs.[22] Furthermore, certain positions, such as the quarterback, defensive backs, and wide receivers, were more likely to sustain concussions.[9,23]

The high incidence of fatal injuries in the late 1960s led to the creation of several institutions to monitor and study traumatic brain injuries and to recommend rules changes to make the sport safer. The National Operating Committee on Standards for Athletic Equipment (NOCSAE), created in 1969, studied the effects of and developed national standards for protective head gear.[23,24] In 1977, The National Collegiate Athletic Association (NCAA) created the forerunner to the present day National Center for Catastrophic Sports Injury Research for the improved understanding of factors related to traumatic injuries and for the proposal of rule changes to improve safety.[23] Through these early mechanisms, fatalities decreased by 74% and the incidence of severe head injuries decreased from 4.25 per 100,000 to 0.68 per 100,000 following the implementation of NOCSAE standards.[23] Today, there is still an estimated incidence of head injuries of 4% to 20% and up to four deaths yearly as a result of TBI in football.[13,25–27] Interestingly, high school football players had a higher incidence of catastrophic head injuries than college players.[22]

From 2003 to the present, the NFL's Committee on Mild Traumatic Brain Injury published a series of papers examining the biomechanics of football related head injuries.[4–8] Impacts to a player's head resulting in a concussion were reconstructed in a laboratory environment using Hybrid III anthropometric test devices (General Motors, Detroit, Michigan) and video analysis of game footage.[5] This allowed for determinations of speed, direction, and location of impact upon the helmet of the players sustaining concussion. Concussed players sustained initial head impacts of 9.3 ± 1.9 m/s, with changes in head velocity of 7.2 ± 1.8 m/s, peak head accelerations of 98 ± 28 g (1 g $= 9/8$ m/s^2), and peak force of 4.4 ± 1.2 kN during a 15-millisecond impact.[5] In contrast, non-concussed players and striking players experienced head velocity changes in the order of 5.0 ± 1.1 m/s and 4.0 ± 1.2 m/s, respectively, and peak head accelerations of 60 ± 24 g.[5] In a prospective study of 38 varsity football players at the Virginia Polytechnic Institute and State University (Virginia Tech) were equipped with accelerometers in their helmets, and impacts identified an average peak head acceleration of 32 ± 25 g in individuals who did not sustain concussions, whereas the lone concussed individual had a peak head acceleration of 81 g.[28]

Although the NFL committee found that translational acceleration sustained by the head with direct facemask or side impacts or impacts to the back of the head during the subsequent fall most strongly correlated with concussions, rotational acceleration of the head closely tracked that of the translational acceleration.[5] Although these results were in contrast with earlier work by Gennarelli and colleagues[14] the authors noted the strong possibility that rotational acceleration of the head may have played a significant role in concussion occurrences.

The NFL committee also examined the location, magnitude, and direction of force sustained by the helmet and head of the concussed player,[6] with the helmet subdivided into different quadrants and analyzed in relation to the these three factors. Oblique impacts to the facemask of the helmet from below the center of gravity of the head, which resulted in translational and rotational accelerations, were most strongly correlated with concussions. While these types of impacts exhibited the highest impact velocities, they also demonstrated the lowest change in velocities and lowest accelerations associated with concussions.[6] Interestingly, unlike in the previous study, there were no significant influence of rotational acceleration upon the occurrence of concussion.[5,6]

The NFL committee also examined the deformation of the brain using a mathematical model and associated it with clinical signs or symptoms of concussion.[4] The Wayne State University head injury model used by the committee incorporated the viscoelastic properties of the brain, surrounding soft tissues, and cranium in a finite element model to study the brain response to certain forces.[29,30] This model demonstrated a low strain response of the brain at the initial impact site early in the course of the impact. During the midphase, there was a migration of the strain response to the contrecoup location. Ultimately, the strain response migrated to the midbrain region during the late-phase of the impact. The largest strain responses were sustained by deep structures, such as the corpus callosum, fornix, and midbrain, during the late phase of the response. These late phase responses correlated with loss of consciousness, cognitive and memory problems, and removal from play for the concussed athlete, whereas early strain responses in the orbital-frontal cortex and temporal lobe correlated with symptoms of dizziness.[4]

RUGBY AND AUSTRALIAN RULES FOOTBALL

To better understand the increasing concussion rates in professional Australian rules football (ARF) and develop safer athletic headgear, McIntosh and colleagues[31] conducted a study of the dynamics of 100 concussive head impacts in professional ARF and rugby matches in 2000. After reviewing video sequences of the impacts and gathering the necessary anthropometric data on the impacting and impacted players, researchers at the University of New South Wales determined the kinematics sustained by the head during the concussive impacts. The majority of concussive impacts occurred in the temporal region and resulted from contact with the striking player's upper limbs, shoulders, or thorax.[31] The mean change in velocity and the energy imparted to the head during the impact were 4 m/s and 56 J, respectively.[31] Although these results were in accordance with results the authors had previously published in concussions sustained by helmeted bicyclists, it is interesting to compare them with those from the NFL (**Table 1**). The discrepancies may be related to differences in protective head and body gear worn in the respective leagues, the nature of the object striking the head, or the differences in tackling techniques.

SOCCER

Although the act of heading the ball in soccer has been controversially associated with cognitive deficits and head injuries, recent studies have emphasized head-to-head or head-to-body impact as a more common cause of concussion.[32–36] Withnall and colleagues[34] recreated various types of impacts with a soccer player's head in a laboratory setting, relating impacts to concussion risk. Sixty-two video-recorded cases of head-to-upper extremity and head-to-head impacts were reviewed, and six upper extremity-to-head and three head-to-head impacts were reconstructed using the Hybrid III anthropometric test device. Experienced volunteer soccer players assisted in the recreation of elbow and hand/wrist impacts to the model's head, while head-to-head impacts were recreated using two Hybrid III models. When comparing the results from the laboratory re-enactments with head injury reference values, Withnall and colleagues[34] determined that the risk of concussions with upper extremity-to-head impacts was low compared with the risk of concussions following head-to-head impacts.

Naunheim and colleagues[37] analyzed the peak accelerations of the head during a standardized heading action in volunteer high school soccer players who were asked to wear a helmet equipped with a triaxial accelerometer. Soccer balls were kicked from 30 yards away, traveling at 39.3 ± 1.8 miles per hour. These results were compared with high school football linemen and hockey players similarly equipped during live games. The average peak accelerations sustained during the heading of a soccer ball were statistically higher than the peak accelerations sustained by the football and hockey players during the course of a game.[37] Whereas the calculated Gadd SI and HIC scores were below the threshold for an impact to cause significant

Table 1
Comparison of study results

Sport	ΔV (m/s)	Translational Acceleration (g)	Rotational Acceleration (rad/s²)	Impulse (kg·m/s)	HIC
Football (NFL)[5]	7.2 ± 1/8	98 ± 28	6596 ± 1866		345 ± 181
Football (college)[23]		81			
Football (high school)[a,32]		29.2 ± 1.0			
ARF/rugby (professional)[b,26]	4 ± 2			29 ± 11	
Soccer (professional)[b,29]		86.7 ± 0.3[c] 79.0 ± 0.1[d]	7033 ± 30		
Soccer (high school)[a,32]		54.7 ± 4.1			48.5 ± 7.0
Boxing (hook)[a,7]		71.2 ± 32.2	9306 ± 4485		
Boxing (straight punch)[a,41]		58 ± 13	6343 ± 1789	25 ± 8	71 ± 49

a Did not result in concussions.
b High likelihood of resulting in concussions.
c Frontal boss to side of head impacts.
d Forehead to rear of head impacts.

brain injury, the scores for soccer were statistically higher than those in football or hockey.[37] These results may support the possibility of repetitive subconcussive head impacts leading to long-term neuropsychological deficits found in some soccer players.[37,38]

BOXING

Few sports are more closely associated with traumatic brain injuries than boxing. Injury and concussion rates have been analyzed with both retrospective reviews and prospective cohort studies.[39,40] Concussions account for 16% to 33% of the injuries sustained during practice and competition.[39,40] Several recent articles have examined the biomechanics of boxing and its associated risk of mild traumatic brain injuries.[7,41] Walilko and colleagues[41] examined the force from straight punches of seven Olympic boxers spanning five different weight classes (112 to 240 lbs.) on the Hybrid III anthropometric models. The average translational acceleration, rotational acceleration, and HIC were 58 ± 13 g, 6343 ± 1789 rad/s^2, and 71 ± 49 respectively.[41] Viano and colleagues[7] also examined the punch force of eleven Olympic boxers weighing 112 to 185 lbs on Hybrid III models. This study not only examined the straight punch, but also the hook and the uppercut. The highest translational and rotational accelerations, 71.2 ± 32.2 g and 9306 ± 4485 rad/s^2 respectively, were recorded with hook punches.[7] When compared with NFL studies, values were similar to those calculated for concussive impacts in the NFL, but the calculated HIC were lower in boxing because of the shorter duration of accelerations.[7] Although both studies determined that the likelihood of concussions were low per punch, neither study examined the cumulative effects of punches sustained by the head during the course of about.

SUMMARY

With the improved conditioning, size, and speed of professional athletes and the rise in the numbers of individuals engaging in sports and recreational activities today, there is potential for rising numbers of traumatic brain injuries throughout the sports world. Fortunately, parallel strides in basic research technology and improvements in computer and video technology have created a new era of discovery in the study of the biomechanical aspects of sports-related head injuries. Although prevention will always be the most important factor in reducing the incidence of sports-related traumatic brain injuries, ongoing studies will lead to the development of newer protective equipment, improved recognition and management of concussions on the field of play, and modification of rules and guidelines to make these activities safer and more enjoyable for all.[34,42–45]

REFERENCES

1. Layden T. The big hit. Sports Illustrated 2007;107(4):52–62.
2. Guskiewicz K, Marshall S, Bailes J, et al. Recurrent concussion and risk of depression in retired professional football players. Med Sci Sports Exerc 2007; 39(6):903–9.
3. Guskiewicz K, Marshall S, Bailes J, et al. Association between recurrent concussion and late-life cognitive impairment in retired professional football players. Neurosurgery 2005;57(4):719–26.
4. Viano D, Casson I, Pellman E, et al. Concussion in professional football: brain responses by finite element analysis: part 9. Neurosurgery 2005;57(5):891–916.

5. Pellman E, Viano D, Tucker A, et al. Concussion in professional football: reconstruction of game impacts and injuries. Neurosurgery 2003;53(4):799–812.
6. Pellman E, Viano D, Tucker A, et al. Concussion in professional football: location and direction of helmet impacts—part 2. Neurosurgery 2003;53(6):1328–40.
7. Viano D, Casson I, Pellman E, et al. Concussion in professional football: comparison with boxing head impacts—part 10. Neurosurgery 2005;57(6):1154–72.
8. Viano D, Pellman E. Concussion in professional football: biomechanics of the striking player—part 8. Neurosurgery 2005;56(2):266–80.
9. Pellman E, Powell J, Viano D, et al. Concussion in professional football: epidemiological features of game injuries and review of the literature—Part 3. Neurosurgery 2004;54(1):81–94.
10. Centers for Disease Control and Prevention. Nonfatal traumatic brain injuries from sports and recreation activities—United States, 2001–2005. MMWR Morb Mortal Wkly Rep 2007;56(29):733–7.
11. Langlois J, Rutland-Brown W, Wald M. The epidemiology and impact of traumatic brain injury: a brief overview. J Head Trauma Rehabil 2006;21(5):375–8.
12. Anderson R, McLean J. Biomechanics of closed head injury. In: Reilly P, Bullock R, editors. Head injury: pathophysiology and management. 2nd edition. London: Hodder Arnold; 2005. p. 26–40.
13. Bailes J, Cantu R. Head injury in athletes. Neurosurgery 2001;48(1):26–46.
14. Holbourn A. Mechanics of head injuries. Lancet 1943;2:438–41.
15. Gennarelli T, Thibault L, Adams J, et al. Diffuse axonal injury and traumatic coma in the primate. Ann Neurol 1982;12(6):564–74.
16. Gurdjian E, Roberts V, Thomas L. Tolerance curves of acceleration and intracranial pressure and protective index in experimental head injury. J Trauma 1966;6: 600–4.
17. Gurdjian E, Lissner H, Webster J, et al. Studies on experimental concussion: relation of physiologic effect to time duration of intracranial pressure increase at impact. Neurology 1954;4(9):674–81.
18. Gadd C. Use of a weighted impulse criterion for estimating injury hazard. Presented at the *10th Stapp Car Crash Conference, Society of Automotive Engineers.* New York, NY, 1966.
19. Versace J. A review of the severity index. Presented at the *15th Stapp Car Crash Conference, Society of Automotive Engineers.* New York, NY, 1971.
20. Kikuchi A, Ono K, Nakamura M. Human head tolerance to lateral impact deduced from experimental head injuries using primates. Presented at the *26th Stapp Car Crash Conference, Society of Automotive Engineers.* Warrendale, PA, 1982.
21. Cantu R, Mueller F. Brain injury-related fatalities in American football, 1945–1999. Neurosurgery 2003;52:846–53.
22. Boden B, Tacchetti R, Cantu R, et al. Catastrophic head injuries in high school and college football players. Am J Sports Med 2007;35(7):1075–81.
23. Levy M, Ozgur B, Berry C, et al. Analysis and evolution of head injury in football. Neurosurgery 2004;55:649–55.
24. Clarke K, Powell J. Football helmets and neurotrauma: an epidemiological overview of three seasons. Med Sci Sports 1979;11:138–45.
25. Gerberich S, Priest J, Boen J, et al. Concussion incidence and severity in secondary school varsity football players. Am J Public Health 1983;73:1370–5.
26. McCrea M, Kelly J, Kluge J, et al. Standardized assessment of concussion in football players. Neurology 1997;48:586–8.
27. Powell J, Barber-Foss K. Traumatic brain injury in high school athletes. JAMA 1999;282:958–63.

28. Duma S, Manoogian S, Bussone W, et al. Analysis of real-time head accelerations in collegiate football players. Clin J Sport Med 2005;15(1):3–8.

29. Zhang L, Yang K, King A. Biomechanics of neurotrauma. Neurol Res 2001;23: 144–56.

30. Zhang L, Yang K, King A. Comparison of brain responses between frontal and lateral impacts by finite element modeling. J Neurotrauma 2001;18:21–30.

31. McIntosh A, McCrory P, Comerford J. The dynamics of concussive head impacts in rugby and Australian rules football. Med Sci Sports Exerc 2000;32(12):1980–4.

32. Matser J, Kessels A, Lezak M, et al. A dose-response relation of headers and concussions with cognitive impairment in professional soccer players. J Clin Exp Neuropsychol 2001;23(6):770–4.

33. Matser J, Kessels A, Jordan B, et al. Chronic traumatic brain injury in professional soccer players. Neurology 1998;51(3):791–6.

34. Withnall C, Shewchenko N, Gittens R, et al. Biomechanical investigation of head impacts in football. Br J Sports Med 2005;39:49–57.

35. Boden B, Kirkendall D, Garrett WJ. Concussion incidence in elite college soccer players. Am J Sports Med 1998;26(2):238–41.

36. Fuller C, Junge A, Dvorak J. A six year prospective study of the incidence and causes of head and neck injuries in international football. Br J Sports Med 2005;39(Suppl 1):i3–9.

37. Naunheim R, Standeven J, Richter C, et al. Comparison of impact data in hockey, football, and soccer. J Trauma 2000;48(5):938–41.

38. Tysvaer A, Lochen E. Soccer injuries to the brain. A neuro-psychologic study of former soccer players. Am J Sports Med 1991;19:56–60.

39. Zazryn T, Cameron P, McCrory P. A prospective cohort study of injury in amateur and professional boxing. Br J Sports Med 2006;40(8):670–4.

40. Zazryn T, Finch C, McCrory P. A 16 year study of injuries to professional boxers in the state of Victoria, Australia. Br J Sports Med 2003;37(4):321–4.

41. Walilko T, Viano D, Bir C. Biomechanics of the head for Olympic boxer punches to the face. Br J Sports Med 2005;39:710–9.

42. Goldberg L, Dimeff R. Sideline management of sport-related concussions. Sports Med Arthrosc 2006;14(4):199–205.

43. Viano D, Pellman E, Withnall C, et al. Concussion in professional football: performance of newer helmets in reconstructed game impacts—Part 13. Neurosurgery 2006;59(3):591–606.

44. Collins M, Lovell M, Iverson G, et al. Examining concussion rates and return to play in high school football players wearing newer helmet technology: a three year prospective cohort study. Neurosurgery 2006;58(2):275–86.

45. Withnall C, Shewchenko N, Wonnocott M, et al. Effectiveness of headgear in football. Br J Sports Med 2005;39(Suppl 1):i40–8.

The Neurophysiology and Assessment of Sports-Related Head Injuries

Mark Lovell, PhD

KEYWORDS

- Head injury • Pathophysiology
- Neurophysiology • Sports

The diagnosis and management of traumatic brain injury is difficult, even under the best of circumstances. The proper diagnosis and management of this injury is challenging particularly for sports medicine practitioners. Team physicians often are called on to make return-to-play decisions based on limited observation of an athlete and after only a brief sideline evaluation. Furthermore, return-to-play decisions often are made under intense pressure from coaches, fans, and players to return an injured athlete to the playing field as quickly as possible.

Over the past 20 years, more than 20 management guidelines have been published to provide guidance regarding return-to-play issues.[1] These guidelines, however, are not evidence-based and largely are based on the opinions of individual physicians or groups of experts rather than on empiric findings.[2] Research within the past 10 years has prompted a re-evaluation and revision of these guidelines with an emphasis on their efficacy in making accurate return-to-play decisions.

This article reviews new developments in the evaluation and management of sports-related concussion and focuses specifically on the integration of evolving scientific research into practical clinical care directives.

EPIDEMIOLOGY

Awareness of sports-related concussion has increased dramatically over the past decade and as public awareness has grown, there has been a corresponding increase in estimates of injuries. The Center for Disease Control recently revised their estimates from approximately 300,000 injuries per year during the 1990s to a current range of 1.6 to 2.3 million per year.[3] Although there are several factors that explain this tenfold increase in injury prevalence, increased awareness at medical and public levels likely

This article originally appeared in *Neurologic Clinics*, Volume 26, Issue 1.
Department of Orthopaedic Surgery, University of Pittsburgh Medical Center for Sports Medicine, 3200 South Water Street, Pittsburgh, PA 15203, USA
E-mail address: lovellmr@upmc.edu

is responsible for increased identification and better reporting of injuries. Given this trend and the high probability that concussion still is under-reported,[4] it is likely that increases in concussion rates over the next decade will continue to be seen.

DEFINITIONS OF CONCUSSION

Definitions of traumatic brain injury (concussion) have undergone substantial change over the past 3 decades as understanding of the brain and its response to injury has continued to evolve. In 1966, the Committee on Head Injury Nomenclature of the Congress of Neurological Surgeons[4] defined concussion as:

> "a clinical syndrome characterized by the immediate and transient post-traumatic impairment of neural function such as alteration of consciousness, disturbance of vision or equilibrium, etc., due to brain stem dysfunction."[5]

More recently, however, other definitions of concussion have been posed. For example, the American Academy of Neurology (AAN)[6] defines concussion as:

> "Any trauma induced alteration in mental status that may or may not include a loss of consciousness."

Authors of the AAN definition believed that the Committee on Head Injury Nomenclature definition may have been too limiting, because other brain structures (eg, cortical areas) commonly are associated with concussion, and the injury is not limited to the brainstem. These guidelines also highlighted that concussion may occur with or without loss of consciousness (LOC).

THE NEUROPHYSIOLOGY OF CONCUSSION

Recent research into the subtle neurometabolic effects of concussion has led to new insights into the pathophysiology of concussion. This area of research was ushered in by Hovda and colleagues at UCLA in the 1990s. Using a rodent model, Hovda and colleagues[7] described metabolic dysfunction that occurred at the intracellular and extracellular levels. They posited that these changes are the result of excitatory amino acid–induced ionic shifts with increased Na/K-ATPase activation and resultant hyperglycolysis.[8] Thus, there is a high-energy demand within the brain shortly after concussive injury. Hovda and colleagues[7] demonstrated further that hyperglycolysis is accompanied by decreased cerebral blood flow resulting in widespread cerebral neurovascular constriction. The resulting "metabolic mismatch" between energy supply and demand within the brain is postulated as leading to cellular vulnerability during the days to weeks after injury.

Given that concussion occurs on a physiologic rather than a structural level, traditional neurodiagnostic techniques (eg, CT scan, MRI, and neurologic examination) almost invariably are normal after concussive insult.[9] It should be stressed, however, that these techniques are valuable in ruling out more serious pathology (eg, cerebral hematoma or skull fracture) that also may occur with head trauma.

Hovda and colleagues' initial research was groundbreaking and led to an increased focus on the pathophysiology of this injury in human subjects. More recent research has examined the potential usefulness of functional MRI (fMRI) as a viable tool for the assessment of neural processes after concussion. The technology is based on the measurement of specific correlates of brain activation, such as cerebral blood flow and oxygenation.[10] fMRI also has promoted the evaluation of specific neuropsychologic test paradigms through which cerebral blood flow changes can be linked to specific tests that measure memory and other cognitive processes. In addition, fMRI involves no exposure to radiation and can be used safely in children. Furthermore, repeat evaluations can be undertaken with minimal risk. This promotes the assessment of changes in neural substrata that may occur with mild concussion, permitting tracking of injured athletes throughout the recovery process. Potentially, one of the most important uses of fMRI scanning is the ability to provide validity data regarding the sensitivity and specificity of neuropsychologic testing for detection of subtle changes in brain function.

Although a promising tool, fMRI has yet to be implemented widely in clinical settings. Few laboratories actively are investigating the use of fMRI in sports-related head injury at present, although this likely will change within the next few years. Notably, Johnston and colleagues[9] at McGill University in Montreal have developed an fMRI protocol that allows the assessment of several components of working memory. In the United States, my laboratory at the University of Pittsburgh represents one of only a handful of research programs structured to collect neuropsychologic and fMRI data in athletes. This multiyear, prospective study relies on the prior baseline neuropsychologic testing (Immediate Post-Concussion Assessment and Cognitive Testing [ImPACT]) of a large cohort (more than 3000) of male and female high school and college athletes. In the event of injury, the athletes undergo repeat testing within 24 to 72 hours and undergo fMRI scanning. An additional fMRI scan and ImPACT testing "in scanner" and "out of scanner" are completed as patients recover, allowing tracking of the correlation between fMRI and neuropsychologic testing. To date, more than 200 athletes have been evaluated within 1 week of injury and again after clinical recovery, and the group with the highest degree of abnormalities on fMRI has demonstrated a significantly longer time to clinical recovery (ie, symptom-free with normal neuropsychologic test performance).[11]

ON-FIELD AND SIDELINE MANAGEMENT OF CONCUSSION

A concussion may occur without direct trauma to the head, and concussed athletes are rendered unconscious infrequently. In addition, athletes may be unaware that they are injured and may not show any obvious immediate signs or symptoms of injury, such as motor incoordination, gross confusion, or amnesia. To complicate the situation further, athletes at all levels of competition may minimize or hide symptoms in an attempt to prevent their removal from the game, creating the potential for re-injury, second concussion, and exacerbation of the original injury.

INITIAL SIDELINE SIGNS AND SYMPTOMS OF EVALUATION AND RETURN TO PLAY

Table 1 provides a summary of common on-field signs and symptoms of concussion. Sideline presentation may vary widely from athlete to athlete, depending on the biomechanical forces involved, athletes' prior history of injury, and many other factors. In reviewing the common signs and symptoms of concussion, it is imperative to understand that an athlete may have only a few signs or symptoms of injury or a constellation of symptomatology. A thorough assessment of all common symptoms associated with concussion should be conducted for concussed athletes.

With regard to the frequency of postconcussion signs and symptoms, headache is the symptom reported most commonly, occurring in approximately 70% of concussed athletes. Although it is true that musculoskeletal headaches and other pre-existing headache syndromes may complicate the assessment of postconcussion headache, any presentation of headache after a blow to the head or body should be managed conservatively. Most frequently, a concussion headache is described as

Table 1
University of Pittsburgh signs and symptoms of concussion

Signs Observed by Staff	Symptoms Reported by Athlete
Appears to be dazed or stunned	Headache
Is confused about assignment	Nausea
Forgets plays	Balance problems or dizziness
Is unsure of game, score, or opponent	Double or fuzzy/blurry vision
Moves clumsily	Sensitivity to light or noise
Answers questions slowly	Feeling sluggish or slowed down
Loses consciousness	Feeling "foggy" or groggy
Shows behavior or personality change	Concentration or memory problems
Forgets events prior to play (retrograde)	Change in sleep pattern (appears later)
Forgets events after hit (posttraumatic)	Feeling fatigue

a sensation of pressure in the skull that most often is localized to the frontotemporal regions of the head. In some athletes (particularly migraineurs), a headache may be unilateral and often is described as throbbing or pulsating. A headache may not develop immediately after injury and may develop over the minutes, or even hours, after injury. It is not unusual for athletes initially to be pain-free, then wake the morning after with headache. Therefore, it is essential to question potentially concussed athletes regarding the development of symptoms beyond the first few minutes or hours after injury. It also is important to prompt family members to observe injured athletes for evolving signs of injury. Another common characteristic of postconcussion headache is that this type of headache often is made worse during physical and cognitive exertion. Athletes frequently report an exacerbation of symptoms after even minor increases in physical activity and after a return to school or activity. Although headache after a concussion does not necessarily constitute a medical emergency, a severe or progressively severe headache, particularly when accompanied by vomiting or rapidly declining mental status, may signal a life-threatening situation, such as a hematoma or intracranial bleed. This should prompt immediate transport to hospital and a CT scan of the brain.

Although headache is the most common symptom of concussion, concussion is possible without headache and other signs or symptoms of injury should be assessed and detailed carefully. For example, athletes often experience blurred vision, changes in peripheral vision, or other visual disturbance. Another common and disabling symptom is fatigue or sluggishness. Fatigue is prominent in concussed athletes especially during the days after injury and may be nearly as frequent as headache. In addition to these symptoms, cognitive or mental status changes commonly are seen immediately after injury. Athletes who have any degree of mental status change should be managed conservatively and a thorough discussion of these issues is warranted.

INITIAL EVALUATION OF CONCUSSION AND MARKERS OF INJURY

Appropriate care of a concussed athlete should begin with the initial on-field evaluation of the athlete (**Box 1**). As with any serious injury, the first priority is evaluating an athlete's level of consciousness and airway, breathing, and circulation. The attending medical staff must be prepared with an emergency action plan in the event that the evacuation of a critically head- or neck-injured athlete is necessary. This plan should

---

Box 1
University of Pittsburgh sideline mental status testing card. On-field cognitive testing

Orientation—ask athlete the following questions:

- What stadium is this?
- What city is this?
- Who is the opposing team?
- What month is it?
- What day is it?

Postraumatic amnesia—ask athlete to repeat the following words:

- Girl, dog, green

Retrograde amnesia—ask the athlete the following questions:

- What happened in the prior quarter or half?
- What do you remember just before the hit?
- What was the score of the game before the hit?
- Do you remember the hit?

Concentration—ask the athlete to do the following:

- Repeat the days of the week backwards, starting with today
- Repeat these numbers backwards: 63, 419

Word list memory

- Ask athlete to repeat the three words from earlier (girl, dog, green)

---

be familiar to all medical staff, with each team member having a role that is defined in advance.

On ruling out more severe injury (eg, traumatic neck injury or acute neurosurgical emergency), the evaluation should continue with assessment of the concussion mental status of the injured athlete. First, a clinician should establish the presence of any LOC. By definition, LOC represents a state of brief coma in which an athlete is unresponsive to external stimuli and the eyes typically are closed. LOC is uncommon and occurs in less than 10% of concussive injuries. Furthermore, athletes who do experience LOC typically are unresponsive for only a brief period (usually seconds). Athletes who have documented LOC should be managed conservatively and return to play is contraindicated, particularly in younger athletes.

Although LOC is uncommon, confusion and amnesia are common sequelae of injury. Confusion (ie, disorientation), by definition, represents impaired awareness and orientation to surroundings and often manifests in athletes who have descriptions of appearing stunned, dazed, or glassy-eyed on the sideline. Confusion frequently presents as difficulties in appropriate play calling, answering questions slowly or inappropriately, or athletes repeating themselves during evaluation (perseveration). Teammates often are the first to recognize a confused athlete during difficulties with running plays or completing assignments. To assess the presence of confusion properly, simple orientation questions can be asked (eg, name, current stadium, city, opposing team, and current month and day).

A careful evaluation of amnesia is of particular importance in the diagnosis and management of concussed athletes. Amnesia may be associated with loss of memory for events preceding (retrograde) or after injury (posttraumatic). Retrograde amnesia is defined as the inability to recall events occurring during the period immediately preceding trauma. To assess on-field retrograde amnesia properly, athletes may be asked questions pertaining to details occurring just before the trauma that caused the concussion. Simple questions posed to an athlete, such as recollection of details of the injury, are a good starting point (**Box 2**). From the point of injury, an evaluator should ask probing questions in an attempt to ascertain the last formed memory before injury. The length of retrograde amnesia typically shrinks over time but an athlete often never regains all of the lost information.

Posttraumatic amnesia typically is represented by the length of time between trauma (eg, helmet-to-helmet contact) and the point at which an individual regains normal continuous memory functioning (eg, standing on the sideline after the hit). As outlined in **Table 1**, on-field posttraumatic amnesia may be assessed through immediate and delayed (eg, 0-, 5-, and 15-minute) memory for three words (eg, girl, dog, and green). In addition, simply asking an athlete to recall specific events that occurred immediately after a trauma is useful (eg, memory of returning to sideline, memory for subsequent plays, and memory of later parts of contest). Any failure to recall these events properly is indicative of posttraumatic amnesia. The presence of posttraumatic amnesia is highly predictive of postinjury neurocognitive and symptom deficit.[12]

THE RETURN-TO-PLAY DECISION-MAKING PROCESS
Return-to-Play Guidelines

During the past 30 years, more than 20 concussion management guidelines have been published with the intent of providing guidance and direction for sports medicine practitioners in making complex return-to-play decisions.[2] The authors of each of these guidelines provided an accompanying grading scale designed to reflect and characterize the severity of an injury. Although these guidelines no doubt have resulted in

---

Box 2

Vienna concussion conference: return-to-play recommendations. Athletes should complete the following step-wise process prior to return to play after concussion

1. Removal from contest if signs/symptoms of concussion

2. No return to play in current game

3. Medical evaluation after injury

    a. Rule out more serious intracranial pathology

    b. Neuropsychologic testing considered cornerstone of proper postinjury assessment

4. Stepwise return to play

    a. No activity and rest until asymptomatic

    b. Light aerobic exercise

    c. Sport-specific training

    d. Noncontact drills

    e. Full-contact drills

    f. Game play

improved care of athletes, these multiple directives have created significant confusion and sparked almost continuous debate. A historical review of all past and current concussion guidelines is beyond the scope of this article; however, brief review is provided.

Cantu[13] originally proposed a grading scale and management guidelines based on clinical experience. Cantu was careful to emphasize, however, that these guidelines were intended to supplement rather than replace clinical judgment. The original Cantu guidelines allowed return to play the day of injury if an athlete were symptom-free at rest and after physical exertion. For athletes who experienced any LOC (eg, grade 3 concussion), a restriction of contact for 1 month was recommended. Athletes who suffered a grade 2 concussion were allowed to return to play in 2 weeks, if asymptomatic for a period of 7 days.

The Colorado guidelines[14] were published in 1991 after the death of a high school athlete from second impact syndrome and were drafted under the auspices of the Colorado Medical Society. These guidelines allowed for same-day return to play if symptoms cleared within 20 minutes of injury. For more severe injury (grade 3 concussion), these guidelines recommended immediate transport to a hospital for further evaluation. These guidelines later were revised under the sponsorship of the AAN.[6] The AAN guidelines allowed return to competition the same day of injury if an athlete's signs and symptoms cleared within 15 minutes of injury. Grade 2 concussions were managed in a manner similar to that of the Colorado guidelines, with return to competition within 1 week, if asymptomatic.

More recently, Cantu has amended his guidelines[15] to emphasize the duration of posttraumatic symptoms in grading the severity of the concussion and making return-to-play decisions. Grade 1 concussion was redefined by an absence of LOC and postconcussion signs or symptoms lasting fewer than 30 minutes. Same-day return to competition was allowed only if athletes were completely asymptomatic after the injury.

Concussion management guidelines reached their zenith of popularity during the 1980s and 1990s; in the late 1990s, sports medicine practitioners and organizations began to question the empiric basis of these guidelines. This trend prompted the American Orthopaedic Society for Sports Medicine (AOSSM) to sponsor a workshop with the purpose of re-evaluating guidelines and establishing practical alternatives.[16] The AOSSM guidelines were the first to emphasize more individualized management of injury rather than applying general standards and protocols.

A particularly important development took place in 2002 under the auspices of the Fédération Internationale de Football Association in conjunction with the International Olympic Committee and the International Ice Hockey Federation. The organizers of this meeting assembled a group of physicians, neuropsychologists, and sports administrators in Vienna, Austria, to continue to explore methods of reducing morbidity secondary to sports-related concussion. The deliberations that took place during this meeting led to the publication of a document outlining recommendations for diagnosis and management of concussion in sports.[17] One of the most important conclusions of this meeting was that none of the previously published concussion management guidelines was adequate to assure proper management of every concussion. Although a complete discussion of these recommendations is beyond the scope of this article, the group emphasized the implementation of postinjury neuropsychologic testing as a cornerstone of proper postinjury management and return-to-play decision making. A second meeting of this group took place in Prague in 2004,[18] and they continued to promote a return-to-play protocol that was based on assessment of signs and symptoms of injury. This statement also continued to avoid the numeric grading system but did suggest the possible classification of concussions as being simple or complex in nature. Although this classification system has yet to be validated, simple concussions were defined as concussions that were followed by improvement within 10 days of injury and not accompanied by convulsions or other obvious signs of brain injury. In addition, athletes who had a past history of concussion automatically were classified as having complex injuries. In contrast, complex concussions were described as taking more than 10 days to recover, being accompanied by convulsions or occurring within the context of a history of multiple injuries.

To date, there has only one study that has investigated the validity of the simple-complex dichotomy. The investigation by Iverson[19] used cognitive function scores in four categories (verbal memory, visual memory, reaction time, and processing speed) and symptoms provided by the ImPACT test battery to investigate the clinical usefulness of the new classification system. Iverson found that within 72 hours of injury, high school athletes who had complex concussions performed worse than baseline on three of four cognitive composite scores (visual memory, processing speed, and reaction time) than those who had simple concussions. Furthermore, the study found that patients who had complex concussions were more likely to report a total symptom score of 40 or greater on the postconcussion scale (a self-report symptom inventory) (**Table 2**). Iverson suggested that low composite scores in two or three of

Table 2
The postconcussion symptom scale

Symptom	None	Minor		Moderate		Severe	
Headache	0	1	2	3	4	5	6
Nausea	0	1	2	3	4	5	6
Vomiting	0	1	2	3	4	5	6
Balance problems	0	1	2	3	4	5	6
Dizziness	0	1	2	3	4	5	6
Fatigue	0	1	2	3	4	5	6
Trouble falling asleep	0	1	2	3	4	5	6
Sleeping more than usual	0	1	2	3	4	5	6
Sleeping less than usual	0	1	2	3	4	5	6
Drowsiness	0	1	2	3	4	5	6
Sensitivity to light	0	1	2	3	4	5	6
Sensitivity to noise	0	1	2	3	4	5	6
Irritability	0	1	2	3	4	5	6
Sadness	0	1	2	3	4	5	6
Nervousness	0	1	2	3	4	5	6
Feeling more emotional	0	1	2	3	4	5	6
Numbness or tingling	0	1	2	3	4	5	6
Feeling slowed down	0	1	2	3	4	5	6
Feeling mentally "foggy"	0	1	2	3	4	5	6
Difficulty concentrating	0	1	2	3	4	5	6
Difficulty remembering	0	1	2	3	4	5	6
Visual problems	0	1	2	3	4	5	6

Adapted from Lovell MR, Collins MW. Neuropsychological assessment of the college football player. J Head Trauma Rehabil 1998;13:9–26; with permission.

the aforementioned cognitive tests may be indicative of a complex concussion or slower recovery.

In addition to investigating the validity of simple-complex distinction, Iverson challenged the assumption that multiple prior concussions were associated with the occurrence of complex concussions. Although poorer presentation and vulnerability of subsequent concussions of three or more concussions is well documented,[20] Iverson[19] found that athletes who have one or two previous concussions do not take longer to recover than those experiencing their first. Iverson's study did not examine, however, the change over the recovery curve or predictive potential of individual symptoms or patterns of symptoms.

In addition to the use of neuropsychologic testing in making return-to-play decisions, a graduated return-to-play protocol was emphasized by the Vienna and Prague groups.[17,18] The specific recommendations of these groups are presented in **Box 2**. It specifically was recommended that each step would, in most circumstances, be separated by 24 hours. Furthermore, any recurrence of concussive symptoms should lead to an athlete dropping back to the previous level. In other words, if an athlete is asymptomatic at rest and develops a headache after light aerobic exercise, the athlete should return to complete rest. The Vienna and Prague groups recognized further that conventional structural neuroimaging studies (eg, CT scan, MRI, and electroencephalogram) typically are unremarkable after concussive injury and should be used only when a structural lesion is suspected. The group suggested further that functional imaging techniques are in the early stages of development but may provide valuable information in the future.

Individual Factors Determining Return to Play

Return-to-play decisions after a concussion can be complicated and are influenced by several factors, including but not limited to an athlete's age, history of prior injury, and particular sport. Making return-to-play decisions, on the field and during postinjury management of injury, can be one of the most complex decisions facing sports medicine physicians and represents a dynamic process. Therefore, a brief review of factors that may affect recovery from concussion follows.

Age

Past concussion guidelines assumed identical return-to-play criteria for athletes regardless of age. Based on these guidelines, it traditionally has been assumed that the speed of recovery is the same at all age groups and athletic levels. Before the mid-1990s, however, there were no published studies examining outcome from concussion in high school athletes or younger populations. Recent research has begun to expose potential differential age-related responses to concussive injury.

Based on research done with more severe mild traumatic brain injury in nonathletes, several theories exist to explain age-related differences to recovery from concussion. One theory is that children may experience more prolonged cerebral swelling after traumatic brain injury, which suggests that they may be at an increased risk for secondary injury.[21] In addition, an immature brain may be more sensitive to glutamate,[22] a neurotransmitter involved in the metabolic cascade after concussion. These factors could lead to a longer recovery period and could increase the likelihood of permanent or severe neurologic deficit should re-injury occur during the recovery period. This research has been used by some to help account for the finding that second impact syndrome has been found to occur only in child and adolescent athletes.[23] Second impact syndrome represents malignant brain swelling that often results in death or serious disability.

One published study has examined directly recovery from concussion in college versus high school aged athletes.[24] Specifically, baseline and postconcussion neurocognitive functioning was measured in a sample of 53 athletes. Even though the college sample had a greater prior incidence of concussion, high school athletes were found to take longer to recover during an in-study concussion. This study suggests more protracted recovery from concussion in high school athletes. Another study examined the issue of the "ding," or mild concussion, in high school athletes ages 13 to 17.[25] This study revealed that high school athletes who had fewer than 15 minutes of on-field symptoms required at least 7 days before full neurocognitive and symptom recovery. These findings suggest that it may be wise to remove concussed high school athletes from play during the contest in which they are injured. One published study examined recovery from concussion in high school and professional football players.[26] This study found that National Football League (NFL) athletes recovered significantly faster than their younger counterparts, many of them performing normally on neuropsychologic testing within 24 to 48 hours of injury. In contrast, the high school group demonstrated significantly longer recovery times.

History of prior injury

In addition to the age of athletes, the concussion history of athletes is identified by some researchers as a potentially important factor in making return-to-play decisions. There is some evidence to suggest there may be cumulative detrimental effects of multiple concussions. In a study of almost 400 college football players, Collins and colleagues[1] found long-term subtle neurocognitive deficits in those suffering two or more concussions. Similarly, Matser and colleagues[27] suggested that cumulative long-term consequences of repetitive blows to the head are seen in professional soccer players. In addition, high school and collegiate athletes suffering three or more concussions seem more vulnerable to subsequent injury than athletes who have no history of injury.[20] More clear-cut deficits are associated with neuropsychologic impairment in boxers.[28,29] Other studies, however, have not found a significant cumulative effect of multiple injuries. In the study by Iverson, there were no significant differences between athletes who had experienced one or two concussions compared with a group that had no concussion history. In addition, Pellman and colleagues did not find evidence of a cumulative neuropsychologic deficit in a sample of NFL athletes.[30] Although research in this area will continue to evolve, it is clear that decisions regarding disqualification from sports should be made based on consideration of a variety of factors, including but not limited to number of injuries.

Time between injuries

Another issue often evaluated in making return-to-play decisions is the time between injuries. Although there is no current research that has investigated this factor formally, most concussion management guidelines contain a provision for restriction of play after multiple concussions within a given season.[6,13] This recommendation is based on the anecdotal experience of many sports medicine physicians that recently concussed athletes are prone to re-injury if a second concussion occurs soon after an initial injury. More research is needed, however, before conclusions can be drawn regarding this factor.

Additional potential factors

The factors discussed previously represent only a partial list of issues that could affect short- and long-term outcome from concussion. There are many other potential factors, however, that deserve further study. For instance, the role of genetic factors is postulated as playing a role in recovery from injury, largely because of preliminary research in boxers and linkage to the ApoE-4 allele, a marker of expression of Alzheimer's disease.[28] In addition, the role of headache history potentially is important. Suffering a blow to the head is a well-known trigger for headaches, and a prior history of migraine and other headache may play a role in protracted recovery from concussion.

THE ROLE OF NEUROPSYCHOLOGIC ASSESSMENT

The use of neuropsychologic testing in sports medicine is a recent development, initially taking place in the mid-1980s. Barth and colleagues at the University of Virginia[31] demonstrated the potential usefulness of neuropsychologic test procedures to document cognitive recovery within the first week after concussion. Although a landmark study, this project initially did not result in the widespread adoption of neuropsychologic testing in organized athletics. In the early 1990s, a series of events transpired that shifted the use of neuropsychologic testing in sports to the clinical arena. First, injuries to several high-profile professional athletes resulted in the implementation of baseline neuropsychologic testing by several NFL teams in the mid-1990s.[32] Similarly, after career-ending injuries in the National Hockey League (NHL), the NHL mandated baseline neuropsychologic testing for all athletes.[33] In addition to the increased use of neuropsychologic testing in professional sports, several large-scale studies of collegiate athletes were completed. These studies[1,34–36] provided further evidence that neuropsychologic testing yielded useful clinical information. Specifically, neuropsychologic testing allowed a baseline/postinjury analysis of the subtle aspects of cognitive function likely affected by concussive injury, thus providing objective data to assist team medical staff members in making return-to-play decisions.

The use of traditional neuropsychologic testing (eg, paper-and-pencil testing) has resulted in a rapid expansion of knowledge regarding concussion. More widespread application of testing within the college ranks, however, has been limited because of practical and economic constraints. Furthermore, neuropsychologic testing at the high school level was limited before the year 2000. This latter fact is disturbing given that the majority of at-risk athletes fall within the high school ranks and below. As a result of these inherent limitations of traditional assessment, and in parallel to the widespread proliferation of the microcomputer, several researchers have developed computer-based neuropsychologic testing procedures.

Computer-based neuropsychologic testing procedures have several advantages and few disadvantages compared with traditional neuropsychologic testing procedures. First, the use of computers allows evaluation of large numbers of student athletes with minimal time and effort. For example, through the program at the University of Pittsburgh, up to 20 athletes routinely are evalutated simultaneously within a high school or college computer laboratory. This promotes the assessment of an entire football team within a reasonable time period using minimal human resources. Second, data acquired through testing easily can be stored in a specific computer or computer network and, therefore, can be accessed at a later date (eg, after injury). This not only promotes efficient clinical evaluation of athletes but also greatly expands the possibilities for research. Third, the use of the microcomputer promotes more accurate measurement of cognitive processes, such as reaction time and information processing speed. Computerized assessment allows for evaluation of response times that are accurate to 0.01 of a second, whereas traditional testing allows for accuracy only to 1 to 2 seconds. This increased accuracy no doubt will increase the validity of test results in detecting subtle changes in neurocognitive processes, in particular deficits in cognitive speed. Fourth, the use of the computer allows for randomization of test stimuli that should help improve reliability across multiple administration periods, minimizing the practice effects that naturally occur with multiple exposures to the stimuli. These practice effects have clouded the interpretation of research studies and presented an obstacle for clinicians evaluating the true degree of neurocognitive deficit after injury. Limiting the influence of practice effects on testing allows a direct interpretation of postinjury data to athletes' baselines to determine whether or not full cognitive recovery has occurred. Finally, a computer-based approach allows for automatic scoring of tests and, therefore, reduces human error in scoring and transcription of test results. The one disadvantage is the lack of opportunity of neuropsychologists to observe athletes directly who are completing an actual test.

APPROACHES TO COMPUTER-BASED NEUROPSYCHOLOGIC TESTING

Currently, there are several computer-based concussion management tools published or under development.[37] Specifically, results from four computer-based models are published in the scientific literature. These include ImPACT,[38] CogState,[39] Headminders,[40] and automated neuropsychological assessment metric.[41] Differences exist between these test batteries and each is at different stages of validation. Issues, such as sensitivity, reliability, and validity, of the respective test batteries should be given careful scrutiny before implementation. In addition, issues regarding test selection, cognitive domains measured, details of the clinical report, and consultation options for each instrument should be given careful review before implementation. A detailed review of these critical issues for each computerized battery is beyond the scope of this article. Readers are urged to evaluate the advantages and disadvantages of each approach.

To help familiarize readers with a popular approach to computerized neuropsychologic testing, the concussion management program at the University of Pittsburgh Center for Sports Medicine is described. It is emphasized, however, that this represents only one model and other approaches also have value.

A CLINICAL MODEL FOR COMPUTERIZED NEUROPSYCHOLOGIC TESTING

The University of Pittsburgh Medical Center (UPMC) Sports Medicine Concussion Program represents a specialized clinical and research program that uses neurocognitive testing to assist in general concussion management issues (eg, determining return-to-play or retirement decisions). This program uses the ImPACT computer-based neuropsychologic testing program.[42,43] This test battery was developed to address the inherent limitations of traditional neuropsychologic assessment and is used widely throughout Canada and the United States. The development and construction of this computer program is detailed elsewhere[38] and is not repeated in this article. The ImPACT neuropsychologic test battery is comprised of six test modules that assess multiple neurocognitive abilities. In the interest of gathering as much neuropsychologic data as possible within an approximate 25-minute administration time, several modules are designed to simultaneously evaluate multiple cognitive domains, including attentional processes, memory, and neurocognitive speed. As an adjunct to the neurocognitive scores provided by a clinical report, a symptom self-report inventory is included within the ImPACT program. This 21-item scale[44] requires athletes to rank symptoms, such as headache, dizziness, and photosensitivity, subjectively. Each symptom is rated on a scale of 0 (no complaint) to 6 (severe symptom). This allows for direct comparison of postconcussion symptoms to preinjury symptom reporting and promotes a more comprehensive understanding of the recovery process for athletes, health care professionals, and other interested individuals, such as parents and coaches. Subjective symptoms and neurocognitive test results do not always correlate and the evaluation of both aspects of recovery is essential.

Although the issue of recovery from concussive injury is complex, I recommend that athletes be symptom-free and cognitively intact at rest and after exertional activity before return to sport participation after concussive injury. The optimal usefulness of this approach is to compare athletes to their own individual baselines. In the absence of baseline data, however, it is necessary to compare an athlete's performance to that of age-matched peers.

UNIVERSITY OF PITTSBURGH MEDICAL CENTER CONCUSSION PROGRAM: PROTOCOL FOR RETURN TO PLAY

Based on recent research regarding recovery from concussion and the Vienna international consensus statement,[17] the UPMC return-to-play protocol involves the graduated return to play of athletes to competition based on their progression through several steps in the recovery process. First and foremost, I believe strongly that athletes who have abnormal neuropsychologic testing results or are symptomatic should not be returned to play after injury until they are asymptomatic and any cognitive difficulties have resolved.

As discussed previously, I also suggest strongly that younger athletes (eg, high school age and below) should not be returned to play during the game in which they are injured. This allows for closer evaluation of evolving signs and symptoms and helps prevent more severe injury. I recommend formal neuropsychologic testing (eg, ImPACT) the day after injury to assess initial neurocognitive status. It is important to re-evaluate athletes regularly with regard to reported at-rest symptoms.

Once athletes are symptom-free at rest, I suggest graduated aerobic exertional testing to examine for return of symptoms, such as headache, dizziness, nausea, or fogginess. When athletes become asymptomatic after exertion, neuropsychologic testing should be completed and athletes' test results compared with their baseline. If preinjury baseline neuropsychologic testing has not been completed previously, athletes' test performance should be compared with normative standards for age and gender. Finally, it should be emphasized that this protocol is based on research with younger, primarily high school–aged subjects, and the management of older athletes (eg, college or professional) may vary. Hopefully, recent large-scale research projects within the NFL and NHL will shed additional light on the management of concussion in professional athletes.

CONCLUSIONS AND FUTURE DIRECTIONS

This article has reviewed current standards for evaluation and management of sports-related concussion. The clinical management of concussion is evolving rapidly and the base of knowledge regarding this injury currently is far from complete. Although concussion management within the 1980s and 1990s largely was dominated by the publication of concussion guidelines, there has been a more recent movement toward the adoption of individualized standards for clinical care. Within this context, the use of neuropsychologic testing has become increasingly popular and is evolving into the standard of care in professional sports. Continued growth in this area is anticipated over the next few years as more researchers become involved directly in the management of sports-related injury.

REFERENCES

1. Collins MW, Grindel SH, Lovell MR, et al. Relationship between concussion and neuropsychological performance in college football players. JAMA 1999;282:964–70.

2. Collins MW, Lovell MR, McKeag D. Current issues in managing sports-related concussion. JAMA 1999;282:2383–5.
3. Center for Disease Control. Heads up and sports concussion. 2006.
4. Delaney JS, Lacroix VJ, Leclerc S, et al. Concussion among university football and soccer players. Clin J Sport Med 2004;12(6):331–8.
5. Congress of Neurological Surgeons. Committee on head injury nomenclature: glossary of head injury. Clin Neurosurg 1966;12:386–94.
6. American Academy of Neurology. Practice parameter: the management of concussion in sports (summary statement). Report of the Quality Standards Subcommittee. Neurology 1997;48:581–5.
7. Hovda DA, Prins M, Becker DP. Neurobiology of concussion. In: Bailes JE, Lovell MR, Maroon JC, editors. Sports related concussion. St. Louis (MO): Quality Medical Publishing; 1999. p. 12–51.
8. Bergschneider M, Hovda DA, Shalmon E. Cerebral hyperglycolsis following severe human traumatic brain injury:a positron emission tomography study. J Neurosurg 2003;86:241–51.
9. Johnston KM, Pitto A, Chankowsky I, et al. New frontiers in diagnostic imaging in concussive head injuries. Clin J Sport Med 2001;11:166–75.
10. McAllister TW, Sparling MB, Flashman LA. Differential working memory load effects after mild head injury. Neuroimage 2001;14:1004–12.
11. Lovell MR, Pardini JE, Welling J, et al. Functional brain abnormalities are related to clinical recovery and time to return-to-play in athletes. Neurosurgery 2007;61(2):352–9.
12. Collins MW, Iverson GL, Lovell MR, et al. On-field predictors of neuropsychological and symptom deficit following sports-related concussion. Clin J Sport Med 2003;13:222–9.
13. Cantu RC. Cerebral concussion in sport: management and prevention. Sports Med 1992;14:64–74.
14. Kelly JP, Nichols JS, Filley CM. Concussion in sports: guidelines for the prevention of catastrophic outcome. JAMA 1991;266:2867–9.
15. Cantu RC. Posttraumatic retrograde and anterograde amnesia: pathophysiology and implications in grading and safe return to play. J Athl Train 2001;36:244–8.
16. Wojyts ED, Hovda D, Landry G, et al. Concussion in sports. Am J Sports Med 1999;27:676–86.
17. Aubry M, Cantu R, Dvorak J, et al. Summary of the first international conference on concussion in sport. Clin J Sport Med 2002;12:6–11.
18. McCrory P, Johnston K, Meeuwisse W, et al. Summary and agreement statement of the 2nd International Conference on Concussion in Sport, Prague 2004. Br J Sports Med 2005;39(4):196–204.
19. Iverson GL. Predicting slow recovery from sport-related concussion: the new simple-complex distinction. Clin J Sport Med 2007;17(1):31–7.
20. Collins MW, Lovell MR, Iverson GL, et al. Cumulative effects of sports concussion in high school athletes. Neurosurgery 2002;51:1175–81.
21. Pickles W. Acute general edema of the brain in children with head injuries. N Engl J Med 1950;242:607–11.
22. McDonald JW, Johnston MV. Physiological and pathophysiological roles of excitatory amino acids during central nervous system development. Brain Res Brain Res Rev 1990;15:41–70.
23. Cantu R, Voy R. Second impact syndrome: a risk in any sport. Clin Sports Med 1998;17(1):37–44.
24. Field M, Collins MW, Lovell MR, et al. Does age play a role in recovery from sports-related concussion? A comparison of high school and collegiate athletes. J Pediatr 2003;142:546–53.

25. Lovell MR, Collins MW, Iverson GL, et al. Recovery from mild concussion in high school athletes. J Neurosurg 2003;98:296–301.
26. Pellman EJ, Lovell MR, Viano D, et al. Concussion in professional football: recovery of NFL and high school athletes by computerized neuropsychological testing-part 12. Neurosurgery 2006;58(2):263–74.
27. Matser E, Kessels A, Lezak M. Neuropsychological impairment in amateur soccer players. JAMA 1999;282:971–4.
28. Jordan BD, Relkin NR, Ravdin LD. Apolipoprotein E e4 associated with chronic traumatic brain injury in boxing. JAMA 1997;278:136–40.
29. Roberts GW, Allsop B, Bruton C. The occult aftermath of boxing. J Neurol Neurosurg Psychiatry 1990;53:373–8.
30. Pellman EJ, Lovell M, Viano DC, et al. Concussions in professional football: neuropsychological testing-part 6. Neurosurgery 2004;55(6):1290–305.
31. Barth JT, Alves WM, Ryan TV, et al. Mild head injury in sports. In: Levin HS, Eisenberg H, Benton A, editors. Mild head injury. Oxford: Oxford University Press; 1989. p. 257–75.
32. Lovell MR. Evaluation of the professional athlete. In: Bailes JE, Lovell MR, Maroon JC, editors. Sports-related concussion. St. Louis (MO): Quality Medical Publishing, Inc.; 1999. p. 200–14.
33. Lovell MR, Burke CJ. Concussion management in professional hockey. In: Cantu RE, editor. Neurologic athletic head and spine injury. Philadelphia: WB Saunders; 2000. p. 109–16.
34. Echemendia RJ, Putukian M, Macklin RS. Neuropsychological test performance prior to and following sports-related mild traumatic brain injury. Clin J Sport Med 2001;11:23–31.
35. Hinton-Bayre AD, Geffen GM, Geffen LB. Concussion in contact sports: reliable change indices of impairment and recovery. J Clin Exp Neuropsychol 1999;21:70–86.
36. Macciocchi SN, Barth JT, Alves W. Neuropsychological functioning and recovery after mild head injury in collegiate athletes. Neurosurgery 1996;39:510–4.
37. Schnirring L. How effective is computerized concussion management? Phys Sportsmed 2001;29:11–6.
38. Maroon JC, Lovell MR, Norwig J. Cerebral concussion in athletes: evaluation and neuropsychological testing. Neurosurgery 2000;47:659–72.
39. Collie A, Maruff P, McStephen M, et al. Psychometric issues associated with computerized neuropsychological assessment of concussed athletes. Br J Sports Med 2003;37(6):556–69.
40. Erlanger D, Kausik T, Cantu R, et al. Symptom-based assessment of the severity of concussion. J Neurosurg 2003;98:34–9.
41. Cernich A, Reeves D, Sun W, et al. Automated metrics sports medicine battery. Arch Clin Neuropsychol 2007;1(Suppl):101–14.
42. vankampen DA, Lovell MR, Pardini JE, et al. The Value added for neurocognitive testing for sports related concussion. Am J Sports Med 2006;34(10):1630–5.
43. Fazio V, Lovell MR, Pardini JE, et al. The relationship between post-concussion symptoms and neurocognitive performance in concussed athletes. Journal of Neurorehabilitation 2007;22(3):207–16.
44. Lovell MR, Collins MW. Neuropsychological assessment of the college football player. J Head Trauma Rehabil 1998;13:9–26.

Spinal Injuries in Sports

Barry P. Boden, MD[a,b,]*, Christopher G. Jarvis, MD[c]

KEYWORDS

- Spinal injury • Pathophysiology
- Operative management • Athletic competition

Athletic competition has been an established cause of spinal injuries for centuries. Approximately 8.7% of all new cases of spinal cord injuries in the United States are related to sports.[1] Athletic injuries are third only to motor vehicle accidents and violence as the most common cause of spinal cord injury in people aged 30 years or younger.[1] A 3-year nationwide survey of all sports in Japan revealed a spinal injury incidence of 1.95 per million per year, with a mean age at injury of 28.5 years, and with 88% occurring in males.[2] Catastrophic spinal cord injuries are much more likely to result from a cervical spinal injury than thoracic or lumbar trauma. Historically, sports at greatest risk for catastrophic spinal injuries have been football, ice hockey, wrestling, diving, skiing, snowboarding, rugby, cheerleading, and baseball.[3]

The most common spine injuries in athletics can be carefully managed with nonoperative treatment. More serious spinal injuries, however, may lead to death, permanent disability, and extreme morbidity. The most common mechanism for injury leading to quadriplegia is an axial compressive force applied to the top of the head while the neck is slightly flexed, leading to loss of the protective cervical lordosis and alignment of the cervical vertebra. Information on catastrophic injuries in sports has been recorded by the National Center for Catastrophic Sports Injury Research (NCCSIR), the National Spinal Cord Injury Statistical Center, the United States Consumer Product Safety Commission (CPSC), and other organizations (**Table 1**). The NCCSIR defines a catastrophic sports injury as any severe spinal, spinal cord, or cerebral injury incurred during participation in any school- or college-sponsored sport. These injuries are further subclassified into direct and indirect, and serious, nonfatal, and fatal for epidemiologic purposes.[4]

In this article, the authors discuss common spinal injuries in the athletic population, typical mechanisms of injury, sport-specific catastrophic injuries and potential preventive measures in these at-risk sports.

This article originally appeared in *Neurologic Clinics*, Volume 26, Issue 1.

[a] The Orthopaedic Center, 9711 Medical Center Drive #201, Rockville, MD 20850, USA

[b] The Uniformed Services University of the Health Sciences, 4301 Jones Bridge Road, Room A1041, Bethesda, MD 20814, USA

[c] Family and Sports Medicine, Building 5979, Desert Storm Avenue, Fort Campbell, KY 42223, USA

* Corresponding author. The Orthopaedic Center, 9711 Medical Center Drive #201, Rockville, MD 20850.

E-mail address: bboden@alum.haverford.edu (B.P. Boden).

Table 1	
Sources of information on sport safety	
American Association of Cheerleading Coaches and Advisors (AACCA)	www.aacca.org
Consumer Product Safety Commission (CPSC)	www.cpsc.gov
The National Collegiate Athletic Association (NCAA)	www.ncaa.org
National Catastrophic Center Sports Injury Research (NCCSIR)	www.unc.edu/dept/nccsi/
National Spinal Cord Injury Statistical Center (NCDDR)	www.ncddr.org
National Center of Injury Prevention and Control (NCIPC), Centers for Disease Control and Prevention (CDC)	www.cdc.gov/ncipc
National Federation of State High School Associations (NFHS)	www.nfhs.org
National Operating Committee on Standards for Athletic Equipment (NOCSAE)	www.nocsae.org
National Spinal Cord Injury Statistics Center (NSCISC)	www.spinalcord.uab.edu
USA Baseball	www.usabaseball.com

COMMON SPINE INJURIES

Common athletic injuries to the spine include strains, muscle spasms, compression fractures, avulsion fractures, and disc herniations, with strains being the most common. Strains can be caused by any low-grade force to the spine, including the sudden extension-flexion mechanism associated with whiplash injuries. These athletes typically present with paravertebral muscle spasm, limited range of motion, and a normal neurologic examination. The loss of normal cervical lordosis or thoracic kyphosis may be seen on plain radiographs. Treatment involves conservative management with relative rest, anti-inflammatories (NSAIDs), muscle relaxants, and physical therapy.

Although compression fractures can occur anywhere along the course of the vertebral column, cervical spine compression fractures typically occur at the lower levels of C4 to C7. Radiologic evaluation with anterior-posterior, lateral, and flexion-extension radiographs are helpful in excluding serious injuries. Occasionally, when radiolographic negative evaluations are negative, CT or MRI may be necessary to further characterize an injury when the clinician has a high suspicion for cervical injury. Isolated compression fractures with less than 25% anterior compression can be conservatively managed with a cervical orthosis. Compression fractures with greater than 50% anterior compression are frequently associated with posterior ligamentous disruption, are usually unstable, and may require surgical fixation. A CT scan is helpful in evaluating fractures of the posterior vertebra and the vertebral elements that, if injured, may compromise spinal stability.

Cervical spinous process avulsion injuries, known as clay shoveler's fractures, usually occur in football players and power lifters at the C7 level (**Fig. 1**). The most widely accepted theory for the mechanism of injury in clay shoveler's fracture is a forceful flexion of the cervical spine, or forceful contraction of the trapezius and rhomboid muscles. These avulsion fractures are quite stable and can usually be treated with cervical orthosis and other symptomatic measures such as pain medications and ice.

Return-to-play decisions for these fractures are usually straight forward. Patients who have a stable, healed compression or spinous process avulsion fracture, full, painless range of motion, and no neurologic deficits may return to contact sports participation.

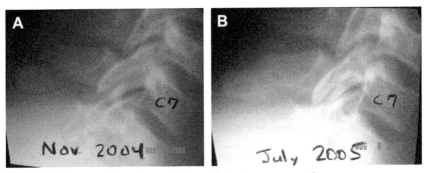

Fig. 1. (A) C7 spinous process fracture. (B) Healed spinous process fracture.

Disc herniation may occur in many sports (**Fig. 2**). Typical symptoms and physical examination findings include pain, restricted range of motion, radicular symptoms, and sensory and motor deficits. A thorough neurologic examination can localize the level of the herniation, but an MRI will confirm the diagnosis and further characterize the extent of disc herniation. Athletes who have a herniated disc frequently respond to conservative, nonoperative modalities such as relative rest, NSAIDS, steroid dose pack, physical therapy, or epidural steroid injections. Only after these conservative measures fail, or if the athlete has a progressive neurologic deficit, is surgical decompression indicated. An anterior cervical discectomy with instrumented fusion is the surgical standard of care for most cervical disc herniations. Far lateral cervical disc herniations usually require a minimally invasive posterior foraminotomy to decompress the nerve root. Rarely, athletes may develop transient quadriplegia or long-tract findings from large central disc herniations. In these cases, urgent surgical management with anterior cervical discectomy and interbody vertebral fusion is recommended.

CATASTROPHIC CERVICAL SPINE INJURIES

Catastrophic cervical spine injuries include unstable fractures or dislocations, cervical cord neuropraxia (CCN or transient quadriplegia), and intervertebral disc herniations.[5] The most frequent causes of catastrophic cervical spine injury, unstable fractures and

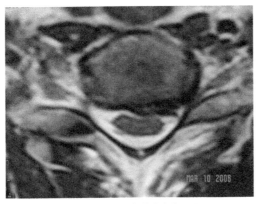

Fig. 2. Axial MRI of patient with C6–C7 left-sided disk herniation.

dislocations, often result in permanent neurologic sequalae and usually occur in the lower cervical spine. In the lower cervical spine, the spinal cord occupies close to 75% of the canal's cross-sectional area as compared with less than half at the level of the atlas.[6]

Cervical injuries resulting in quadriplegia typically occur following application of an axial force to the top of the head while the neck is slightly flexed.[7] The neutrally positioned neck has a protective lordotic curve, and most of the energy is dissipated by the paravertebral muscles and the intervertebral discs during an impact. When the neck is forward flexed about 30°, the cervical spine straightens, allowing the forces to be transmitted to the aligned cervical column. Once maximum compressive forces are reached, the spine fails. This occurs in either a flexion (flexion teardrop) or pure compression (burst fracture) mode with a resultant fracture, dislocation, or subluxation. This injury sequence may cause vertebral fragments or the intervertebral disc to retropulse into the spinal canal causing spinal cord damage.

CCN is an acute, usually transient neurologic injury, associated with sensory changes and possible weakness or paralysis in at least two extremities.[7–9] Despite these findings, the cervical spine bony elements are usually uninjured and the patient is pain-free at the time of injury, with full range of motion. CCN is classified based on the neurologic deficit, duration of neurologic symptoms, and the pattern of injury.[10] Injury grading is based on the duration of symptoms: Grade I, less than 15 minutes; Grade II, 15 minutes to 24 hours; and Grade III, longer than 24 hours. The pattern of injury is classified as quadriplegia, upper only, lower only, or hemiplegia. A prevalence of seven per 10,000 football participants has been previously estimated.[7] Symptoms typically resolve within 10 to 15 minutes. Cervical stenosis is theorized to be the primary predisposing factor to CCN.[9] Previously, the postulated mechanism of injury was either a hyperflexion or hyperextension of the neck causing a pincer-type spinal cord compression injury;[7] however, new data have revealed that no one position particularly predisposes to CCN, and that various mechanisms, including axial forces, can be causative.[11]

An episode of CCN is not an absolute contraindication to return to contact sports. It is unlikely that athletes who have had previous CCN injuries are at increased risk for permanent quadriplegia with further contact activities. Rather, poor technique using the top of the head for tackling is the primary risk factor for quadriplegia. Currently, there are no reports of any previously CCN-injured athlete sustaining a quadriplegic event after returning to contact sports; however, because the number of athletes returning to play after a CCN injury is low, no definitive conclusions can be made. Although complete resolution of symptoms is the rule with CCN, mild permanent neurologic deficits have been rarely reported.[12,13]

Athletes who sustain a CCN injury need to be counseled on the known and potential risks of injury with return to contact sports. Specifically, there is a 50% overall risk of a recurrent CCN episode with return to football, which varies individually based on the canal diameter size—the smaller the canal diameter, the greater the risk of recurrence.[9] Athletes who have any ligamentous instability, neurologic symptoms lasting longer than 36 hours, recurrent episodes, or MRI evidence of cord defect, cord edema, or minimal functional reserve should be excluded from return to contact sports.[7]

SCREENING

Currently only athletes who have a previous history of CCN should undergo screening for spinal cord stenosis. Radiation risk and cost make screening all athletes prohibitive. During the pre-participation physical examination (PPEs) providers should screen all athletes for any previous history of neck injury because this may obviate further questioning and screening. The Pavlov-Torg ratio for assessing cervical spinal stenosis involves measuring the cervical canal diameter and dividing it by the antero-posterior width of the vertebral body.[7] A ratio of less than 0.8 potentially indicates significant cervical stenosis; however, this is a poor screening tool, because many football players have normal canal dimensions but large vertebral bodies, artificially decreasing this ratio below 0.8.[14] A functional spinal stenosis may be a more accurate way of looking for athletes at risk of CCN. This is seen when there is a loss of the normal amount of cerebrospinal fluid around the spinal cord on MRI or CT myelography.[15]

SPORT-SPECIFIC CONSIDERATIONS FOR CATASTROPHIC SPINE INJURIES
Football

Because of large participation numbers and a high incidence of catastrophic injuries, football is associated with the highest number of severe cervical injuries per year for any high school or collegiate sport.[4,16,17] Though head-related fatalities declined in the early 1970s as a result of better protective helmets, the number of cervical quadriplegia cases increased, likely because tacklers began hitting opponents using the crown of the head because of decreased fear of head injury. Torg and colleagues[18] were instrumental in reducing the rate of quadriplegia as a result of cervical injury once they demonstrated that spearing, or tackling another player using the top of the head, was the major cause of permanent cervical quadriplegia (**Fig. 3**). Spear tackling injuries typically occur to defensive players, especially defensive backs, as they attempt to tackle an offensive player.[8,10] Special team players are especially susceptible because the speed at the time of collision is extremely high.[11] After intentional spearing was banned in 1976, the rate of catastrophic cervical injuries dropped 80% from 1976 to 1987.[7] This decline continued, and the incidence of quadriplegic injuries at the high school and college levels remained stable in the 1990s and early

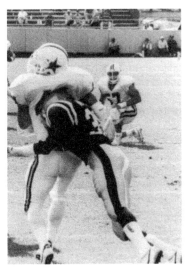

Fig. 3. Photograph of athlete spear-tackling with the top of his head. (*From* Torg, JS, Guille, JT, Jaffe, S. Current concepts review: injuries to the cervical spine in American football players. J Bone Joint Surg Am 2002;84:112–22; with permission.)

2000s at 0.52 per 100,000 participants per year.[10] In a recent review of over 500,000 high school football injuries of the 2005–2006 season, 4.1% of all injuries involved the neck or cervical spine, further defining this at-risk population.[19]

Despite significant decreases in quadriplegia incidence during the late 1970s and 1980s, there has been no significant further decline in the 1990s and early 2000s. This led the NCAA in 2005 to further strengthen its rule banning spear tackling. The revised rule removed the word "intentional," which makes it easier for referees to call spearing penalties. The previous rule made it difficult to prove intent, and the penalty was rarely called as a result. The NCAA has publicized the spearing rule change via posters in locker rooms, slide presentations, and a video of the risks, mechanism of injury, the concept of axial loading, and preventive measures by adopting safe tackling technique.[20] Only future incidence data will reveal if this new rule can further reduce catastrophic cervical injury in football.

Education is the key to preventing catastrophic cervical injuries in football. Identification of spear tackling as the primary culprit leading to quadriplegic injuries has had a profound effect on reducing this catastrophic injury. Coaches need to continually reinforce proper tackling and blocking techniques with the head up. Players should never be allowed to tackle with the head down (**Box 1**).

Ice Hockey

In one study of injury data from the 2001–2002 NCAA ice hockey season, 9% of all hockey injuries occurred to the spine.[21] When compared with other sports, the overall number of catastrophic injuries in high school and college ice hockey players is lower, but the incidence is comparatively higher.[4] These injuries generally occur in the cervical region, especially at the C-5 through C-7 levels.[22] Checking from behind is the most common cause of injury; the player being checked is looking down and not anticipating the check, which sends him hurtling crown first into the boards, axially loading the cervical spine (**Fig. 4**).[22,23] Impact velocities as slow as 1.8 m/s provide 75% of the axial compressive load necessary for cervical spine failure.[24] By comparison, skating speeds exceed 12 m/s and the speed of a sliding skater can be as high as 6.7 m/s,[25] with either situation able to create the force necessary to cause cervical axial load compression failure in a vulnerable player.

A longitudinal survey of Canadian hockey injuries from 1966 to 1993 demonstrated 241 spinal fractures and dislocations.[23] Unfortunately, the incidence of major spinal injuries worldwide in ice hockey began increasing in the early 1980s,[26] likely because of the increased size and speed of players and more emphasis on checking as a part of the game. Data from the Canadian ThinkFirst-SportSmart Sports and Recreational Injuries Research and Prevention Center registry demonstrated an average of 17 cases per year, peaking in 1995 with 26 injuries.[26]

There have been some successful preventive strategies enacted in ice hockey. The International Ice Hockey Federation changed its rules book in 1994, making it a penalty to push or check from behind (**Fig. 5**),[27] dramatically decreasing the incidence of severe spinal injuries occurring in international play.[26] As in football, the introduction of head and face protection in the 1980s may have led greater aggression, resulting in an increased risk of catastrophic spinal injuries.[28] Research into the use of padded boards as another strategy for preventing these injuries may be beneficial.

Wrestling

The vast majority of catastrophic injuries in wrestlers are caused by cervical fractures or major cervical ligament injuries, and the annual catastrophic injury rate is about 1 per 100,000 high school and collegiate wrestlers.[29] Most injuries occur during match

---

Box 1
"Keep the head out of football" coaches' checklist

Keep the head up.

Discuss risk of injury.

Keep the head out of contact.

Explain how serious injuries can occur.

Involve parents in early season meeting.

Have a set plan for coaching safety.

Clearly explain and demonstrate safe techniques.

Provide best medical care possible.

Monitor blocking and tackling techniques every day.

Repeat drills which stress proper and safe techniques.

Admonish or discipline users of unsafe techniques.

Receive clearance by doctor for athlete to play following head trauma.

Stress safety every day.

Don't glorify head hunters.

Support officials who penalize for illegal helmet contact.

Don't praise or condone illegal helmet contact.

Provide conditioning to strengthen neck muscles.

Entire staff must be "tuned in" to safety program.

Check helmet condition regularly.

Improper technique causes spinal cord injuries.

Helmet must fit properly.

Be prepared for a catastrophic injury.

The game doesn't need abusive contact.

Player safety is your responsibility.

It's a game—not a job—for the players.

Data from University Scholastic League, Austin, TX.

---

competitions in the low and middle weight classes.[29] The most common wrestling maneuver associated with these injuries was the takedown of a standing opponent in a defensive position.[29] Wrestlers are typically injured by one of three mechanisms: (1) the wrestler is thrown to the mat while both arms are being held, preventing him from being able to protect himself and resulting in the wrestler landing on his head; (2) the wrestler is landed upon by the full weight of the top wrestler midway through an attempted roll; or (3) the wrestler sustains an axial compression force to the cervical spine while attempting to "shoot" on an opponent as a result of hitting heads, a knee, or another hard surface.

Prevention strategies for catastrophic spine injuries in wrestling encompass actions by referees, coaches, and athletes. Referees should strictly enforce penalties for slams, which are throws involving the use of excessive force. Particularly, referees should observe for wrestlers in a vulnerable defensive position who may be off balance, have one or both arms held, or may have the potential for having their opponent

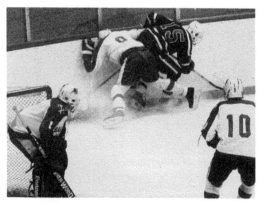

Fig. 4. Illustration of ice hockey player checked from behind and thrown into boards head first. (*Courtesy of* JS Torg, MD, Philadelphia, PA.)

land on top of them while their necks are flexed and their heads are against or moving toward the mat. More stringent penalties for intentional slams are encouraged, and the referee should have a low threshold for stopping a match during potentially dangerous situations. Coaches can assist in injury prevention by emphasizing safe, legal wrestling techniques such as the head-up position during any takedown maneuver, and proper rolling. Wrestlers can help avoid injuries by practicing safe, controlled takedowns, proper rolling, and avoidance of excessive force when on the offensive. More research toward understanding which holds and maneuvers are most dangerous may help prevent injuries in the future.

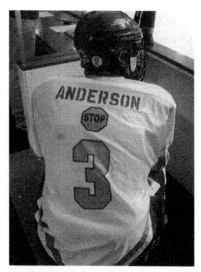

Fig. 5. Safety Toward Other Players (STOP) patch worn on the back of an amateur hockey player as a visual reminder for players not to hit an opponent from behind. (*From* Waninger, KN. Management of the helmeted athlete with suspected cervical spine injury Am J Sports Med 2004;32:1334; with permission.)

Diving

Most swimming-associated catastrophic spinal injuries occur with race diving into the shallow end of a pool.[4] This occurs when a swimmer sustains a cervical axial compression injury after diving head-first into the shallow end of a pool (**Fig. 6**). The national high school and collegiate associations have implemented rules to prevent injuries during the racing dive. At the high school level, swimmers must start the race in the water if the water depth at the starting end is less than 3.5 feet. If the water depth is 3.5 feet to less than 4 feet at the starting end, the swimmer may start in the water or from the deck. If the water depth at the starting end is 4 feet or more, the swimmer may start from a platform up to 30 inches above the water surface. College rules require a minimum water depth of 4 feet at the starting end of the pool. During practice sessions where platforms may not be available, swimmers are advised to only dive into the deep end of the pool or to jump into the water feet first.

Many recreational diving injuries go unreported, hampering attempts at improved awareness and water safety. In a retrospective review of traumatic spinal cord injuries presenting to a trauma center in Germany, 7.7% were caused by diving accidents.[30] Ninety-seven percent of the injured patients were male. Inadequate supervision, alcohol use, shallow water, and inexperienced divers are all risk factors for injury.[31]

Preventive strategies for swimmers include not diving head-first into shallow or unknown waters, removing the high board in favor of a water slide, maintaining adequate supervision of inexperienced swimmers and divers, and avoiding alcohol and other judgment-affecting substances to reduce the incidence of spinal cord injuries.

Downhill Skiing/Snowboarding

The incidence of severe spinal cord injury is 0.01 injuries per 1,000 skier-days.[32] These injuries are evenly distributed at all spinal levels.[33] These injuries have been increasing among skiers during the last 2 decades, especially in young males. They occur during falls as a result of poorly groomed slopes, equipment failures, unfavorable weather conditions, overcrowding, skier error, or loss of control. Of significance is that injury

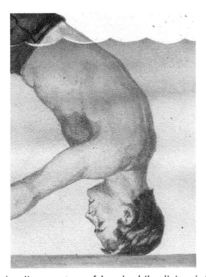

Fig. 6. Diagram of diver landing on top of head while diving into shallow end of pool. (*Courtesy of* JS Torg, MD, Philadelphia, PA.)

rates increase late in the day, suggesting fatigue as a risk factor. Overall, fatality rates are estimated at one per 1.5 million skier-days for downhill skiers, and fatalities occur when reckless skiers collide with stationary objects such as trees.[32] Although spinal injuries are not the etiology of all skiing fatalities, they have been well-documented as a significant cause of death in skiers.[32]

Spinal injuries in snowboarders have been reported to be three- to fourfold higher than in skiing, and this ratio seems to be increasing as snowboarding grows in popularity.[34,35] Snowboard injuries typically occur in two basic populations: inexperienced snowboarders having falls, and expert and intermediate snowboarders involved in jumping accidents.[35] Snowboard jumping causes up to 80% of spinal injuries, which usually affect the thoracolumbar region in these athletes.[33–35]

Prevention strategies include the enforcement of safe skiing by the ski patrol, regulating downhill runs to prevent overcrowding of the slopes, and possibly separation of snowboarders from skiers on the slopes. Also, snowboarders need to be educated concerning the potentially injurious effects of high-risk jumping practices.

Rugby

Like football, rugby has an aggressive style of play, but without protective gear, resulting in a high rate of cervical injury. Ten percent of serious injuries in rugby involve the cervical spine, and spinal cord contusions constitute one fourth of these injuries.[36,37] Cervical spine injuries most frequently occur during a scrum, when the opposing sides of tightly bound players come forcibly together (engagement).[38] The hooker, or the central player on the front row of the scrum suffers the most injuries (**Fig. 7**). During engagement, each side of the scrum may generate weights up to 1.5 tons: the hooker may encounter almost 50% of this weight. If engagement does not occur properly or the hooker employs the head as a weapon with the neck flexed during contact, a severe cervical injury may result.

Preventive methods include avoiding a mismatch in physical size of the hookers, not allowing unskilled players to participate on the front row, restricting spear tackling and

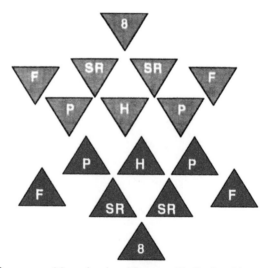

Fig. 7. Diagram of scrum positions: hooker (H), prop (P), flanker (F), second row (SR), and eightman (8). (*From* Wetzler, MJ, Akpata, T, Laughlin, W, et al. Occurrence of cervical spine injuries during the rugby scrum. Am J Sports Med 1998;26:178; with permission.)

stiff-arming,[39] and changing the rules of engagement. Sequential engagement or having the front rows engage separately from the pack prevents the second and third rows from thrusting unprepared front-row players into their opponents. An uncontested scrum in which the offensive team is allowed to win the scrum has also been shown to be an effective preventive strategy.[38] There are insufficient data to determine if use of protective headgear changes the rates of cervical spine injury.

Cheerleading

Recently cheerleading has evolved from a motivational support role into an activity demanding high levels of skill, athleticism, and complex gymnastic maneuvers. Though the incidence of cheerleading injuries is relatively low compared with other sports, it carries a high risk of catastrophic injury. Cheerleaders have accounted for more than half of the catastrophic injuries that occurred in high school and college female athletes from 1982 to 2005.[4] College athletes are five times more likely than high school athletes to sustain a catastrophic injury. This is likely because of the increased complexity of stunts at the college level.[40] In 2000 the CPSC documented a total of 1814 neck injuries, including 76 cervical fractures, in cheerleaders who presented to emergency departments.[41]

Pyramid formations with the cheerleader on the top and the basket toss, in which a cheerleader is thrown into the air to heights of 6 to 20 feet and then caught before landing on the ground, are the most common stunts to result in catastrophic injury.[40] Other less common mechanisms of injury involve advanced floor tumbling routines, participating on a wet surface, or performing a mount. The vast majority of injuries occur when an athlete lands on a hard surface.[40]

Various associations have attempted to reduce pyramid injuries by reducing the height and limiting the complexity of pyramid stunting, and by specifying required positions for spotters. Currently pyramids are limited to no more than two levels in high school and 2.5 body lengths in college. Cheerleaders on top of pyramids must be supported by one or more individuals (base) in direct weight-bearing contact with the performing surface. A minimum of one spotter per person extended above shoulder level must be present. Any suspended persons are also not allowed to be inverted or to rotate on dismount.

Some safety measures already instituted for the basket toss include limiting the basket toss to four throwers, beginning the toss from the ground level, and having one of the throwers behind the flyer during the toss. Flyers are also trained to be directed vertically and not allow their heads to drop backward out of alignment with the torso, or below a horizontal plane with their body.

Several injuries have been reported during rainy conditions; therefore all stunts should be restricted when wet conditions are present. Tumbling injuries may be prevented with proper supervision, only progressing to complex tumbling when simple maneuvers are mastered, and using spotters as necessary. Any apparatus used to propel a participant through the air, such as a mini-trampoline or springboard, has been prohibited at or below the collegiate level since the late 1980s.

Cheerleading coaches need to place at least as much time and attention on practicing safe technique and attentiveness of spotters in practice as on simply accomplishing the stunts. The advanced cheerleading techniques of pyramids and basket tosses should be limited to experienced cheerleaders who have mastered all other skills, and should not be performed without qualified spotters and appropriate landing mats.[40] All coaches should be trained in gymnastics and partner stunting.[4]

Other preventive measures have been recommended by various bodies, and these include: assuring pre-participation health of all cheerleaders by mandating a preseason PPE; physician or athletic trainer to be available at all competitions, games, and practices; cheerleader removal from participation if any previous injury should preclude continued cheerleading activities; and certification of all coaches in a certified safety course, such as the one currently offered by The American Association of Cheerleading Coaches and Advisors.[4]

Baseball

Although baseball has a low noncatastrophic injury rate, it has a relatively high catastrophic injury incidence compared with other sports, with 1.95 catastrophic injuries per year, or 0.43 injuries per 100,000 participants.[42] Severe head injuries are more common than cervical spine injuries. Catastrophic spine injuries in baseball most commonly occur as a result of a collision between a base runner and a fielder, typically the catcher.[42] A typical mechanism is when a base runner dives head-first into a catcher, sustaining an axial compression cervical injury.[42] Although rarely enforced, baseball rules state that the fielder has the right of way to the base path and that the runner should avoid the fielder, especially when it involves the catcher at home plate. Because the speed of head-first sliding has not been shown to be statistically different from feet-first sliding and the risk of catastrophic injury is high with head-first sliding, the rules regarding the head-first slide needs to be reassessed at the high school and collegiate levels.[43] In Little League Baseball, head-first sliding is never allowed.

Preventive measures include enforcing the rules regarding base path right of way, and instituting or enforcing feet-first sliding only in all baseball below the professional leagues.

SUMMARY

Athletic participation is an excellent way to encourage physical fitness in all ages, to promote teamwork, camaraderie, and to support self esteem. Although there is an extremely low risk of catastrophic spine injuries in organized sports, the physical, mental, and financial cost of a catastrophic injury to injured athletes, their families, and to society can be tremendous. Not withstanding the decreased quality of life for the injured athlete, the lifetime cost for a quadriplegic injury individual can easily surpass 2 million dollars.[44] The annual aggregate cost of sports-related spinal cord injuries in the United States in 1995 was close to $700 million.[44] Primary preventive strategies are the most effective means of reducing the incidence and costs associated with catastrophic spine injuries. Continued research into the epidemiology and mechanisms of catastrophic spine injuries is critical to the future prevention of these injuries.

REFERENCES

1. National Spinal Cord Injury Statistical Center. Spinal cord injury: facts and figures. University of Alabama; 2006. Available at: www.spinalcord.uab.edu. Accessed January, 2007.
2. Katoh S, Shingu H, Ikata T, et al. Sports-related spinal cord injury in Japan (from the nationwide spinal cord injury registry between 1990 and 1992). Spinal Cord 1996;34:416–21.
3. Boden BP, Prior C. Catastrophic spine injuries in sports. Curr Sports Med Rep 2005;4:45–9.
4. Mueller FO, Cantu RC. National Center for Catastrophic Sports Injury Research: Twenty-Third Annual Report, Fall 1982–Spring 2005. Chapel Hill (NC): National Center for Catastrophic Sports Injury Research; 2005.

5. Banerjee R, Palumbo MA, Fadale PD. Catastrophic cervical spine injuries in the collision sport athlete, part 1: epidemiology, functional anatomy, and diagnosis. Am J Sports Med 2004;32:1077–87.

6. Parke WW. Correlative anatomy of cervical spondylotic myelopathy. Spine 1988; 13:831–7.

7. Torg JS, Guille JT, Jaffe S. Current concepts review: injuries to the cervical spine in American football players. J Bone Joint Surg Am 2002;84:112–22.

8. Torg JS, Pavlov H, Genuario SE, et al. Neuropraxia of the cervical spinal cord with transient quadriplegia. J Bone Joint Surg Am 1986;68:1354–70.

9. Torg JS, Naranja RJ Jr, Pavlov H, et al. The relationship of developmental narrowing of the cervical spinal canal to reversible and irreversible injury of the cervical spinal cord in football players. An epidemiological study. J Bone Joint Surg Am 1996;78:1308–21.

10. Torg JS, Corcoran TA, Thibault LE, et al. Cervical cord neurapraxia: classification, pathomechanics, morbidity, and management guidelines. J Neurosurg 1997;87: 843–50.

11. Boden BP, Tacchetti RL, Cantu RC, et al. Catastrophic cervical injuries in high school and college football players. Am J Sports Med 2006;34:1223–32.

12. Brigham CD, Adamson TE. Permanent partial cervical spinal cord injury in a professional football player who had only congenital stenosis. J Bone Joint Surg Am 2003;85:1553–6.

13. Cantu RV, Cantu RC. Guidelines for return to contact sports after transient quadriplegia. J Neurosurg 1994;80:592–4.

14. Herzog RJ, Wiens JJ, Dillingham MF, et al. Normal cervical spine morphometry and cervical spinal stenosis in asymptomatic professional football players: plain film radiography, multiplanar computed tomography, and magnetic resonance imaging. Spine 1991;16:S178–86.

15. Cantu RC. Functional cervical spinal stenosis: a contraindication to participation in contact sports. Med Sci Sports Exerc 1993;25:1082–3.

16. Cantu RC, Mueller FO. Catastrophic football injuries: 1977–1998. Neurosurgery 2000;47:673–7.

17. Boden BP. Direct catastrophic injury in sports. J Am Acad Orthop Surg 2005;13: 445–53.

18. Torg JS, Vegso JJ, O'Neill MJ, et al. The epidemiologic, pathologic, biomechanical, and cinematographic analysis of football-induced cervical spine trauma. Am J Sports Med 1990;18:50–7.

19. Shankar PR, Collins CL, Dick RW. Epidemiology of high school and collegiate football injuries in the United States, 2005–2006. Am J Sports Med 2007;35:1295–303.

20. Available at: www.ncaa.org/health-safety. Accessed January, 2007.

21. Flik K, Lyman S, Marx RG. American collegiate men's ice hockey: an analysis of injuries. Am J Sports Med 2005;33:183–7.

22. Molsa JJ, Tegner Y, Alaranta H, et al. Spinal cord injuries in ice hockey in Finland and Sweden from 1980 to 1996. Int J Sports Med 1999;20:64–7.

23. Tator CH, Carson JD, Edmonds VE. Spinal injuries in ice hockey. Clin Sports Med 1998;17:183–94.

24. Bishop PJ, Wells RP. Cervical spine fractures: mechanism, neck load, and methods of prevention. In: Castaldi CR, Hoerner EF, editors. Safety in ice hockey, vol. 2. ASTM STP 1050. Philadelphia: American Society for Testing and Materials; 1989. p. 71–83.

25. Sim FH, Chao EY. Injury potential in modern ice hockey. Am J Sports Med 1978; 15:30–4.

26. Biasca N, Wirth S, Tegner Y. The avoidability of head and neck injuries in ice hockey: an historical review. Br J Sports Med 2002;36:410–27.
27. International Ice Hockey Federation (IIHF). Official rule book 1994. Zurich: IIHF; 1994.
28. Stuart MJ, Smith AM, Malo-Ortiguera SA, et al. A comparison of facial protection and the incidence of head, neck, and facial injuries in junior A hockey players: a function of individual playing time. Am J Sports Med 2002;30:39–44.
29. Boden BP, Lin W, Young M, et al. Catastrophic injuries in wrestlers. Am J Sports Med 2002;30:791–5.
30. Schmitt H, Gerner HJ. Paralysis from sport and diving accidents. Clin J Sport Med 2001;11:17–22.
31. Cooper MT, McGee KM, Anderson DG. Epidemiology of athletic head and neck injuries. Clin Sports Med 2003;22(3):427–43.
32. Morrow PL, McQuillen EN, Eaton LA Jr, et al. Downhill ski fatalities: the Vermont experience. J Trauma 1998;28(1):95–100.
33. Levy AS, Smith RH. Neurologic injuries in skiers and snowboarders. Semin Neurol 2000;20:233–45.
34. Tarazi F, Dvorak MF, Wing PC. Spinal injuries in skiers and snowboarders. Am J Sports Med 1999;27(2):177–80.
35. Yamakawa H, Murase S, Sakai H, et al. Spinal injuries in snowboarders: risk of jumping as an integral part of snowboarding. J Trauma 2001;50:1101–5.
36. Scher AT. Rugby injuries to the cervical spine and spinal cord: a 10 year review. Clin Sports Med 1998;17(1):195–206.
37. Scher AT. Rugby spinal cord concussion in rugby players. Am J Sports Med 1991;19(5):485–8.
38. Wetzler MJ, Akpata T, Laughlin W, et al. Occurrence of cervical spine injuries during the rugby scrum. Am J Sports Med 1998;26:177–80.
39. Dec KL, Cole SL, Metivier S. Screening for catastrophic neck injuries in sports. Curr Sports Med Rep 2007;6:6–19.
40. Boden BP, Tacchetti R, Mueller FO. Catastrophic cheerleading injuries. Am J Sports Med 2003;31:881–8.
41. Available at: www.cpsc.gov. Accessed January, 2007.
42. Boden BP, Tacchetti R, Mueller FO. Catastrophic injuries in high school and college baseball players. Am J Sports Med 2004;32:1189–96.
43. Kane SM, House HO, Overgaard KA. Head-first versus feet-first sliding: a comparison of speed from base to base. Am J Sports Med 2002;30:834–6.
44. DeVivo MJ. Causes and costs of spinal cord injury in the United States. Spinal Cord 1997;35:809–13.

Recognition and Management of Spinal Cord Injuries in Sports and Recreation

Charles H. Tator, MD, PhD, FACS, FRCSC

KEYWORDS
- Spinal cord injury • Sport • Recreation
- Injury prevention

In developed countries, sports and recreation often rank as the second most common cause of acute spinal cord injury (SCI), just behind motor vehicle crashes and ahead of injuries at work and falls at home.[1] In some countries, sports-related SCI comprises 20% or more of the cases of SCI.[2,3] It has been estimated that the frequency of SCI in sports and recreation in various countries ranges from 4.5 to 95 cases per 100,000 population.[4] In some sports, such as football and hockey, there has been a decline in the incidence of spinal injuries[5] because of specific prevention efforts, but in other sports, such as alpine skiing and snowboarding, there has been an increase in most countries.[6] There are some differences in the pathophysiology and clinical management of SCI attributable to sports and recreation compared with the other causes of SCI.[7] Most of the injuries occur acutely, but many athletes have chronic progressive syndromes, such as chronic cervical myelopathy, after prolonged participation or "overuse" in impact sports, such as tennis. Injury prevention is one of the most important considerations in SCI attributable to sports and recreation, given that virtually all these injuries are avoidable. Another important issue relates to the guidelines for return to play after SCI incurred in sports or recreation.

CLINICAL MANIFESTATIONS
General Features

Worldwide, diving is the most common cause of acute SCI in sports and recreation.[8–10] The injuries in diving are almost always to the cervical spine, and there is a high incidence of complete SCI. These injuries occur most often in the setting of unsupervised recreation at the lakeside, the ocean, or in private pools, and less often in a supervised setting such as a pool at a school. Trained divers seldom sustain SCI.

This article originally appeared in *Neurologic Clinics*, Volume 26, Issue 1.
Toronto Western Hospital, University of Toronto, Suite 4W-433, 399 Bathurst Street, Toronto, Ontario, M5T 2S8, Canada
E-mail address: charles.tator@uhn.on.ca

Phys Med Rehabil Clin N Am 20 (2009) 69–76
doi:10.1016/j.pmr.2008.10.013

With respect to organized sports, football in the United States and hockey in Canada are the team sports with the highest incidence of acute SCI.[11,12] These sports also cause a high incidence of accelerated degenerative spinal changes that can lead to chronic myelopathy and radiculopathy. In the U.S. and in Canada, registries have been developed that provide systematic reporting of the incidence of SCI related to football[13] and hockey.[14] Major prevention programs have been developed to deal with some of the identified causes of these injuries, such as "clotheslining" and "spearing" in football and hitting from behind into the boards in hockey. Other organized sports with a high incidence of spinal injury or SCI are gymnastics (including the trampoline), wrestling, skiing, hang gliding, mountain climbing, rugby, and horseback riding.[15-17] Bicycling and motor sports, including snowmobiles, all-terrain vehicles, dirt bikes, and motor cycle racing, also are responsible for large numbers of SCI in specific regions of many countries that have terrain and facilities suitable for these recreational activities.[7]

In almost all types of sports and recreation, approximately 80% of the SCIs are sustained by male participants, and this is true for organized and unorganized activities. Horseback riding is one of the major exceptions in North America, because female participants are affected more often than male participants, likely reflecting the higher numbers of female participants. In sports and recreation, the SCI victims are usually young, with children occasionally affected.[18] Indeed, in such sports as hockey, football, and rugby, teenagers often sustain SCI. In general, children younger than 10 years of age have a lower incidence of SCI but are prone to ligamentous injuries, especially of the upper cervical spine. In contrast, older children have injuries in the middle and lower segments of the cervical spine similar to adults.[19]

Sideline Evaluation

It is safe and best practice to assume that until proved otherwise, all unconscious athletes have an unstable cervical, or other spinal level, fracture or dislocation of the spine. This implies a "no movement" policy for the unconscious player with strict attention directed to immobilization of the neck and back. The one exception to this rule is that the patient may need to be moved to establish an adequate airway and breathing. The same precaution holds for concussed athletes who may not have lost consciousness because they may also have sustained a concomitant spinal injury. Caution is also required in removing the helmet of football or hockey players; in general, it is best to leave the helmet in place until adequate help is available. Once prepared, it is best to remove the helmet and shoulder pads together as a unit to avoid the tendency for extension of the neck if the helmet is removed while the shoulder pads remain in place.

Level, Severity, and Type of Spinal Cord and Spinal Injuries

In general, cervical SCI is much more common in sports and recreation than thoracic or thoracolumbar injury.[10] In certain activities, such as diving, SCIs are almost exclusively cervical. Motor sports, such as those involving all-terrain vehicles and snowmobiles, and horseback riding cause a large number of thoracic and thoracolumbar injuries.[20] Similar to the findings in nonathletic injuries, approximately 60% of SCIs in sports and recreation are incomplete injuries, with American Spinal Injury Association (ASIA) grades of B, C, and D. In some sports, however, notably diving, complete spinal cord injuries occur more often than incomplete injury. SCIs without spinal fracture are frequent in sports and recreation, especially related to acute disc herniations, which can occur at any level of the spinal column.

Many of the sports and recreational injuries of the spine involve a combination of high speed and axial loading, and this is especially true in football and hockey, in which burst fractures and compression fractures frequently occur. The combination of flexion and axial loading, or extension and axial loading, can lead to fracture-dislocation with or without associated disc rupture. Bilateral locked facets in the cervical region with anterior dislocation or fracture-dislocation are common injuries sustained in diving, whereas young gymnasts have a propensity for fractures of the pars interarticularis in the lumbar region.[18] In children, the mechanisms of injury reflect those in adults, although there are significant differences, such as a greater tendency for SCI without fracture or dislocation of the spine.[18]

Overuse spinal injuries accelerate the onset and magnify the severity of such conditions as degenerative disc disease, cervical spondylosis, and spinal osteoarthritis.[21,22] These conditions may occur at a much earlier age in athletes than in the general population because of repetitive loading of the spine, as in wrestling, weightlifting, and gymnastics. There are several risk factors that make the adolescent spine susceptible to stress fractures manifesting as spondylolysis. The neurologic sequelae of these spinal diseases present as radiculopathy or myelopathy. Activities in which these chronic spinal conditions frequently become significantly symptomatic include running/jogging, tennis, and squash.

Repetitive lifting of heavy weight can also worsen preexisting degenerative spinal conditions. Practitioners should caution participants approaching middle age that high-impact activities may have to be tailored back or abandoned for lower impact or nonimpact activities, such as fast walking or swimming. Similar advice should be given about limiting the amount of weight to be lifted.

TREATMENT
Acute Injuries

It is important for physicians associated with sports teams or athletic or recreational events to have the necessary training and equipment to provide first aid safely and effectively. In general, the first aid and subsequent hospital management of the athlete with an acute SCI are identical to the management of other patients with these injuries. There should be preparation for the management of a catastrophic spinal injury,[23] with special attention to airway, breathing, and circulation—the "ABC's" of resuscitative trauma management. The attending physician or trainer should quickly obtain a thorough history of the injury, inquiring specifically for spinal pain, muscle weakness, and sensory loss, followed by an examination of the nervous system, including assessment of power and sensation. The examiner should gently palpate the entire spine for detection of crepitus, tenderness, or deformity. It is essential to ensure absolute immobilization of the entire spine during examination, and before any required transfers and transport. Effective treatment includes the prevention of secondary injuries, such as pressure sores, and administration of appropriate resuscitative measures. These measures prevent worsening of neurologic deficits or the initiation of a neurologic deficit in persons without an initial deficit who have an unstable spinal injury. There should be complete documentation of any previous injuries, because this information is essential for inclusion in the deliberations regarding return to play.

Helmet removal of injured players requires specific attention in sports like football and hockey sports in which players are also wearing shoulder pads.[5] In these cases, the helmet should not be removed first. If there is a problem with airway management, only the facemask should be removed, and this can be accomplished with heavy wire cutters. Removal of the helmet first in a player wearing shoulder pads may cause extension of the neck because of the thickness of the shoulder pads. In these players, the shoulder pads and helmet should be removed simultaneously while maintaining the neck in axial alignment with the trunk.[24,25] Spinal injuries in athletes require complete imaging, preferably by a combination of CT and MRI to detect evidence of current and previous injury to the spine and spinal cord, including ligamentous injury, and to detect spinal instability and intracanalicular space-occupying lesions, such as with herniated vertebral discs. MRI is especially useful for the detection of ligamentous injury, disc herniation, and presence of subtle signal changes in the injured cord. The details of management and the choice of surgical versus nonsurgical management are beyond the scope of this article, except that there is a greater tendency toward recommendations for operative fusion in athletes because of the high level of impact forces, especially in contact sports.

Chronic Injuries

The management of athletes with chronic injuries is no different from that of nonathletes with similar injuries, except for the importance of changing to lower impact or nonimpact activities and avoidance of lifting heavy weights.

RETURN-TO-PLAY GUIDELINES

The issue of return to play presents a specific management challenge in athletes. In general, the treatment team should use the same return-to-play guidelines for professional and amateur athletes, although professionals often treat themselves differently from the general population. The practitioner should be prepared for resistance from some relatives, coaches, trainers, league officials, and players' agents and should be prepared for a higher percentage of noncompliance from professional athletes.

Many factors need to be considered when advising athletes about return to play after spinal injuries. Although there have been good attempts to develop return-to-play guidelines for spinal injuries,[26–29] there is still a great deal of uncertainty. The decision about return to play depends primarily on the nature of the injury and the nature of the activity in which the athlete is engaged (**Table 1**).

The Nature of the Injury

Athletes with neurologic and spinal column injuries pose special problems compared with those with spinal column injuries alone. After a permanent SCI, it is best to advise no return to contact sports. MRI findings of extensive T2 signal change or syrinx should also preclude return to play. If the cord injury has been transient, however, or if the injury involves only a root injury and there is no significant spinal column injury or MRI abnormality, the athlete may be eligible to return to play. The nature of the spinal column injury is the next most important variable. If the spinal column injury is stable, such as with a spinous process or transverse process fracture, or a mild compression fracture, the athlete can probably be allowed to return to play, with or without surgical treatment. In the case of an unstable injury, the athlete should not be permitted to return to play unless stability can be restored by conservative or operative means. Athletes who have had an operative fusion involving one spinal motion segment or who have undergone a single corpectomy for burst fracture may be eligible for return to play in 6 to 12 months. Most athletes who have had a radiculopathy attributable to a herniated disc can be allowed to return to play after successful conservative or operative treatment. Instability should be assessed by flexion-extension views of the spine. Congenital or acquired lesions, such as atlantoaxial dislocation or severe cervical spondylosis or stenosis, should preclude return to play (see **Table 1**).

Table 1
Spinal injuries in sports: criteria and guidelines for return/nonreturn to play in contact and other high-risk sports and recreational activities

	Allow Return to Play	Advise Never to Return to Play
Neurologic injury	• No persisting neurologic symptoms or deficit attributable to cord injury • Neurologic deficit that recovers to normal • Persisting neurologic deficit related to root injury only • Single transient SCI or spinal cord concussion	• Residual neurologic deficit related to SCI • Repeated transient cord injury or spinal cord concussion • Chronic myelopathy
Spinal column injury	• Stable spinal column • Spinal column stability restored by conservative or operative treatment • Minor fracture (eg, spinous process, single body compression fracture) • No instability in flexion-extension radiographs	• Unstable spinal column • Major fracture (eg, burst fracture with canal compromise) • Instability present in flexion-extension radiographs
Congenital lesions	• Minor spinal stenosis • Congenital or operative fusion of one motion segment	• Major spinal stenosis • Atlantoaxial dislocation • Congenital or operative fusion of two or more motion segments
Acquired lesions	• Mild cervical spondylosis or other arthropathy	• Severe cervical spondylosis or other arthropathy
MRI findings	• Normal cord signal	• T2 signal changes in cord • Syrinx

The Nature of the Sport or Recreational Activity

With contact sports, such as hockey, football, or rugby, the potential for recurrent injury may be much greater, and athletes with significant neurologic or spinal column injuries can seldom return to play. Caution must also extend to sports with potential for high-impact forces, such as skiing, horseback riding, and baseball. Less caution is required for noncontact sports, such as tennis.

Athletes who require surgery, such as cervical or lumbar fusion, are permitted to return to activity gradually, beginning with walking only in the first month and progressing to floor exercises and bicycling. In the second month, postoperative weight training can begin and swimming is encouraged. In the third month, treadmill workouts can be allowed, with return to aerobic exercise the fourth month. With respect to contact sports, athletes should not participate until the next season after a cervical or lumbar fusion or after disc removal (see **Table 1**).

In summary, players should not return to play if there is persisting neurologic deficit or spinal column instability. In patients developing neurologic deficit, return to play may be permitted only when there has been full neurologic recovery and a stable spinal column. In those without neurologic deficit, return to play may be permitted if the spinal column is stable. All these possibilities are tempered by the nature of the activities involved, and the discretion of the attending physician is always critical.

INJURY PREVENTION

Unfortunately, screening of participants is of limited value in terms of prevention for SCI in sports and recreation. Routine radiologic examination of the spine in all athletes is not cost-effective, although there are specific exceptions to this rule. For example, atlantoaxial dislocation is a recognized complication in Down's syndrome[30] and in people with Klippel-Feil syndrome and other congenital anomalies;[31] all such patients should have flexion-extension views before participation. Fortunately, the incidence of SCI in the Special Olympics is low.[32] The issue of routine radiologic screening in high-risk sports, such as football and hockey, has not been settled. There is no definite evidence that certain presumed radiologic indicators for stenosis, such as the ratio of the diameter of the spinal canal to the vertebral body, other measures of spinal stenosis, or the features of the so-called "spear tackler's spine," are proved contraindications to play.[28,29,33,34] Lumbar spondylolisthesis has been shown to be present in a high proportion of gymnasts,[35,36] but it has not been shown that this is a proved contraindication to their participation, although the continuing pain associated with this condition may limit participation. The same is true of progressive degenerative spondyloarthropathies in sports like hockey and football. The pain and neurologic deficits associated with disc protrusions and osteophytes, which produce radiculopathy or myelopathy, may prevent return to play. There is a need for further study of the effectiveness of prevention strategies for spinal injuries in sports.[37]

The education of players, coaches, trainers, referees, and the administrators of sports leagues and associations is an important aspect of injury prevention. There should be an emphasis on respect for the health and safety of all players, including opponents. Awareness of the specific risk factors inherent in individual sports is essential. Repeated safety messages can be given by means of coaching sessions, videotapes, posters, and specialized educational sessions. Players should be warned about highly dangerous maneuvers, such as tackling with the "head into the numbers" in football and checking from behind in hockey. There is mounting evidence that these prevention measures have helped to reduce the incidence of SCI in football and hockey.[11–17] There should be screening of the participants in sports like rugby to exclude small-stature players from vulnerable positions. Proper conditioning also has value, especially neck muscle conditioning in young athletes with poorly developed neck muscles who play contact sports, such as hockey and football. Adherence to appropriate return-to-play guidelines as outlined in this article can also help to reduce the incidence of catastrophic spinal injury.

Prevention can also be promoted by attention to the structural and physical aspects of the sports venue and by the use of special equipment that has been developed to enhance sports safety. For example, breakaway goal posts in hockey and padded goal posts in football are strongly advocated, although absolute proof of their effectiveness is lacking. There is a need for improved helmet design in many sports. More research is required to determine the best shape and padding for energy deflection and energy absorption, respectively. It should be noted that there is no definite evidence that helmets have led to an increase in SCI in sports like hockey or that improved helmets can actually reduce the incidence of SCI. It may be true that "helmets can neither cause nor prevent serious neck injuries."[4] Nevertheless, it is the view of this author that proper helmet design and use can reduce the incidence and severity of SCI in certain sports, such as hockey.

SUMMARY

Spinal injuries and SCIs in sports and recreation represent frequent and important causes of injury and disability. These injuries are virtually all preventable through strict adherence to the codes of conduct of the rules and regulations for sports and recreation and through an attitude of respect for one's own welfare and the welfare of the opponents or other participants. Adherence to guidelines for return to sport after injury can help to prevent worsening of deficits and the onset of new deficits.

REFERENCES

1. Tator CH. Sports and recreation as causes of spinal cord injury: epidemiology, screening, injury management, and return to play. In: Tator CH, Benzel EC, editors. Contemporary management of spinal cord injury: from impact to rehabilitation. Park Ridge (IL): American Associaion of Neurological Surgeons; 2000.
2. Kraus JF, Franti CE, Riggins RS, et al. Incidence of traumatic spinal cord lesions. J Chronic Dis 1975;28(9):471–92.
3. Tator CH, Duncan EG, Edmonds VE, et al. Changes in epidemiology of acute spinal cord injury from 1947 to 1981. Surg Neurol 1993;40(3):207–15.
4. Clarke K, Jordan B. Sports neuroepidemiology. In: Jordan B, Tsairis P, Warren R, editors. Sports neurology. 2nd edition. Philadelphia: Lippincott-Raven; 1998. p. 3–13.
5. Bailes JE, Petschauer M, Guskiewicz KM, et al. Management of cervical spine injuries in athletes. J Athl Train 2007;42(1):126–34.
6. Ackery A, Hagel B, Provvidenza C, et al. An international review of head and spinal cord injury in alpine skiing and snowboarding. Injury Prevention 2007; 13(6):368–75.
7. Banerjee R, Palumbo MA, Fadale PD. Catastrophic cervical spine injuries in the collision sport athlete, part 1: epidemiology, functional anatomy, and diagnosis. Am J Sports Med 2004;32(4):1077–87.
8. Katoh S, Shingu H, Ikata T, et al. Sports-related spinal cord injury in Japan (from the nationwide spinal cord injury registry between 1990 and 1992). Spinal Cord 1996;34(7):416–21.
9. Kurtzke JF. Epidemiology of spinal cord injury. Exp Neurol 1975;48:163–236.
10. Tator CH. Diving. In: Jordan BD, Tsairis P, Warren RF, editors. Sports neurology. 2nd edition. Philadelphia: Lippincott-Raven Press; 1998. p. 375–80.
11. Mueller F, Zemper ED, Peters A. American football. In: Caine DJ, Caine CG, Lindner KJ, editors. Epidemiology of sports injuries. Champaign (IL): Human Kinetics; 1996. p. 41–62.
12. Tator C, Carson J, Cushman R. Spinal injuries in Canadian ice hockey players, 1966–1996. In: Cantu R, editor. Neurologic athletic head and spine injuries. Toronto (Canada): WB Saunders Company; 2000. p. 289–96.
13. Mueller FO, Blyth CS. An update on football deaths and catastrophic injuries. Physician Sportsmed 1986;14:139–42.
14. Tator CH, Edmonds VE, Lapczak L, et al. Spinal injuries in ice hockey players, 1966–1987. Can J Surg 1991;34(1):63–9.
15. Bruce DA, Schut L, Sutton LN. Brain and cervical spine injuries occurring during organized sports activities in children and adolescents. Prim Care 1984;11(1): 175–94.
16. Keene JS, Albert MJ, Springer SL, et al. Back injuries in college athletes. J Spinal Disord 1989;2(3):190–5.

17. Cooper MT, McGee KM, Anderson DG. Epidemiology of athletic head and neck injuries. Clin Sports Med 2003;22(3):427–43, vii.
18. Jagannathan J, Dumont AS, Prevedello DM, et al. Cervical spine injuries in pediatric athletes: mechanisms and management. Neurosurg Focus 2006; 21(4):E6.
19. McGrory BJ, Klassen RA, Chao EY, et al. Acute fractures and dislocations of the cervical spine in children and adolescents. J Bone Joint Surg Am 1993;75(7): 988–95.
20. Siebenga J, Segers MJ, Elzinga MJ, et al. Spine fractures caused by horse riding. Eur Spine J 2006;15(4):465–71.
21. Micheli LJ, Curtis C. Stress fractures in the spine and sacrum. Clin Sports Med 2006;25(1):75–88, ix.
22. Barile A, Limbucci N, Splendiani A, et al. Spinal injury in sport. Eur J Radiol 2007; 62(1):68–78.
23. Leidholt JD. Spinal injuries in athletes: be prepared. Orthop Clin North Am 1973; 4(3):691–707.
24. Ford M. Neck, spinal cord and back. In: Bull R, editor. Handbook of sports injuries. New York: McGraw-Hill; 1999. p. 55–71.
25. Palumbo MA, Hulstyn MJ, Fadale PD, et al. The effect of protective football equipment on alignment of the injured cervical spine. Radiographic analysis in a cadaveric model. Am J Sports Med 1996;24(4):446–53.
26. Bailes JE, Hadley MN, Quigley MR, et al. Management of athletic injuries of the cervical spine and spinal cord. Neurosurgery 1991;29(4):491–7.
27. Rapaport L, Cammisa FJ, O'Leary P. Fractures and dislocations of the cervical spine. In: Jordan B, Tsairis P, Warren R, editors. Sports neurology. 2nd edition. Philadelphia: Lippincott-Raven; 1998. p. 157–79.
28. Torg J, Glasgow S. Criteria for return to contact sports following cervical spine injury. Clin J Sport Med 1991;1:12–26.
29. Eddy D, Congeni J, Loud K. A review of spine injuries and return to play. Clin J Sport Med 2005;15(6):453–8.
30. Chang F. The disabled athlete. In: Stanitski C, deLee J, Drez D, editors, Pediatric and adolescent sports medicine, vol. 3. Philadelphia: WB Saunders; 1994. p. 48–76.
31. Pizzutillo P. Klippel-Feil syndrome. In: The Cervical Spine Research Society Editorial Committee, editor. The cervical spine. 2nd edition. Philadelphia: JB Lippincott; 1987. p. 258–71.
32. Robson HE. The Special Olympic Games for the mentally handicapped—United Kingdom 1989. Br J Sports Med 1990;24(4):225–30.
33. Torg JS, Pavlov H. Cervical spinal stenosis with cord neurapraxia and transient quadriplegia. Clin Sports Med 1987;6(1):115–33.
34. Torg JS, Sennett B, Pavlov H, et al. Spear tackler's spine. An entity precluding participation in tackle football and collision activities that expose the cervical spine to axial energy inputs. Am J Sports Med 1993;21(5):640–9.
35. Caine D, Lindner K, Mandelbaum B, et al. Gymnastics. In: Caine D, Caine C, Lindner K, editors. Epidemiology of sports injuries. Champaign (IL): Human Kinetics; 1996. p. 213–46.
36. Sward L. The thoracolumbar spine in young elite athletes. Current concepts on the effects of physical training. Sports Med 1992;13(5):357–64.
37. McIntosh AS, McCrory P. Preventing head and neck injury. Br J Sports Med 2005; 39(6):314–8.

Peripheral Nerve Injuries Attributable to Sport and Recreation

Cory Toth, MD, FRCPC

KEYWORDS

• Peripheral nerve • Nerve entrapment • Sport • Recreation

The scope of sports-related injuries is extensive and most commonly involves the musculoskeletal system. There are numerous and varied peripheral nervous system (PNS) injuries that depend on the nature of the sporting activity, age of the participants, and intensity of play, however. The type of sport may vary from recreational games, such as bowling or lawn darts, to spectator sports, such as professional football. The physician may be confronted with symptoms and signs reflecting injury to several neurologic levels, including the peripheral nerve, spinal roots, and brachial plexus. The recognition of specific injury and its relation to specific sporting activities may assist the physician with the rapidity of diagnosis, cessation of offending activities, and possible therapy.

This article highlights injuries to peripheral nerves attributable to particular sporting or recreational activities. As possible, only those peripheral nerve injuries associated with a clear clinical presentation or supporting laboratory data have been included. Peripheral nerve injuries have been classified based on the sporting or recreational activity, although tables are provided to classify by individual peripheral nerves and by individual sporting activities. Some peripheral nerve injuries have been covered in other articles in this issue and have not been reiterated here. Sporting activities associated with known peripheral nerve injuries are listed in **Box 1**, whereas peripheral nerve injuries are organized by sport in **Box 2** and anatomically in **Box 3**.

ARCHERY

The use of an archery bow can lead to compression of the digital nerves.[1] Compression of the median nerve at the wrist and at the pronator teres intersection[1] can also occur with repeated drawing of the bow. Finally, an isolated long thoracic nerve palsy has also occurred in an archer.[2] The action of repeated drawing of the bow leading to relative hypertrophy of shoulder and periscapular muscles may play a role in

This article originally appeared in *Neurologic Clinics*, Volume 26, Issue 1.
Department of Clinical Neurosciences, University of Calgary, Room 155, Heritage Medical Research Building, 3330 Hospital Drive NW, Calgary, Alberta, Canada T2N 4N1
E-mail address: corytoth@shaw.ca

Box 1
Sporting activities associated with PNS injury categorized by sport

Archery
Arm wrestling
Australian rules football
Auto racing
Ballet dancing
Baseball
Basketball
Bicycling
Bodybuilding
Bowling
Boxing
Cheerleading
Cross-country skiing
Dancing
Football
Frisbee
Golf
Gymnastics
Handball
Hiking
Ice hockey
Judo
Karate
Kickboxing
Mountain climbing
Racquetball
Rodeo
Running
Scuba diving
Shooting
Skating
Snowmobiling
Soccer
Softball
Squash
Surfing
Swimming
Tae kwon doe
Tennis

Volleyball

Weightlifting

Wheelchair basketball

Wrestling

Yoga

compression of these nerves. Archery safety may be improved with switching to the use of a light-weight bow, proper forearm flexor muscles conditioning, and modifications in the procedure of drawing the bowstring.[1]

ARM WRESTLING

The action of arm wrestling can lead to humeral shaft fractures, particularly during the end of a match, when full force is being exerted to win the match or to change momentum. In 23% of these fractures in arm wrestlers, concurrent radial nerve palsy occurs.[3]

AUTO RACING

Auto racing is obviously dangerous because of its acute injuries, but peripheral nerve injuries are likely rare. The brachial plexus of race car drivers is at risk because of the unique positioning of a tight fastening of the arm to the helmet to prevent excessive centrifugal force; in this position, the sciatic and peroneal nerves can be compressed as a result of the small size of the car cockpit and this position, which is maintained for several hours during a race.[4]

BALLET OR PROFESSIONAL DANCING

Peripheral nerve injuries in dancers may occur within the upper and lower extremities. As in other sports in which an overhead motion is performed repetitively, suprascapular neuropathy may occur in dancers as a result of repetitive forceful movements of the arm with external rotation and abduction, leading to painless isolated weakness of external rotation attributable to denervation of the infraspinatus.[5] Entrapment of the suprascapular nerve at the spinoglenoid notch seems to be the most likely anatomic localization. In one patient, a near-complete recovery of muscle function occurred after 4 months of cessation of dancing.[5] Entrapment of the femoral nerve can occur in dancers who perform repeated simultaneous hip extension and knee flexion (the "Horton hinge").[6] Peroneal and sural neuropathies attributable to compression of these nerves by excessively tightened ribbons and elastics in dancing shoes are also possible.[7] Entrapment of the dorsal cutaneous nerve of the foot rarely occurs in dancers who sit on their feet, placing pressure on the dorsum of the foot.[7] As may occur in joggers, dancers can occasionally present with a Morton's neuroma of the plantar nerves.[8]

BASEBALL

In addition to suprascapular, axillary, and ulnar nerve injuries identified in baseball players (as described in the article by Cummins and Schneider elsewhere in this issue), other peripheral nerve injuries are rarely seen. During the biomechanics of throwing the baseball, the humerus is whipped with a maximum torque of 14,000 pounds-force inch,[9] placing significant muscular force and great stress on musculoskeletal and

Box 2
PNS injuries by sport

Archery

    Digital nerve compression

    Median neuropathy at wrist

    Median neuropathy at pronator teres

    Long thoracic nerve palsy

Arm wrestling

    Radial nerve palsy

Auto racing

    Brachial plexopathy

    Sciatic neuropathy

    Peroneal neuropathy

Ballet dancing

    Suprascapular neuropathy

    Femoral neuropathy

    Peroneal neuropathy

    Sural neuropathy

    Dorsal cutaneous neuropathy

    Morton's neuroma

Baseball

    Suprascapular neuropathy

    Radial neuropathy

    Ulnar neuropathy

    Musculocutaneous neuropathy

    Median neuropathy at pronator teres

    Thoracic outlet syndrome

    Axillary neuropathy with quadrilateral space syndrome

    Digital neuropathy at thumb

    Brachial plexopathy (pitcher's arm)

Basketball

    Suprascapular neuropathy

    Stinger

    Median neuropathy at the wrist (wheelchair athletes)

    Ulnar neuropathy at the wrist (wheelchair athletes)

Bicycling

    Ulnar neuropathy at Guyon's canal

    Ulnar neuropathy at the elbow

Median neuropathy at the wrist

Pudendal neuropathy

Posterior cutaneous nerve of the thigh neuropathy

Sciatic nerve palsies (unicyclists)

Bodybuilding/weightlifting

Ulnar neuropathy at the deep motor branch

Ulnar neuropathy at flexor carpi ulnaris

Ulnar neuropathy at the deep palmar branch

Ulnar neuropathy at the elbow

Posterior interosseous neuropathy

Medial pectoral neuropathy

Suprascapular neuropathy

Median neuropathy at the wrist

Long thoracic neuropathy

Lateral antebrachial cutaneous neuropathy

Musculocutaneous neuropathy

Femoral neuropathy

Thoracodorsal neuropathy

Dorsoscapular neuropathy

Stinger

Rectus abdominis syndrome with rhabdomyolysis

Bowling

Digital neuropathy of the thumb

Boxing

Stinger

Cheerleading

Digital neuropathy

Median neuropathy at the palmar branch

Football

Stinger

Upper trunk brachial plexopathy

Radiculopathy of C5, C6, L5, or S1 roots

Axillary neuropathy with or without dislocated shoulder

Suprascapular neuropathy

Ulnar neuropathy at the elbow

Median neuropathy at the wrist

Long thoracic neuropathy

Radial neuropathy

(continued on next page)

Box 2
(*continued*)

    Thoracic outlet syndrome

    Iliohypogastric neuropathy

    Peroneal neuropathy with knee dislocation

    Sciatic nerve (hamstring syndrome)

Frisbee

    Posterior interosseous neuropathy

Golf

    Median neuropathy distal to wrist

    Carpal tunnel syndrome (CTS)

    Ulnar neuropathy at flexor carpi ulnaris

Gymnastics

    Posterior interosseous neuropathy

    Lateral femoral cutaneous neuropathy

    Femoral neuropathy

Handball

    Handball goalie's elbow

Hockey

    Stinger

    Axillary neuropathy

    Tibial neuropathy attributable to tarsal tunnel syndrome

    Peroneal neuropathy

In-line skating, rollerskating, and skateboarding

    Superficial peroneal neuropathy

Judo, karate, and kickboxing

    Morton's neuroma of a plantar nerve

    Ulnar neuropathy at trauma site

    Axillary neuropathy at trauma site

    Spinal accessory neuropathy at trauma site

    Long thoracic neuropathy at trauma site

    Peroneal neuropathy at trauma site

Mountain climbing, hiking

    Tarsal tunnel syndrome

    Rucksack paralysis—brachial plexopathy (upper and middle trunks)

    Suprascapular neuropathy

    Axillary neuropathy

    Long thoracic neuropathy

Rugby/Australian rules football

    Axillary neuropathy

    Obturator neuropathy

Running

    Peroneal neuropathy

    Lateral femoral cutaneous neuropathy

    Tibial neuropathy at the tarsal tunnel

    Posterior tibial neuropathy

    Morton's neuroma of a plantar nerve

    Interdigital neuropathies

    Plantar neuropathies

    Calcaneal neuropathy

    Sural neuropathy

    Superficial peroneal neuropathy

    Saphenous neuropathy

    Rhabdomyolysis

Scuba diving

    Lateral femoral cutaneous neuropathy

Shooting

    Long thoracic neuropathy

Skiing, snowboarding, sledding, and ski jumping

    Femoral neuropathy (cross-country skiing)

    Ulnar neuropathy (cross-country skiing)

    Brachial plexus injury (snowboarding)

Snowmobiling and all-terrain vehicle riding

    Brachial plexopathy

    Ulnar neuropathy at Guyon's canal

Soccer

    Peroneal neuropathy

Surfing

    Common peroneal neuropathy

    Saphenous neuropathy

Swimming

    Thoracic outlet syndrome

Tennis/racquetball

    Posterior interosseous neuropathy at the arcade of Frohse

    Suprascapular neuropathy

    Long thoracic neuropathy

(continued on next page)

Box 2
(continued)

    Lateral antebrachial cutaneous neuropathy

    Radial neuropathy secondary to fibrous arches at lateral head of triceps

    Digital neuropathy

    Superficial radial neuropathy attributable to constrictive sweatband

    Thoracic outlet syndrome

Volleyball

    Suprascapular neuropathy

    Axillary neuropathy

    Long thoracic neuropathy

Wrestling

    Stinger

    Brachial plexopathy

    Axillary neuropathy

    Ulnar neuropathy

    Median neuropathy at the wrist

    Long thoracic neuropathy

    Suprascapular neuropathy

Yoga

    Sciatic neuropathy

---

nervous elements. Windmill pitching used by softball pitchers, in which an underhand pitch is delivered after rotation and posterior extension, has been associated with radial neuropathy at different anatomic sites.[10] Humeral shaft fractures in softball[11] and baseball[12] pitchers have been associated with radial nerve palsies. In adults with humeral fractures associated with throwing a baseball, 16% of patients had concurrent radial nerve palsy.[12] Ulnar neuropathy at the elbow is common among baseball pitchers.[6,13–17] In one study of 72 professional baseball players undergoing arthroscopic or open elbow surgery, ulnar neuropathy was diagnosed in 15%.[13] Of adult baseball players with ulnar nerve entrapment undergoing surgical correction with an anterior transfer of the nerve and placement of the nerve deep to the flexor muscles, approximately 50% of players have sufficient recovery to return to playing.[14] Pitchers are also subject to pronator syndrome within the proximal forearm associated with entrapment of the median nerve by fibrous bands of the pronator teres.[6] The controversial entity of thoracic outlet syndrome has presented as numbness within the throwing hand fingers of a college baseball player; compression of the neurovascular bundle was demonstrated using magnetic resonance angiography while the arm was held in abduction.[18–20] Baseball pitchers are also subject to the acute onset of musculocutaneous neuropathy, with clinical presentations of abrupt onset of pain in the pitching arm, followed by weakness and atrophy of the biceps and coracobrachialis along with numbness over the lateral antebrachial nerve territory.[21]

    Possibly complicating our assessment of peripheral nerve injuries in pitchers is the notion of a "pitcher's arm" noted during electrodiagnostic testing. Professional and amateur baseball pitchers have had reduced sensory nerve action potentials in an asymptomatic throwing arm, with no definite impact on player performance. Although uncertain, the phenomenon of a pitcher's arm may be a repetitive use syndrome affecting the brachial plexus.[22]

Unlike baseball pitchers, batters are susceptible to developing a traumatic neuroma of the ulnar digital nerve of the thumb.[23]

BASKETBALL

Only a small number of basketball injuries seem to be neurologic in nature, with even fewer affecting peripheral nerves. Suprascapular neuropathy in the absence of shoulder girdle trauma may have developed in a basketball player as a result of repeated nerve traction over the coracoid notch during dunking of the basketball.[24] A complete recovery took place after 3 weeks of cessation of basketball.[24] The burner, or stinger, most commonly described in football players, has rarely presented in basketball players.[25] Compression neuropathies of the arms are common injuries in wheelchair basketball players; 30% of world-class wheelchair basketball players have symptoms consistent with CTS, with 70% of these cases having electrodiagnostic confirmation.[26,27] In addition, 12% of wheelchair basketball players have abnormal electrophysiology of the ulnar nerve at the wrist.[26,27]

BICYCLING

Peripheral nerve injuries attributable to recreational and competitive cycling have been described in the article by Kennedy elsewhere in this issue.

BODYBUILDING/WEIGHTLIFTING

Bodybuilding can be associated with a range of entrapment neuropathies, as described in the article by Busche elsewhere in this issue.

BOWLING

Bowling is rarely associated with injury to the PNS. The repetitive nature of bowling can lead to injuries to the digital nerve of the thumb, which is placed inside the 10-pin bowling ball holes[28] (also called "cherry pitter's thumb"). Perineural fibrosis of the digital nerve of the thumb[28] and thumb neuroma may occur as a result of chronic trauma attributable to bowling.[29]

BOXING

Although boxing is associated with obvious head and brain injury, the lone PNS lesion is one usually seen in football players—the burner, or stinger.[25]

CHEERLEADING

Cheerleading can rarely be associated with median palmar digital neuropathy, perhaps related to chronic trauma to the palm during repeated cheerleading activities.[30]

DIVING AND SCUBA DIVING

Lateral femoral cutaneous neuropathy attributable to compression of the diver's weight belt on the nerve has been reported in a single case.[31]

Box 3
Injuries of the PNS attributable to sport organized by anatomic location

Digital nerves

    Archery

    Baseball

    Bowling

    Cheerleading

    Tennis

Median nerve

    Wrist

        Archery

        Basketball (wheelchair)

        Bicycling

        Bodybuilding/weightlifting

        Football

        Golf

        Wrestling

    Palmar branch

        Cheerleading

        Golf

    Pronator teres

        Archery

        Baseball

Ulnar nerve

    At the elbow

        Baseball

        Bicycling

        Bodybuilding/weightlifting

        Judo, karate, and kickboxing

        Cross-country skiing

        Wrestling

    At the wrist

        Basketball (wheelchair)

        Bicycling

        Football

        Cross-country skiing

        Snowmobiling

At flexor carpi ulnaris

    Bodybuilding/weightlifting

    Golf

At the deep motor branch

    Bodybuilding/weightlifting

Radial nerve

  Arm wrestling

  Baseball

  Football

  Tennis/racquetball

Posterior interosseous neuropathy

  Bodybuilding/weightlifting

  Frisbee

  Gymnastics

  Tennis/racquetball

Superficial radial nerve

  Tennis/racquetball

Axillary nerve

  Baseball

  Football

  Hiking

  Hockey

  Judo, karate, and kickboxing

  Rugby

  Volleyball

  Wrestling

Spinal accessory nerve

  Judo, karate, and kickboxing

Musculocutaneous nerve

  Bodybuilding/weightlifting

  Baseball

Lateral antebrachial cutaneous neuropathy

  Bodybuilding/weightlifting

  Tennis

Thoracic outlet syndrome

  Baseball

  Football

(continued on next page)

Box 3
(*continued*)

    Swimming

    Tennis

Long thoracic nerve

    Archery

    Bodybuilding/weightlifting

    Football

    Judo, karate, and kickboxing

    Hiking

    Shooting

    Tennis/racquetball

    Volleyball

    Wrestling

Thoracodorsal neuropathy

    Bodybuilding/weightlifting

Dorsoscapular nerve

    Bodybuilding/weightlifting

Suprascapular nerve

    Ballet dancing

    Baseball

    Basketball

    Bodybuilding/weightlifting

    Football

    Hiking

    Tennis/racquetball

    Volleyball

    Wrestling

Medial pectoral neuropathy

    Bodybuilding/weightlifting

Brachial plexus

    Auto racing

    Baseball

    Football (upper trunk)

    Hiking (upper and middle trunk)

    Snowmobiling

    Snowboarding

    Wrestling

Stinger
  Basketball
  Bodybuilding/weightlifting
  Boxing
  Football
  Hockey
  Wrestling

Cervical radiculopathy
  Football

Femoral nerve
  Ballet dancing
  Bodybuilding/weightlifting
  Gymnastics
  Cross-country skiing

Obturator nerve
  Rugby/Australian rules football

Peroneal nerve
  Auto racing
  Ballet dancing
  Football
  Hockey
  Judo, karate, and kickboxing
  Running
  Soccer
  Surfing

Pudendal nerve
  Bicycling

Iliohypogastric nerve
  Football

Sciatic nerve
  Auto racing
  Bicycling
  Football (hamstring syndrome)
  Yoga

Superficial peroneal nerve
  Running

(*continued on next page*)

Box 3
(continued)

Interdigital nerves of foot

    Running

Tibial nerve

    At tarsal tunnel

        Hockey

        Hiking

        Running

Sural nerve

    Ballet dancing

    Running

Lateral femoral cutaneous nerve

    Gymnastics

    Running

    Scuba diving

Posterior cutaneous nerve of the thigh

    Bicycling

Superficial peroneal nerve

    Rollerskating

    Running

Saphenous nerve

    Surfing

    Running

Dorsal cutaneous nerve of foot

    Ballet dancing

Lumbar radiculopathy

    Football

Morton's neuroma of plantar nerve

    Ballet dancing

    Judo, karate, and kickboxing

    Running

Plantar nerves of feet

    Running

Calcaneal neuropathy

    Running

Rhabdomyolysis

    Bodybuilding/weightlifting

    Running

FOOTBALL

American and Canadian football is an aggressive sport with high rates of injury, serious injury, and neurologic injury. Most injuries affecting the nervous system seem to be head and spinal injuries in nature, but there are risks to the PNS.

Brachial plexus injury may be one of the most common forms of peripheral nerve injury in football. In Canadian varsity football players, brachial plexus injuries were the third most common specific diagnosis in football injuries,[32] and the rate was even higher (49%) at two university centers.[33] The incidence of plexus injury has been reported to be as high as 2.2 cases per 100 players.[34] This high incidence of injury to the brachial plexus frequently includes the burner, or stinger, which some investigators believe represents a C5 or C6 radiculopathy,[35] whereas others believe it to be brachial plexus upper trunk dysfunction.[36,37] Initially called a nerve pinch syndrome, this phenomenon is estimated to comprise approximately 36% of all neurologic upper extremity injuries related to football.[38] Patients describe pain and paresthesias shooting down the arm into fingers associated with transient weakness and prompt recovery over minutes. There are rare cases in which weakness may persist several months,[39] suggesting axonotmesis of the upper trunk brachial plexus; this is supported by electromyography,[33] which documents abnormality in 12% of players with such injuries.[36] Electromyographic abnormalities in such injuries best correlate with the presence of weakness at 72 hours after injury.[40] More persistent cervical plexus injuries have included upper trunk brachial plexopathies and C5 or C6 radiculopathies.[38,41] Thoracic outlet syndrome has been controversially associated in the throwing arm of football quarterbacks.[19,20]

Peripheral nerve injuries in football may also occur as a result of blocking or tackling techniques. In one study, football was the most common sport to cause injury in patients referred for electrodiagnostic testing.[41] Mononeuropathies reported in upper limbs of football players include axillary neuropathy,[41,42] suprascapular neuropathy,[41] ulnar neuropathy,[41] median neuropathy at the carpal tunnel,[41] long thoracic neuropathy,[41] and radial neuropathy.[41] Axillary neuropathy can occur in shoulder dislocation[41,43] or as a result of direct trauma to the anterolateral deltoid region.[42] Most athletes with axillary neuropathy (91%) return to pre-injury levels of professional sports activities.[42] The syndrome of "footballer's hernia" with lower abdominal bulging may rarely lead to iliohypogastric neuropathy.[31] Peroneal neuropathy occurs in 24% of football players in whom complete knee dislocation and ligamentous injury have taken place.[41,44] Sciatic neuropathy may also occur but may present as the controversial "hamstring syndrome".[31] Lumbosacral radiculopathies related to football injury seem to be quite uncommon.[41]

FRISBEE

The lone reported peripheral nerve lesion in active frisbee players is a posterior interosseous nerve syndrome, thought to be attributable to repeated elbow and wrist extension.[45]

GOLF

Mononeuropathies in golfers are often atypical. A new golfer presented with an unusual form of median neuropathy, with evidence of segmental demyelination found 2 to 3 cm distal to the wrist crease on nerve conduction studies. The clinical presentation of sensory deficit within the distal median nerve distribution, including the palmar branch, suggested the unusual localization.[46] Golf-induced CTS affecting the median nerve at the wrist is less clear, but repetitive gripping and sustained hyperflexion and hyperextension may contribute.[47] A professional golf instructor was reported to have ulnar neuropathy localized as a focal conduction block in the distal forearm approximately 7 cm proximal to the ulnar styloid, perhaps attributable to enlargement of the flexor carpi ulnaris and subsequent compression of the adjacent ulnar nerve; similar pathologic findings were demonstrated at surgery.[48]

GYMNASTICS

The difficult maneuvers and body postures of a gymnast place the body at risk for injury, including peripheral nerves. Gymnasts seem to be susceptible to femoral neuropathy as a result of iliacus hematoma or hemorrhage within the femoral nerve sheath.[49,50] Lateral femoral cutaneous neuropathy occurred in a female gymnast who entered an intensive program of jumping rope, with the repetitive hip flexion and extension thought to be causative.[51] Distal posterior interosseous neuropathy has been attributed to repetitive wrist dorsiflexion in a gymnast.[52]

HANDBALL

Handball is a popular European sport that combines skills of basketball and soccer. Some goalkeepers in this sport present with "handball goalie's elbow," with radiating pain or numbness within the ulnar territory of the forearm in addition to local elbow pain, mimicking ulnar neuropathy. Electrophysiologic assessment is negative, however, leading most to believe that this is musculoskeletal in nature because of repetitive forced hyperextensions of the elbow rather than ulnar neuropathy.[53]

HOCKEY

Ice hockey nervous system injuries most commonly consist of concussions and spinal cord injuries, with peripheral nerve injuries much less common. Although more common in football players, the stinger may also occur in hockey players.[25] Shoulder dislocation leading to axillary neuropathy has been reported in two hockey players related to player contact trauma.[42,54] An interesting form of compression neuropathy is demonstrated with a case of tarsal tunnel syndrome secondary to the use of inflatable ice hockey skates in a male recreational hockey player, with significant clinical and electrophysiologic improvement after cessation of wearing the skates.[55] Peroneal neuropathy has rarely occurred in hockey players in situations of laceration of the nerve with a skate blade or attributable to direct blunt nerve trauma.[56,57]

IN-LINE AND ROLLER SKATING

The wearing of tight roller skates has led to entrapment of the superficial peroneal nerve.[58]

JUDO/KARATE/KICKBOXING AND RELATED SPORTS

Although the martial arts have been associated with numerous injuries, neurologic injuries, usually involving the head and neck, seem to be relatively uncommon.[59] Peripheral nerve injury can occur in the martial arts as a result of direct blows leading to nerve contusions affecting the ulnar, axillary, spinal accessory, long thoracic, and peroneal nerves.[60,61] Morton's neuroma may occur in karate enthusiasts, presumably because of repeated irritation of the ball of the foot from fighting stances.[61]

MOUNTAIN CLIMBING/HIKING

Mountain climbers and hikers can be subject to unique forms of peripheral nerve injury. Tarsal tunnel syndrome attributable to repetitive dorsiflexion of the ankle can occur in mountain climbers.[6] Hikers' use of a backpack has been associated with a unique condition called "rucksack paralysis," a syndrome presenting with injury of the brachial plexus at the upper and middle trunk and, occasionally, the suprascapular, axillary, and long thoracic nerves.[62–64] Brachial plexus traction seems to be causative, and one predisposing factor for this condition is the use of a pack without waist support.[63] Often, rucksack paralysis presents with painless arm paresthesias. Electrophysiology can demonstrate conduction block or axonal loss in some patients with rucksack paralysis, with axonal loss associated with a poorer prognosis for recovery.

RODEO

Rodeo injuries are most common for participants in bull riding, bareback riding, and "saddle bronc" events,[65] in which concussions account for most neurologic injuries.[65] Little has been reported about PNS injury, although it may occur. The author has seen two cases of axillary neuropathy secondary to shoulder dislocation and radial neuropathy secondary to humeral fracture.

RUGBY AND AUSTRALIAN RULES FOOTBALL

Rugby and Australian rules football are both highly subject to cerebral concussion, with some occurrence of peripheral nerve injuries.[66] Australian rules football players can develop obturator neuropathies[67,68] as a result of fascial entrapment of the obturator nerve at the short abductor muscle of the thigh. Obturator neuropathy may be responsive to surgical neurolysis.[67,68]

Direct trauma to the anterolateral deltoid without shoulder dislocation has been reported as a cause of axillary neuropathy in rugby players, likely attributable to nerve contusion.[54]

RUNNING

Peripheral nerve injuries attributable to running have been covered in the article by McKean elsewhere in this issue.

SHOOTING

Long thoracic neuropathy has been reported in a world class marksman, probably attributable to positional stress on the shoulder during repetitive shooting postures.[69]

SKIING (CROSS-COUNTRY)

Cross-country skiing has been associated with mononeuropathies. Isolated femoral neuropathy may occur in cross-country skiers as a result of vigorous hip flexion-extension movements.[70] Ulnar neuropathy has developed in cross-country skiers, thought to be attributable to forceful poling; cessation of activity led to clinical improvement.[71]

SNOWBOARDING

Most nervous system injuries to snowboarders consist of spinal and head injuries. Falls placing the shoulder in a compromised position have led to brachial plexus injuries, however. Landing on the snow with the shoulder held in hyperextension and internal rotation is predisposing to upper or lower plexus injuries.[72]

SNOWMOBILING AND ALL-TERRAIN VEHICLE RIDING

Peripheral nerve injuries attributable to snowmobiling are common; brachial plexus injuries occur in 4.8% of snowmobile accident victims.[73] Often, the brachial plexus injury is severe in such cases—complete brachial plexopathy occurs in 67% of patients with brachial plexus injury who have had snowmobile accidents. These brachial plexus injuries are often associated with orthopedic shoulder injury.[74] Supraclavicular injuries affecting the brachial plexus seem to be more common and more severe than infraclavicular injuries.[73] The author has seen one patient with bilateral ulnar neuropathies at Guyon's canal after a full day of snowmobiling when he fastened his hands to the handlebars with duct tape to prevent excessive hand vibration.

SOCCER

Peripheral nerve injury is rare in soccer players. Peroneal nerve compression at the fibular neck has been attributed to excessive play in one soccer player only.[75] The author has seen two soccer players who sustained kicks to their lower legs leading to tibiafibula fractures with concomitant individual peroneal and tibial nerve palsies.

SWIMMING

The controversial neurogenic thoracic outlet syndrome may develop in association with hypertrophied pectoralis minor muscles in swimmers.[19,20]

SURFING

Repetitive microtrauma attributable to prolonged wave-surfing has been associated with common peroneal neuropathy and saphenous neuropathy in boys and young men.[76,77] These may occur as a result of riding the surfboard for a prolonged duration of time and the subsequent compression on the inner leg and stretching of the peroneal nerve attributable to prolonged leg abduction.

TENNIS AND OTHER RACQUET SPORTS

Tennis and other related racquet sports involve repetitive arm swinging, which can lead to several musculoskeletal difficulties that may mimic a nerve entrapment syndrome. Specific nerve entrapments are possible in tennis players, however. Posterior interosseous nerve entrapment is relatively common in tennis players because of compression at the arcade of Frohse and presents with weakness of the wrist extensors and metacarpophalangeal extensors.[6,78] Suprascapular neuropathy also occurs in tennis players, likely because of repetitive overhead swinging during serving, with compression at the suprascapular or supraglenoid notches, and possibly with an associated ganglion cyst.[79,80] Long thoracic neuropathy, possibly attributable to stretching of the nerve with prolonged serving, can occur in the tennis player.[81] Radial nerve palsy may also occur as a result of compression from fibrous arches at the lateral head of the triceps.[82,83] Compression of the lateral cutaneous nerve of the forearm has also been seen in a tennis player thought to have excessive use of the forehand swing.[84] Tennis players wearing a constrictive wrist band or a racquetball strap have been reported to develop superficial radial neuropathy.[85] Digital nerve injuries have also occurred in highly active tennis players.[86] Shoulder pain with radiation caused by neurogenic thoracic outlet syndrome has been documented within the serving arm of tennis players.[19,20]

VOLLEYBALL

Volleyball is one of the safest competitive and recreational sports played by high-school and collegiate athletes,[87] but peripheral nerve injuries seem to be relatively common in volleyball players. The most frequent form of peripheral nerve entrapment is an isolated entrapment of the suprascapular nerve occurring at the spinoglenoid notch, which presents with painless weakness of dominant arm external rotation and with evidence of infraspinatus atrophy on examination.[88,89] This neuropathy only occurs in the serving, or dominant, arm of the volleyball player.[88] In international-level volleyball players, the overall prevalence of suprascapular neuropathy was high, ranging from 33% to 45%, based on combined clinical and electrophysiologic examination.[90,91] In addition to those clinically affected, another 12% of volleyball players have subclinical suprascapular neuropathy,[88] with electromyography in these subclinical cases demonstrating denervation and loss of motor units restricted to the infraspinatus muscle.[89] Increased range of motion of the shoulder joint may be associated with the development of isolated suprascapular neuropathy.[92] An alternative explanation may be that the medial tendinous margin between the infraspinatus and supraspinatus muscles impinges on the lateral edge of the scapular spine, producing compression of the infraspinatus branch of the suprascapular nerve;[93] this hypothesis is favored by the positive response of elite volleyball players to a spinoglenoid notchplasty procedure.[93] Isolated mononeuropathies of the axillary nerve and long thoracic nerve may also occur in younger volleyball players; a quadrilateral space syndrome may be related in the case of axillary mononeuropathies.[94,95]

WRESTLING

Amateur wrestling is an aggressive sport with frequent spinal injury.[87] Brachial plexus injury occurs relatively commonly in wrestling compared with other sports; such injury takes place as a result of holds that place the opposing wrestler's head in far lateral flexion, such as with a full- or half-Nelson hold.[96] Burners, or stingers, account for 37% of all head and neck injuries in competitive wrestlers.[25,97] Other forms of peripheral nerve injuries rarely reported in wrestlers include axillary neuropathy,[41] ulnar neuropathy,[41] CTS,[41] long thoracic neuropathy,[41] and suprascapular neuropathy.[41]

YOGA

The author has seen two yoga participants who maintained a crossed-leg posture for a long duration of time, one of whom fell asleep for several hours in this position. Both developed bilateral foot drop on attempting to stand and were found to have bilateral sciatic neuropathies based on combined clinical and electrophysiologic assessments. These patients had a near-complete recovery after 12 months of cessation of sitting in this yoga position.

SUMMARY

Sporting disciplines can lead to a range of peripheral nerve injuries. Even apparently benign sporting activities, such as bowling, cheerleading, golf, and dancing, have been associated with peripheral nerve injuries. The literature probably underreports the incidence of injury in many sports because of lack of recognition and the presence of scattered case reports as opposed to prospective studies as have been performed to examine concussion in professional football. For the health care professional faced with diagnosing injuries in the athlete, it is hoped that this article assists in the recognition of sport-specific injuries, particularly for those physicians who encounter athletes with unique or difficult problems.

REFERENCES

1. Rayan GM. Archery-related injuries of the hand, forearm, and elbow. South Med J 1992;85(10):961–4.
2. Shimizu J, Nishiyama K, Takeda K, et al. [A case of long thoracic nerve palsy, with winged scapula, as a result of prolonged exertion on practicing archery]. Rinsho Shinkeigaku 1990;30(8):873–6.
3. Ogawa K, Ui M. Humeral shaft fracture sustained during arm wrestling: report on 30 cases and review of the literature. J Trauma 1997;42(2):243–6.
4. Trammell TR, Olivary SE. Crash and injury statistics from Indy-Car racing 1985–1989. 34th Annual Conference. Scotsdale, AZ. Association for Advancement of Automotive Medicine Proceedings. 329–35. 1991. Ref Type: Conference Proceeding.
5. Kukowski B. Suprascapular nerve lesion as an occupational neuropathy in a semi-professional dancer. Arch Phys Med Rehabil 1993;74(7):768–9.
6. Lorei MP, Hershman EB. Peripheral nerve injuries in athletes. Treatment and prevention. Sports Med 1993;16(2):130–47.
7. Sammarco GJ, Miller EH. Forefoot conditions in dancers: part II. Foot Ankle 1982; 3(2):93–8.
8. Wang FC, Crielaard JM. [Entrapment neuropathies in sports medicine]. Rev Med Liege 2001;56(5):382–90 [in French].
9. Gainor BJ, Piotrowski G, Puhl J, et al. The throw: biomechanics and acute injury. Am J Sports Med 1980;8(2):114–8.
10. Sinson G, Zager EL, Kline DG. Windmill pitcher's radial neuropathy. Neurosurgery 1994;34(6):1087–9.
11. Kuschner SH, Lane CS. Recurrent fracture of the humerus in a softball player. Am J Orthop 1999;28(11):654–6.
12. Ogawa K, Yoshida A. Throwing fracture of the humeral shaft. An analysis of 90 patients. Am J Sports Med 1998;26(2):242–6.
13. Andrews JR, Timmerman LA. Outcome of elbow surgery in professional baseball players. Am J Sports Med 1995;23(4):407–13.
14. Del Pizzo W, Jobe FW, Norwood L. Ulnar nerve entrapment syndrome in baseball players. Am J Sports Med 1977;5(5):182–5.
15. Hang YS. Tardy ulnar neuritis in a little league baseball player. Am J Sports Med 1981;9(4):244–6.
16. Hirasawa Y, Sakakida K. Sports and peripheral nerve injury. Am J Sports Med 1983;11(6):420–6.
17. Wojtys EM, Smith PA, Hankin FM. A cause of ulnar neuropathy in a baseball pitcher. A case report. Am J Sports Med 1986;14(5):422–4.
18. Esposito MD, Arrington JA, Blackshear MN, et al. Thoracic outlet syndrome in a throwing athlete diagnosed with MRI and MRA. J Magn Reson Imaging 1997; 7(3):598–9.
19. Karas SE. Thoracic outlet syndrome. Clin Sports Med 1990;9(2):297–310.
20. Strukel RJ, Garrick JG. Thoracic outlet compression in athletes: a report of four cases. Am J Sports Med 1978;6(2):35–9.

21. Hsu JC, Paletta GA Jr, Gambardella RA, et al. Musculocutaneous nerve injury in major league baseball pitchers: a report of 2 cases. Am J Sports Med 2007;35(6): 1003–6.
22. Long RR, Sargent JC, Pappas AM, et al. Pitcher's arm: an electrodiagnostic enigma. Muscle Nerve 1996;19(10):1276–81.
23. Belsky M, Milleander LH. Bowler's thumb in a baseball player. Orthopedics 1980; 3:122.
24. Tsur A, Shahin R. [Suprascapular nerve entrapment in a basketball player]. Harefuah 1997;133(5–6):190–2, 247 [in Hebrew].
25. Feinberg JH. Burners and stingers. Phys Med Rehabil Clin N Am 2000;11(4): 771–84.
26. Jackson DL, Hynninen BC, Caborn DN, et al. Electrodiagnostic study of carpal tunnel syndrome in wheelchair basketball players. Clin J Sport Med 1996;6(1): 27–31.
27. Burnham RS, Steadward RD. Upper extremity peripheral nerve entrapments among wheelchair athletes: prevalence, location, and risk factors. Arch Phys Med Rehabil 1994;75(5):519–24.
28. Viegas SF, Torres FG. Cherry pitter's thumb. Case report and review of the literature. Orthop Rev 1989;18(3):336–8.
29. Kisner WH. Thumb neuroma: a hazard of ten pin bowling. Br J Plast Surg 1976; 29(3):225–6.
30. Shields RW Jr, Jacobs IB. Median palmar digital neuropathy in a cheerleader. Arch Phys Med Rehabil 1986;67(11):824–6.
31. McCrory P, Bell S. Nerve entrapment syndromes as a cause of pain in the hip, groin and buttock. Sports Med 1999;27(4):261–74.
32. Meeuwisse WH, Hagel BE, Mohtadi NG, et al. The distribution of injuries in men's Canada West university football. A 5-year analysis. Am J Sports Med 2000;28(4): 516–23.
33. Clancy WG Jr, Brand RL, Bergfield JA. Upper trunk brachial plexus injuries in contact sports. Am J Sports Med 1977;5(5):209–16.
34. Clarke KS. Prevention: an epidemiologic view. In: Torg JS, editor. Athletic injuries in the head, neck and face. Philadelphia: Lea and Febiger; 1982. p. 15–26.
35. Poindexter DP, Johnson EW. Football shoulder and neck injury: a study of the "stinger." Arch Phys Med Rehabil 1984;65(10):601–2.
36. Markey KL, Di Benedetto M, Curl WW. Upper trunk brachial plexopathy. The stinger syndrome. Am J Sports Med 1993;21(5):650–5.
37. Di Benedetto M, Markey K. Electrodiagnostic localization of traumatic upper trunk brachial plexopathy. Arch Phys Med Rehabil 1984;65(1):15–7.
38. Krivickas LS, Wilbourn AJ. Peripheral nerve injuries in athletes: a case series of over 200 injuries. Semin Neurol 2000;20(2):225–32.
39. Chrisman O, Snook G, Tanitis JM, et al. Lateral-flexion neck injuries in athletic competition. JAMA 1965;192:613–5.
40. Speer KP, Bassett FH III. The prolonged burner syndrome. Am J Sports Med 1990;18(6):591–4.
41. Krivickas LS, Wilbourn AJ. Sports and peripheral nerve injuries: report of 190 injuries evaluated in a single electromyography laboratory. Muscle Nerve 1998; 21(8):1092–4.
42. Perlmutter GS, Leffert RD, Zarins B. Direct injury to the axillary nerve in athletes playing contact sports. Am J Sports Med 1997;25(1):65–8.
43. Kessler KJ, Uribe JW. Complete isolated axillary nerve palsy in college and professional football players: a report of six cases. Clin J Sport Med 1994;4:272–4.

44. Yu JS, Goodwin D, Salonen D, et al. Complete dislocation of the knee: spectrum of associated soft-tissue injuries depicted by MR imaging. AJR Am J Roentgenol 1995;164(1):135–9.

45. Fraim CJ, Peters BH. Unusual cause of nerve entrapment. JAMA 1979;242(23): 2557–8.

46. Hsu WC, Chen WH, Oware A, et al. Unusual entrapment neuropathy in a golf player. Neurology 2002;59(4):646–7.

47. Murray PM, Cooney WP. Golf-induced injuries of the wrist. Clin Sports Med 1996; 15(1):85–109.

48. Campbell WW. AAEE case report #18: ulnar neuropathy in the distal forearm. Muscle Nerve 1989;12(5):347–52.

49. Brozin IH, Martfel J, Goldberg I, et al. Traumatic closed femoral nerve neuropathy. J Trauma 1982;22(2):158–60.

50. Giuliani G, Poppi M, Acciarri N, et al. CT scan and surgical treatment of traumatic iliacus hematoma with femoral neuropathy: case report. J Trauma 1990;30(2): 229–31.

51. Goldberg MJ. Gymnastic injuries. Orthop Clin North Am 1980;11(4):717–26.

52. Aulicino PL. Neurovascular injuries in the hands of athletes. Hand Clin 1990;6(3): 455–66.

53. Rise IR, Dhaenens G, Tyrdal S. Is the ulnar nerve damaged in 'handball goalie's elbow'? Scand J Med Sci Sports 2001;11(4):247–50.

54. Perlmutter GS, Apruzzese W. Axillary nerve injuries in contact sports: recommendations for treatment and rehabilitation. Sports Med 1998;26(5):351–61.

55. Watson BV, Algahtani H, Broome RJ, et al. An unusual presentation of tarsal tunnel syndrome caused by an inflatable ice hockey skate. Can J Neurol Sci 2002; 29(4):386–9.

56. MacDonald PB, Strange G, Hodgkinson R, et al. Injuries to the peroneal nerve in professional hockey. Clin J Sport Med 2002;12(1):39–40.

57. Shevell MI, Stewart JD. Laceration of the common peroneal nerve by a skate blade. CMAJ 1988;139(4):311–2.

58. Dewitt LD, Greenberg HS. Roller disco neuropathy. JAMA 1981;246(8):836.

59. NEISS data highlights. United States Consumer Product Safety Commission. 1985;12–1.

60. Bjerrum L. [Scapula alata induced by karate]. Ugeskr Laeger 1984;146(27):2022 [in Danish].

61. Nieman EA, Swann PG. Karate injuries. Br Med J 1971;1(5742):233.

62. Corkill G, Lieberman JS, Taylor RG. Pack palsy in backpackers. West J Med 1980;132(6):569–72.

63. Goodson JD. Brachial plexus injury from light tight backpack straps. N Engl J Med 1981;305(9):524–5.

64. Johnson RJ. Anatomy of backpack-strap injury. N Engl J Med 1981;305(26):1594.

65. Butterwick DJ, Hagel B, Nelson DS, et al. Epidemiologic analysis of injury in five years of Canadian professional rodeo. Am J Sports Med 2002;30(2):193–8.

66. Orchard J, Wood T, Seward H, et al. Comparison of injuries in elite senior and junior Australian football. J Sci Med Sport 1998;1(2):83–8.

67. Bradshaw C, McCrory P. Obturator nerve entrapment. Clin J Sport Med 1997; 7(3):217–9.

68. Bradshaw C, McCrory P, Bell S, et al. Obturator nerve entrapment. A cause of groin pain in athletes. Am J Sports Med 1997;25(3):402–8.

69. Woodhead AB III. Paralysis of the serratus anterior in a world class marksman. A case study. Am J Sports Med 1985;13(5):359–62.

70. Muellner T, Ganko A, Bugge W, et al. Isolated femoral mononeuropathy in the athlete. Anatomic considerations and report of two cases. Am J Sports Med 2001; 29(6):814–7.
71. Fulkerson JP. Transient ulnar neuropathy from Nordic skiing. Clin Orthop Relat Res 1980;153:230–1.
72. Ogawa T, Ochiai N, Hara Y. Brachial plexus injury in snowboarding. J Hand Surg [Br] 2006;31(6):661–2.
73. Midha R. Epidemiology of brachial plexus injuries in a multitrauma population. Neurosurgery 1997;40(6):1182–8.
74. Braun BL, Meyers B, Dulebohn SC, et al. Severe brachial plexus injury as a result of snowmobiling: a case series. J Trauma 1998;44(4):726–30.
75. Leach RE, Purnell MB, Saito A. Peroneal nerve entrapment in runners. Am J Sports Med 1989;17(2):287–91.
76. Fabian RH, Norcross KA, Hancock MB. Surfer's neuropathy. N Engl J Med 1987; 316(9):555.
77. Watemberg N, Amsel S, Sadeh M, et al. Common peroneal neuropathy due to surfing. J Child Neurol 2000;15(6):420–1.
78. Kaplan PE. Posterior interosseous neuropathies: natural history. Arch Phys Med Rehabil 1984;65(7):399–400.
79. Daubinet G, Rodineau J. [Paralysis of the suprascapular nerve and tennis. Apropos of 3 groups of professional players]. Schweiz Z Sportmed 1991;39(3):113–8 [in French].
80. Romeo AA, Rotenberg DD, Bach BR Jr. Suprascapular neuropathy. J Am Acad Orthop Surg 1999;7(6):358–67.
81. Pasternack JS, Veenema KR, Callahan CM. Baseball injuries: a Little League survey. Pediatrics 1996;98(3 Pt 1):445–8.
82. Prochaska V, Crosby LA, Murphy RP. High radial nerve palsy in a tennis player. Orthop Rev 1993;22(1):90–2.
83. Streib E. Upper arm radial nerve palsy after muscular effort: report of three cases. Neurology 1992;42(8):1632–4.
84. Felsenthal G, Mondell DL, Reischer MA, et al. Forearm pain secondary to compression syndrome of the lateral cutaneous nerve of the forearm. Arch Phys Med Rehabil 1984;65(3):139–41.
85. Rettig AC. Neurovascular injuries in the wrists and hands of athletes. Clin Sports Med 1990;9(2):389–417.
86. Naso SJ. Compression of the digital nerve: a new entity in tennis players. Orthop Rev 1984;13:47.
87. Powell JW, Barber-Foss KD. Traumatic brain injury in high school athletes. JAMA 1999;282(10):958–63.
88. Ferretti A, Cerullo G, Russo G. Suprascapular neuropathy in volleyball players. J Bone Joint Surg Am 1987;69(2):260–3.
89. Montagna P, Colonna S. Suprascapular neuropathy restricted to the infraspinatus muscle in volleyball players. Acta Neurol Scand 1993;87(3):248–50.
90. Eggert S, Holzgraefe M. [Compression neuropathy of the suprascapular nerve in high performance volleyball players]. Sportverletz Sportschaden 1993;7(3): 136–42 [in German].
91. Holzgraefe M, Kukowski B, Eggert S. Prevalence of latent and manifest suprascapular neuropathy in high-performance volleyball players. Br J Sports Med 1994;28(3):177–9.
92. Witvrouw E, Cools A, Lysens R, et al. Suprascapular neuropathy in volleyball players. Br J Sports Med 2000;34(3):174–80.

93. Sandow MJ, Ilic J. Suprascapular nerve rotator cuff compression syndrome in volleyball players. J Shoulder Elbow Surg 1998;7(5):516–21.
94. Distefano S. Neuropathy due to entrapment of the long thoracic nerve. A case report. Ital J Orthop Traumatol 1989;15(2):259–62.
95. Paladini D, Dellantonio R, Cinti A, et al. Axillary neuropathy in volleyball players: report of two cases and literature review. J Neurol Neurosurg Psychiatr 1996; 60(3):345–7.
96. Snook G. A survey of wrestling injuries. Am J Sports Med 1980;8(6):450–3.
97. Estwanik JJ, Bergfield JA, Collins HR, et al. Injuries in interscholastic wrestling. Physical Sports Medicine 1980;8:111–21.

Muscle Physiology in Healthy Men and Women and Those with Metabolic Myopathies

Michaela C. Devries, BSc, MSc[a], Mark A. Tarnopolsky, MD, PhD, FRCPC[a,b,*]

KEYWORDS

• Muscle physiology • Carbohydrates • Exercise • Fatigue

Carbohydrate (CHO) and fat constitute the main fuels used during endurance exercise, while amino acid oxidation (protein) contributes a small amount to total substrate use. The relative contribution and source of the fuels used during endurance exercise is dependent on the intensity and the duration of the exercise bout.[1–5] Additionally, the relative contribution of CHO, fat, and amino acids to fuel endurance exercise can be influenced by training status,[6–14] sex,[8] and diet.[6,15–17] As such, much work has been done to investigate the potential performance enhancing effect of manipulating training and dietary interventions in athletes.

Given that acute exercise represents a metabolic challenge to intermediary metabolism, it is often a trigger of symptoms for individuals with disorders of carbohydrate and fat oxidation. Because the mitochondria are the final common pathway for oxidative metabolism of all metabolic substrates, patients with primary mitochondrial cytopathies also display symptoms of exercise intolerance.[18–21] Pre-exercise carbohydrate ingestion is of therapeutic benefit for people with McArdle's disease[22] and fat oxidation defects,[23] while carbohydrate loading strategies are helpful in the symptomatic treatment of fat oxidation defects.[24] Conversely, triglyceride infusion can improve exercise capacity in patients with a complex I deficiency;[25] yet a higher fat diet does not appear to benefit patients with mitochondrial complex I deficiency.[26]

This article originally appeared in *Neurologic Clinics*, Volume 26, Issue 1.

This work was supported by National Sciences and Engineering Research Council of Canada, Canadian Institutes of Health Research, and donations from Warren Lammert and Kathy Corkins and Giant Tiger Stores.

[a] Pediatrics & Medicine, Division of Neurology, McMaster University, McMaster University Medical Center, 1200 Main Street West, Hamilton, ON, Canada L8N 3Z5

[b] Neurometabolic, Neuromuscular Clinic, McMaster University, 1200 Main Street West, HSC-2H26, Hamilton, ON, Canada L8N 3Z5

* Corresponding author. Neurometabolic, Neuromuscular Clinic, McMaster University, 1200 Main Street West, HSC-2H26, Hamilton, ON, Canada L8N 3Z5.

E-mail address: tarnopol@mcmaster.ca (M.A. Tarnopolsky).

Endurance exercise training is of significant benefit to those with McArdle's disease[27,28] and mitochondrial cytopathies.[18,29–31] Resistance exercise training may also be of benefit for people with sporadic mitochondrial cytopathies.[18,32] Finally, with the benefits of resistance exercise training being well documented in older adults,[33–35] all patients with metabolic myopathies may derive benefits that counter the age-associated loss of muscle mass and strength.

CARBOHYDRATE OXIDATION DURING ENDURANCE EXERCISE

Carbohydrates are one of the main sources of fuel used during moderate to higher intensity endurance exercise.[2,4] CHO are a versatile fuel, contributing at both aerobic and anaerobic power outputs.[36] The CHO stores used during endurance exercise include plasma glucose and muscle glycogen.[2,4] Muscle glycogen stores represent the major source of carbohydrates used during exercise under most circumstances,[2,4] and are depleted by 1 to 2 hours of moderate to higher intensity exercise.[37] Plasma glucose is derived endogenously from liver glycogen stores or from gluconeogensis in the liver and kidneys, with exogenous sources possible from dietary ingestion. The relative contribution of plasma glucose and muscle glycogen is influenced by exercise duration and intensity, training status, sex, and diet (see below). The uptake of plasma glucose into skeletal muscle is mediated by the facilitated transporters, GLUT-1 and GLUT-4.[38] GLUT-1 is constitutively expressed at the sarcolemma, while GLUT-4 is translocated to the sarcolemma and transverse tubules via stimulation by insulin or exercise.[38–40] Once glucose has entered the muscle it is phosphorylated by hexokinase II to glucose-6-phosphate (G6P),[40] and can either undergo glycogen synthesis or enter glycolysis (**Fig. 1**).

Glycogen synthesis begins with the conversion of G6P to glucose-1-phosphate by phosphoglucomutase, which is then converted into UDP-glucose by UDP-glucose pyrophosphorylase.[41] UDP-glucose donates a glucosyl group, which glycogen synthase (GS, the rate-limiting enzyme in glycogen synthesis) and branching enzymes add to the glycogen granule via α-1,4- and α-1,6-glycosidic linkages, respectively.[42] At the core of the glycogen granule is a protein primer, glycogenin, which acts as a primer for GS to form new glycogen granules.[43] Skeletal muscle glycogen is stored in two main forms called pro- and macroglycogen,[43–45] with proglycogen representing smaller units of glycogen with a relatively high associated protein content, while macroglycogen represents larger particles with a relatively high carbohydrate-to-protein content.[44] Glycogen degradation begins with the conversion of glycogen to glucose-1-phosphate, catalyzed by glycogen phosphorylase and debranching enzyme, which cleave the α-1,4- and α-1,6-glycosidic linkages, respectively.

During endurance exercise, plasma glucose uptake increases because of increased translocation of GLUT-4 to the sarcolemma and T-tubules.[46] The mechanisms of exercise-stimulated GLUT-4 translocation are unknown; however, they are different from insulin stimulated GLUT-4 translocation,[47–49] and although still controversial, it is likely that AMP-activated protein kinase[50,51] and calcium[52] are involved. During exercise, most of the glucose that enters the muscle is routed toward glycolysis, which results in the production of pyruvate.[53,54] Glycolysis is primarily regulated by phosphofructokinase (PFK), which is allosterically modified by activators such as inorganic phosphate and AMP, and inhibited by high levels of adenosine 5'-triphosphate.[55] During exercise, pyruvate is either shunted into the tricarboxylic acid cycle by pyruvate dehydrogenase (PDH) under aerobic conditions,[56] or toward lactate formation by lactate dehydrogenase when the rate of glycolysis exceeds that of PDH entry into the tricarboxylic acid cycle (such as at the onset of exercise or under ischemic

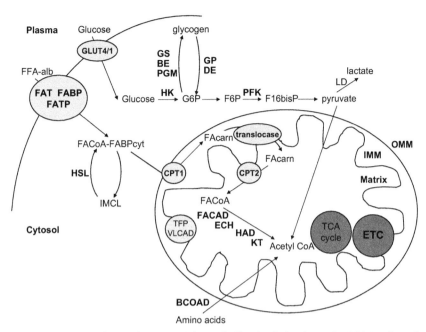

Fig.1. Schematic CHO, fat, and amino acid metabolism in skeletal muscle. BCOAD, branched chain 2-oxoacid dehydrogenase; BE, branching enzyme; CPT1, carnitine palmitoyl transferase 1; CPT2, carnitine palmitoyl transferase 2; DE, debranching enzyme; ECH, Enoyl-CoA hydratase; FABP, fatty acid binding protein; FAcarn, fatty acyl carnitine; FACoA, fatty acyl-CoA; FACAD, fatty acyl-CoA dehydrogenase; FAT, fatty acid transporter; FATP, fatty acid transport protein; FFAalb, free fatty acid albumin; F16bisP, fructose-1,6-bisphosphate; F6P, fructose-6-phosphate; G6P, glucose-6-phsophate; GLUT-4, -1, glucose transporter 4 or 1; GP, glycogen phosphorylase; GS, glycogen synthase; HAD, hydroxyacyl-CoA dehydrogenase; HK, hexokinase; HSL, hormone sensitive lipase; IMM, inner mitochondrial membrane; KT, ketothiolase; LD, lactate dehydrogenase; PFK, phosphofructokinase; PGM, phosphogluco-mutase; OMM, outer mitochondrial membrane; TCA, tricarboxylic acid cycle; TP, trifunctional protein; VLCAD, very long chain acyl-CoA dehydrogenase.

conditions).[57] The PDH complex is activated by a phosphatase and inhibited by a ki-nase (PDK).[56] Dichloroacetate is an activator of PDH and has been used in some cases of mitochondrial cytopathy to reduce lactate levels.[58,59]

LIPID OXIDATION DURING ENDURANCE EXERCISE

Lipid oxidation contributes maximally during moderate-intensity exercise (40%–65% maximal oxygen consumption per unit time or VO_2max; see the section on exercise intensity during endurance exercise, below), representing between 40% and 60% of total energy expenditure.[4] Of this, plasma free fatty acids (FFA) contribute between 40% and 60% of total fat oxidation;[2,4] other fat sources, intramyocellular lipids (IMCL, **Fig. 2**) and lipoprotein-derived triacylglycerol (TG), provide the remainder.

Under normal dietary conditions, the contribution of lipoprotein-derived TG during exercise is less than 10%,[60] implying that IMCL supplies the remaining 30% to 50% of fat oxidation during moderate intensity endurance exercise. However, the use of IMCL during endurance exercise is controversial. Numerous studies have found that IMCL is an important substrate during moderate-intensity endurance exercise,[4,61–65]

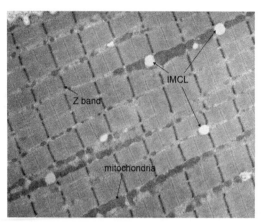

Fig. 2. Electron micrograph of the *vastus lateralis* muscle taken at 6500 magnification, showing IMCL and mitochondria.

whereas other studies have not found this.[66] Additionally, several studies have found that only women use IMCL during endurance exercise.[62,67] However, although it is plausible for women to use more IMCL during a bout of endurance exercise (see section below describing the effect of sex on substrate selection during endurance exercises), it is unlikely that men do not use any IMCL as a fuel source during endurance exercise.[62,67,68]

The most likely cause of the aforementioned discrepancy relates to methodologic limitations associated with quantifying IMCL content. There are several methods used to quantify IMCL content, including biochemical extraction, stable isotope infusion, light microscopy, electron microscopy, and proton magnetic resonance spectroscopy (^{1}H-MRS).[4] It is generally accepted that when using the biochemical method, there can be significant contamination from extramyocellular lipids.[69] The majority of studies that have not shown a decrease in IMCL following a bout of endurance exercise have used the biochemical method,[67,70–72] whereas studies using stable isotope tracers,[2–4,15,73] electron microscopy (EM),[74] and ^{1}H-MRS,[61,63–65,75] consistently show a decrease in IMCL following a bout of endurance exercise for men and women. Furthermore, MRS and EM appear to show similar findings when directly compared.[76] The use of more sophisticated methodologies (^{1}H-MRS and EM) has decreased the confusion regarding the use of IMCL during endurance exercise and it is now generally accepted that IMCL are an important fuel source during endurance exercise.

Free fatty acids are chaperoned in the plasma by albumin.[77] There are three fatty acid binding proteins (fatty acid binding protein of the plasma membrane or FABPpm, fatty acid translocase or FAT/CD36, and fatty acid transporter or FAT) that are responsible for the uptake of FFA into the muscle.[78] Once in the muscle, FFA are chaperoned by FABPcytosol[79] (once charged with a CoA group, FACoA) and can be esterified into IMCL for storage and hydrolyzed when needed. During exercise there is an increase in plasma FFA uptake by the muscle[67,80] as well as an increased IMCL hydrolysis mediated by hormone sensitive lipase (HSL),[36,81–83] which is stimulated by epinephrine.[36,82,83]

It is important to note that although there is a net decrease in IMCL during a bout of endurance exercise, IMCL hydrolysis and FFA esterification are in a state of continual flux during exercise.[84] To be oxidized, FACoA must enter the mitochondria where they undergo β-oxidation (see **Fig. 1**). While short and medium chain FACoAs can diffuse into the mitochondria, long chain FACoAs (LCFACoA) require modification by carnitine palmitoyl transferase I and II (CPT I and CPT II) to enter the mitochondrial matrix.[85] The activity of CPT I is inhibited by malonyl CoA,[86] which is involved in FA synthesis. New research also suggests that FAT/CD36 might also play a role in LCFACoA transport into the mitochondrial matrix.[87] Once in the mitochondrial matrix, the FACoA can undergo β-oxidation, which is a sequence of steps resulting in the formation of acetyl CoA and a FACoA with two less carbons (see **Fig. 1**). The acetyl CoA formed during each turn of β-oxidation then enters the citric acid cycle and the FACoA returns to the start of β-oxidation. Very long chain FAs undergo a special form of β-oxidation using very long chain acyl CoA dehydrogenase (VLCAD) and trifunctional protein at the inner mitochondrial membrane (see **Fig. 1**). VLCAD initiates β-oxidation and trifunctional protein combines the functions of the remaining three enzymes of β-oxidation with long chain specificity.[88]

AMINO ACID OXIDATION DURING ENDURANCE EXERCISE

During endurance exercise there is an increase in leucine oxidation,[89–92] contributing approximately 2% to 3% of total substrate oxidation during the exercise bout.[92] Leucine is oxidized by branched-chain 2-oxoacid dehydrogenase (BCOAD) within the mitochondria (see **Fig. 1**).[93] BCOAD is the rate-limiting enzyme in branched-chain amino acid (leucine, isoleucine, valine) oxidation and is activated upon dephosphorylation by a specific phosphatase and inactivated by BCOAD kinase.[94] During endurance exercise, the activity of BCOAD increases[95] because of increased dephosphorylation of the enzyme, and returns to baseline within 10 minutes after cessation of exercise.[96] The mechanism by which BCOAD activity increases with exercise is unclear. It has been proposed that with muscle stimulation there is an increase in the concentration of α-ketoisocaproic acid,[95] which inhibits BCOAD kinase by interrupting the protein-protein interaction between itself and BCOAD,[97] allowing increased BCOAD activity. In addition to the branched chain amino acids, alanine, asparagine, aspartate, glutamate, and lysine also appear to be oxidized in skeletal muscle.[98] The magnitude of increase in the oxidation for lysine during endurance exercise is not as great as that seen for leucine.[99]

EXERCISE INTENSITY AND DURATION IMPACT SUBSTRATE SELECTION DURING ENDURANCE EXERCISE

Altering exercise intensity has a profound effect on substrate selection during endurance exercise. At low exercise intensities (up to approximately 48% VO_2max), fat is the primary fuel used to sustain exercise.[2,3,5] In a study conducted by Romijn and colleagues[2] during exercise at 25% VO_2max, fat oxidation accounted for 86% of total substrate oxidation. Similarly, when exercise was performed at approximately 40% VO_2max, fat oxidation contributed 55% to total substrate oxidation, while CHO oxidation contributed 45%.[5] As exercise intensity increases from mild to moderate, the rate of fat oxidation also increases,[2,3,5] reaching a maximum between 48% VO_2max and 65% VO_2max, after which the rate of fat oxidation declines.[2,3,5]

Venables and colleagues[5] found that the maximal rate of fat oxidation occurred at 48% VO_2max, and this roughly coincided with the "crossover point" of substrate use, where CHO becomes the predominant fuel used to support endurance exercise. Whereas fat oxidation reaches a maximum and then declines at higher exercise intensities, CHO oxidation continues to increase, with increasing exercise intensities contributing approximately 70% to total substrate oxidation at 85% VO_2max.[2,3]

Exercise intensity not only alters the relative contribution of fat and CHO to total substrate oxidation, it also influences the source of fat and CHO that are used during endurance exercise. At low exercise intensities where fat oxidation predominates, plasma fuel sources (FFA and glucose) are the main contributors to fuel use, while muscle stores (IMCL and glycogen) are not significant contributors.[2,3] As exercise intensity increases, CHO sources contribute more to substrate oxidation, there is an increased reliance on muscle substrate stores, while the contribution of plasma stores remains fairly constant.[1–3]

The mechanism behind the shift in fuel use with increasing exercise intensity remains unclear. However there are several putative mechanisms that may explain these changes, including changes in adipose tissue blood flow, cell signaling molecule phophorylation, muscle pH, and interactions between CHO and fat metabolism. The effect of exercise duration on substrate selection during endurance exercise is more straightforward. During low intensity exercise (25% VO_2max) the relative contribution of fat and CHO remains constant, with plasma FFA being the main source of fuel used to fuel a 120 minute exercise bout.[2] During moderate intensity exercise (65% VO_2max), there is a shift to a greater fat oxidation as exercise duration increases because of a reduction in muscle glycogen stores as exercise progresses.[100,101] Additionally, as exercise duration increases there is an increased reliance on plasma FFA and glucose and a decreased reliance on IMCL and muscle glycogen.[2]

EFFECT OF ENDURANCE TRAINING ON SUBSTRATE SELECTION DURING ENDURANCE EXERCISE

Endurance exercise training increases the reliance on lipid oxidation during exercise at any given absolute workload.[1,8,9,12,73,102–106] Evidence as to the source of the increased reliance on lipid during endurance exercise following training is controversial. Several studies have found that training increases the reliance on plasma FFA.[1,107] Alternatively, several studies have shown that endurance training results in an increased oxidation of nonplasma FFA sources (presumably IMCL,[11]) or greater IMCL depletion.[102,105,109] Additionally, several studies have found that endurance training decreases plasma FFA Rd,[73,103,105] and thus plasma FFA oxidation. Likewise, endurance training did not change adipose tissue lipolytic response to epinephrine infusion[109] and also did not increase whole-body lipolytic response when exercise was performed at the same absolute intensity.[103]

A potential reason for the increased reliance on plasma FFA following training seen in the aforementioned study[1] could be the timing of testing. While this study tested subjects in the postabsorptive state,[1] most studies finding an increased reliance on IMCL following training tested subjects following an overnight fast.[11,73,103] However, similar to studies finding that training increased the reliance on IMCL following training, one study finding increased plasma FFA oxidation after training was also performed following an overnight fast.[107] Further work is needed in this area to elucidate whether endurance training increases plasma FFA or IMCL oxidation or both.

Endurance training increases IMCL content[71,108,110–116] and this is thought to be one of the early responses to endurance training.[114] A recent study using electron microscopy identified that training-induced increases in IMCL content were the result of an increase in the number of IMCL droplets in a given area, not an increase in IMCL size.[110] Metabolically, the effect of endurance training to increase IMCL number and not IMCL size is logical, as this would increase the surface area of IMCL available to interact with mitochondria. An additional finding of the aforementioned study[110] was that endurance training increased the percent of IMCL in direct contact with mitochondria. These findings support the theory that there is an increased reliance on IMCL during endurance exercise following training.

An increased reliance on lipid stores following training is supported by the finding that endurance training increases the capacity of numerous enzymes important in lipid oxidation and mitochondrial function. Endurance training in humans increased the activity of enzymes involved in β-oxidation, including β-hydroxyacyl-CoA dehydrogenase[71,107,110,117–120] and CPT I,[121] as well as the protein content of several enzymes involved in β-oxidation, including VLCAD[11] and medium chain acyl-CoA dehydrogenase (MCAD).[11] Endurance training also enhanced FFA uptake capacity by the muscle, as evidenced by an increased FABPpm[106] and FAT/CD36[122] protein content in rats. Additionally, endurance training in humans increased mitochondrial function by increasing mitochondrial content,[110,112] citrate synthase,[71,104,107,110,117–119,123] malate dehydrogenase,[120] succinate cytochrome c oxidoreductase (CII and CIII),[117] cytochrome c oxidase (COX),[117,124] dehydrogenase (CII),[113] and nicotinamide adenine dinucleotide H cytochrome c oxidoreductase (CI and CIII)[104] enzyme activities. Together, these findings provide the molecular basis for the increased reliance on lipid stores in trained individuals when subjects are tested at the same absolute exercise intensity.

Endurance training also increases muscle glycogen content at rest.[7,71,118,125–127] This elevated resting muscle glycogen content is caused by an increased rate of glycogen accumulation following a bout of endurance exercise when carbohydrate is provided.[125,128,129] The rate of accumulation of glycogen is two times greater in trained, as compared with untrained individuals, during the first 6 hours following a bout of glycogen-depleting exercise.[128] Additionally, 48 and 72 hours after the exercise bout, glycogen levels are 66% higher in trained individuals.[128] The molecular mechanism behind the increased rate of glycogen accumulation with endurance training is thought to be mediated via increased GLUT-4 protein content. A cross-sectional study has shown that GLUT-4 protein content is three times higher in trained versus untrained individuals.[128] In humans and rats, endurance training increased GLUT-4 protein content[118,123–125,127,130–133] and insulin stimulated glucose uptake,[123] with no effect on insulin receptor function.[124] Specifically, with endurance training in rats, there is an increased number of glucose transporters and GLUT-4 protein content at the plasma membrane, not the microsomal membrane.[131] Whether this distributional change is seen in humans is yet to be determined. The increase in GLUT-4 protein content is a very early response to endurance training, occurring within 7 days of training onset.[132] The effect of detraining on GLUT-4 protein content and insulin stimulated glucose uptake occurs even more rapidly, being reversed within a few days of inactivity.[123]

Endurance training not only increases glucose transport into the muscle at rest, but also glucose phosphorylation, as evidenced by an increased hexokinase II activity with endurance training.[119,120,123,133] Following glucose phosphorylation, G6P can be routed toward glycolysis or storage as glycogen. The impact of endurance training on GS activity is at odds with several studies finding no effect of training on GS activity.[125,128,134] Thus, it appears that endurance training increases glycogen accumulation by its effect on GLUT-4 and perhaps hexokinase II activity.

As there is an increased reliance on lipid sources following training, there is a reciprocal effect of endurance training on CHO use during exercise. Numerous studies have found that during exercise at the same absolute intensity there is a decreased reliance on CHO following a period of endurance training.[1,7,8,11,12,53,67,71,105,110,135–137] Despite an increased GLUT-4 protein content[123–125,130–133] and an increased insulin stimulated glucose uptake[123] at rest following a period of endurance training,[8,12,53,127] glucose uptake during a bout of endurance exercise is lower. Specifically, training results in a lower glucose Ra,[7,8,135,137,138] Rd,[7,8,53,135,137,138] and metabolic clearance rate (MCR),[8,53,135,137,138] as well as decreasing net glucose uptake across the working limb[7] during moderate intensity exercise. As a result of this lower glucose uptake, there is a lower oxidation of plasma glucose in the trained state, as evidenced by a reduced rate of plasma glucose oxidation.[135] The effects of training on glucose Ra, Rd, and MCR are seen as soon as 10 days of training and continue to become more pronounced with increased training duration, up to 12 weeks of training.[137] The decreased glucose Ra during exercise in the trained state is mainly the result of a decreased rate of hepatic glycogenolysis, but there is also an effect of endurance training on decreasing the rate of hepatic gluconeogenesis as well.[138] Mechanistically, the decreased glucose uptake during exercise in the trained state is mainly the result of decreased GLUT-4 translocation to the sarcolemma, and thus a lower glucose uptake capacity.[127]

Endurance training attenuates the use of muscle glycogen during a bout of moderate intensity exercise.[7,71] However, during high intensity exercise the use of muscle glycogen is the same between trained and untrained individuals.[118] This finding suggests that, although CHO is spared during exercise performed in the trained state, when exercise intensities increase and lipid is no longer the preferred fuel to support exercise, muscle glycogen begins to compensate for the increased metabolic demand. Support for this notion comes from the finding that plasma glucose uptake remains blunted in trained individuals during high intensity exercise,[53] and that plasma glucose contributes less to total CHO oxidation following a period of endurance training.[135] Endurance exercise training also reduces the proportionate oxidation of leucine during acute endurance exercise for both men and women.[104] This latter effect is associated with a marked attenuation of the exercise-mediated activation of the BCOAD enzyme activity, in spite of an increase in total BCOAD enzyme content.[104] Recently, it has been shown that the training induced attenuation of BCOAD activation and leucine oxidation is associated with an increase in the BCOAD kinase protein content, implying enzyme inactivation.[94] The reduction in BCOAD activation is associated with higher total muscle glycogen levels[104] and lower glycogenolysis[139] after training.

EFFECT OF SEX ON SUBSTRATE SELECTION DURING ENDURANCE EXERCISE

Numerous studies have found that women have a lower respiratory exchange ratio (RER) during endurance exercise as compared with men.[3,5,8,92,140–143] More specifically, women, as compared with men, use less muscle glycogen,[142,144] have higher glycerol turnover,[8] higher plasma FFA concentration,[80,145] lower glucose Rd,[140] lower leucine oxidation,[92,99,104] and higher IMCL oxidation[67,68] during endurance exercise. It has been suggested that these sex differences during exercise are because of differences in estrogen concentration and activity.[146,147] In fact, estrogen supplementation studies in animals and humans have supported the aforementioned findings of higher fat oxidation for women during endurance exercise.

One of the major limiting factors affecting sex comparative studies comes from the ability to accurately match women and men. Men typically have lower percent body fat and a higher maximum oxygen consumption (VO$_2$max), thus subject selection based on body composition and VO$_2$max is not advisable. As such, it is suggested that men and women be selected based on training status, training quantity, and VO$_2$ per kilogram fat free mass, as these are better determinants of fuel use.[117,141] Additionally, as menstrual cycle phase can impact fuel selection during exercise,[144] it is important to take this into consideration when testing eumenorrheic women. Habitual dietary intake can also influence substrate use, with high fat diets increasing fat oxidation[148–150] and high CHO diets increasing CHO oxidation[143,151,152] during exercise. As such, sex differences in nutrient consumption can influence fuel use during exercise, impacting the ability to detect an effect of sex on fuel use during exercise. However, dietary differences do not likely impact the aforementioned sex differences, for several studies that have looked at habitual dietary intake in men and women have not found any differences in the relative contribution of CHO, fat, and protein to total energy intake.[8,92,104]

A higher abundance of type I muscle fibers in women is likely a significant contributor to the observed sex differences in exercise metabolism.[153] A sex difference in metabolism during endurance exercise was first suggested when women began to out perform men during ultra-endurance events.[154] During these events women can sustain a higher %VO_2max for a longer period of time, as compared with equally trained men.[154] Since then, numerous studies have shown that women rely on a greater proportion of lipid to fuel endurance exercise,[5,8,62,65,92,99,104,141–145,155–157] thus sparing carbohydrate stores, which allows women to maintain a higher %VO_2max.[155] The sources of the increased reliance on lipid and decreased reliance on CHO by women during exercise remains controversial. It is generally accepted that women have a lower glucose Ra,[67,144,158] Rd,[67,144,158] and MCR[8,144] during moderate intensity endurance exercise as compared with men, implying a decreased rate of liver glycogenolysis/gluconeogenesis during exercise in women. However, the effect of sex on muscle glycogen use during exercise yields conflicting results. To date only two studies have found that women have a lower net use of muscle glycogen as compared with men,[142,144] while others have found no effect of sex on muscle glycogen use.[65,67,143] Differences in the exercise protocol used (running versus cycling) and the menstrual cycle phase the women were tested in may have contributed to the finding of decreased muscle glycogen use in the aforementioned studies.[142,144]

The source of the increased reliance on lipid by women during exercise remains an area of controversy. A lower RER, thus a greater reliance on lipid stores during exercise, in women is confirmed by studies finding that women have a greater glycerol Ra and Rd, a marker of whole body lipolysis, as compared with men.[8,80] However, whether the increased reliance on lipid stores by women during exercise is plasma- or muscle-derived is a matter of debate.

The effect of sex on IMCL use during exercise is also controversial. It has been consistently shown that women have a greater IMCL content as compared with men.[62,67,68,110,159] Additionally, using the EM technique the authors' laboratory has shown that before and after a period of endurance training women have a higher number of IMCL in a given area of muscle, but not a greater lipid size, as compared with men, and this greater number of IMCL contributed to the increased IMCL content in women.[160] Thus, women have an increased availability of IMCL to use as a substrate source during exercise; however, whether this indeed occurs is a matter of controversy. Because the use of IMCL during endurance exercise is controversial, sex differences in IMCL use during exercise are hard to determine. Several studies have found that women use more IMCL during a bout of moderate intensity endurance exercise as compared with men;[62,67,68] however, these later studies also found that men do not use any IMCL during the exercise bout.[67,68] The results of the aforementioned studies[62,67,68] may be influenced by the use of the biochemical method to determine IMCL content and net use. A study using ^{1}H-MRS found that men used more IMCL than women during exercise,[65] but these findings are confounded by the fact that the men were more trained than the women, which would result in increased IMCL use during exercise. Other studies using ^{1}H-MRS[64] and EM[161] and using equally trained men and women have found no sex difference in IMCL use during exercise or no difference in IMCL use between the sexes. Collectively, these findings suggest that when men and women are equally trained there is no difference in net IMCL use during a bout of endurance exercise at 65% VO_2max.

If the increased reliance on lipids by women during exercise is not a result of increased IMCL use, it is reasonable to assume that it is plasma derived. Yet, several studies have found no effect of sex on plasma FFA Ra uptake and oxidation during exercise performed at 25%,[3] 45%,[162] 65%,[3] and 85%[3] VO_2max. However, one study did find that during the last 30 minutes of a 90 minute cycling bout at 50% VO_2max, women oxidized more plasma FFA as compared with men.[80] Additionally, although not significant, another study found that during the last hour of a 90 minute exercise bout at 60% VO_2max, women oxidized 32% more plasma FFA as compared with men.[67] The results of these two studies are complicated by the fact that during that time point there was no difference in RER between the sexes. Thus, the impact of sex on plasma FFA oxidation during exercise remains controversial.

Perhaps sex differences in lipoprotein-derived TG use exist. To date no study has investigated the effect of sex on lipoprotein-derived TG use during a bout of endurance exercise. However, a recent study showed that at rest in both the fasted and the fed state, women had a greater uptake of serum TG across the leg, as compared with men.[163] Whether or not this would result in greater lipoprotein-derived TG use during a bout of endurance exercise in women is yet to be determined. Additionally, because lipoprotein-derived TG contribute only approximately 10% to total fat oxidation during exercise,[60] the physiologic importance of this finding needs to be determined.

Few studies have been conducted investigating the molecular mechanism behind the observed sex differences in metabolism during exercise. From a mechanistic standpoint, the increased reliance on lipids by women during endurance exercise appears to be an increased capacity for women to uptake plasma FFA into the muscle, as evidenced by the finding of increased mRNA expression of FAT/CD36 and FABPpm (untrained only), as well as an increased FAT/CD36 protein content (untrained and trained) in muscle from women as compared with men.[81] However, no sex difference in plasma FFA uptake during exercise has been observed.[3,67,161]

Women also rely to a lesser extent on amino acid oxidation during endurance exercise as compared with men.[92,99,104] Specifically, men have a higher rate of protein oxidation at rest and during exercise,[99,104] and a higher leucine flux,[104] while women have a higher rate of nonoxidative leucine metabolism.[99] Combining data from six studies investigating the relative contribution of protein to total substrate oxidation during exercise,[92,99,104,142,143,157] the authors' laboratory has found that protein contributes 2.1% of total energy during exercise in women, while in men it contributes 5.5% ($P = .02$).

The observed sex difference in metabolism is mediated by differences in estrogen concentration between the sexes. Supplementation trials of 17-β-estradiol (E2) in animals[147,164,165] and humans[90,166–169] have shown that short-term administration of E2 can modify fuel selection during endurance exercise. In humans, short term E2 supplementation decreased glucose Ra,[166–168] Rd,[166–168] MCR,[166] and RER,[90,167] with no effect of glycerol Ra and Rd.[166,168] E2 supplementation also lowered resting muscle glycogen stores[167] with no effect on muscle glycogen use.[167,169] However, there does not appear to be an effect of E2 supplementation on performance during exercise lasting 1 to 2 hours.[168] Collectively these data suggest that E2 has a primary action on liver glycogenolysis and glucose release, while muscle glycogenolysis is not affected by short term E2 supplementation. Additionally, these studies suggest that at the level of substrate use E2 has a greater impact on

CHO, as opposed to lipid, metabolism. To date only one E2 supplementation study has been conducted investigating the effects of E2 on amino acid metabolism during endurance exercise.[90] In this study, 8 days of high dose E2 supplementation (1 mg per day for 2 days; 2 mg per day for 6 days) to men lowered leucine oxidation at rest and during exercise.[90] Additionally, E2 supplementation resulted in a less negative protein balance.[90] However, there was no effect of E2 supplementation on leucine flux, protein synthesis, or protein breakdown.[90]

Fluctuations in ovarian hormones across the menstrual cycle can also influence substrate use during exercise;[144,170–172] however, this has not been corroborated in all studies.[173–177] Women in the luteal phase of the menstrual cycle have a lower RER,[170–172] CHO oxidation,[170,172] glucose Ra,[144,170] Rd,[144,170] and muscle glycogen use,[144,171,172] as well as higher lipid oxidation.[170] However, not all studies have demonstrated a lower glucose Ra and Rd during the luteal phase of the menstrual cycle,[175] a finding that may be explained by differences in the exercise intensity used or whether subjects were tested in the fed or fasted state. Additionally, it has been consistently shown that women in the luteal phase of the menstrual cycle use less muscle glycogen.[144,171,172] The effect of the menstrual cycle on lipid metabolism is unclear. Several studies have found a lower RER[170] as well as higher lipid oxidation[170] during exercise performed by women in the luteal phase of the menstrual cycle. However, to date no effect of menstrual cycle phase has been found on glycerol[173,174] or palmitate flux.[174] To the best of the authors' knowledge, no study to date has investigated the impact of menstrual cycle phase on IMCL content and use during exercise. Thus, the effect of menstrual cycle phase on lipid metabolism during exercise requires further research.

EFFECT OF DIET ON SUBSTRATE SELECTION DURING ENDURANCE EXERCISE
Carbohydrate Loading

Dietary intake can also impact fuel use during endurance exercise. In a series of classic experiments, Hultman, Bergstrom, and colleagues first demonstrated that muscle glycogen levels can be manipulated by diet and exercise.[178–180] They also observed that following a period of low carbohydrate intake, the resynthesis of muscle glycogen was greater in a leg that had undergone a bout of continuous exercise as compared with a leg that had not exercised,[180] resulting in supercompensated muscle glycogen levels. Subsequently, these investigators determined the effect of consuming a high CHO diet following a bout of glycogen depleting exercise on subsequent muscle glycogen content and exercise performance.[178] A 3-day high CHO diet again resulted in supercompensated muscle glycogen levels and increased time to exhaustion,[178] findings which resulted in a new dietary regime to improve athletic performance. The traditional CHO loading method involved a 6-day taper-diet regime, where on the first 3 days subjects consume moderate CHO (approximately 50% of total calories) and undergo moderate training, followed by three days of high CHO (approximately 70% of total calories) and minimal training.[181,182] This taper-diet regime can increase muscle glycogen levels by approximately 25% as compared with a normal diet.[181,182] More recently shorter regimes (1–4 days), with or without prior bouts of glycogen lowering exercise,[143,183–187] have been developed and found to increase muscle glycogen stores by 23% to 89%. Thus, there are a multitude of dietary strategies by which muscle glycogen stores can be elevated but they all involve a precompetition phase of high intakes of carbohydrates.

How long muscle glycogen levels remain elevated following supercompensation and what type of CHO is best to supercompensate glycogen stores are important factors for athletes preparing for competition. Following a traditional CHO loading regime (with the initial low CHO phase), CHO levels remain elevated for at least 3 days following the cessation of a high CHO diet and abstinence of physical activity.[188] From a practical standpoint, these findings are important because they imply that athletes can elevate their glycogen stores in the days prior (ie, before having to travel to the event) to a competition and maintain these levels as long as they are not training in the meantime. Whether supercompensated muscle glycogen stores remain elevated beyond 3 days following the cessation of high CHO, and whether other loading regimes also result in glycogen stores that remain elevated for at least 3 days following the cessation of the dietary intervention needs to be determined.

Both simple and complex CHO can be used to supercompensate muscle glycogen stores by 44% to 74%.[189] It is more difficult for women to supercompensate muscle glycogen stores when compared with men: men showed increases in muscle glycogen stores and performance time when consuming a loading protocol with a diet containing 75% CHO and 3 days of reduced intensity tapering of training, but women did not.[143] Other investigators have reported that women do not appear to carbohydrate load with the same magnitude to that seen in men.[190] Subsequent studies found that when the amount of CHO was increased to greater than 8 g/kg per day for both sexes, muscle glycogen content increased for both men and women,[186] yet the women still had a relatively lower magnitude of increase.[187] From a practical perspective, most women will have to increase their energy intake during the loading phase to achieve a CHO intake of greater 8 g/kg per day.

Increased muscle glycogen following a period of CHO loading increases the amount of glycogen available to be used during endurance events and can thus improve performance; however, the effect of CHO loading on performance is controversial, with some studies finding improved performance[143,178,190,191] while others find no change in performance.[181,182,185,192] One study finding no effect of CHO loading on performance in women[192] did not measure muscle glycogen stores and thus, as it is more difficult to increase glycogen stores in women, these subjects may not have had elevated muscle glycogen stores at the onset of exercise and this may explain the lack of effect on performance. The additional studies finding no effect of CHO loading on performance used dietary strategies, where subjects consumed between 61% and 70% CHO, whereas studies finding an effect of CHO loading on performance have used dietary strategies where at least 75% of energy comes from CHO.[143,190] These findings suggest that at least 75% of energy from CHO is needed in men (and likely women) to improve performance.

Carbohydrate Drinks During Exercise

In addition to CHO loading before an event, athletes can consume CHO during an event in order to increase CHO availability to the muscle to sustain high levels of CHO oxidation. CHO ingestion during endurance exercise appears to spare liver glycogen stores[193,194] while increasing the reliance on plasma CHO.[193–195] However, there does not appear to be an effect of CHO ingestion during exercise on muscle glycogen use.[193,194] Traditionally, glucose, sucrose, or glucose polymers have been consumed, resulting in CHO oxidation rates of 1 gram per minute;[196] however, recent research has found that a combination of glucose and fructose, glucose and sucrose, glucose, fructose and sucrose, and maltodextrin and fructose can increase CHO oxidation rates up to 1.75 grams per minute because they use different transporters.[197–202] To improve performance, 30 g to 60 g of CHO per hour are required, which translates to approximately 0.5 g/kg to 1 g/kg per hour.[196] Not only can CHO ingestion during exercise extend cycle endurance capacity in events greater than 1 hour, but recent research has shown that CHO ingestion during exercise also increases performance by increasing work output or decreasing the amount of time needed to complete a fixed amount of work,[203] as well as improving performance in events lasting less than 1 hour.[204]

High Fat Diets

Short-term high fat diets can alter substrate use during endurance exercise, increasing lipid oxidation at rest and during exercise.[149,205–212] Specifically, high fat diets lasting longer than 3 days increase IMCL content[213,214] and use,[214] carnitine acyltransferase activity[207] and HSL activity,[149] and decrease pyruvate dehydrogenase activity,[149] thus shifting metabolism to more favorably increase lipid use during exercise. Additionally, several studies,[149,207,211] but not all,[213] have found that high fat diets decrease muscle glycogenolysis during exercise. The theory behind increasing fat intake to improve performance is that a high fat intake decreases muscle glycogen stores[205] and increases IMCL content, shifting metabolism toward an increased reliance on fat oxidation. Thus, when muscle glycogen stores are acutely replenished before exercise they are spared, prolonging the ability to maintain a higher VO_2max.[208] Therefore, the strategy for high fat diets is to increase fat intake for several days before an event, followed by CHO repletion the day before the event to increase fat oxidation and spare glycogen, thus improving performance.

However, the effect of high fat diets on performance is equivocal, with athletes showing an improvement,[212] no change,[148,205,207,208,213,215] or a detriment[208] in performance. Additionally, in untrained individuals a period of training while consuming a high fat diet has no effect on[210] or can be detrimental[206,209] to endurance. Thus, although high fat diets increase lipid oxidation during exercise, they have little effect on athletic performance.

EXERCISE METABOLISM AND NUTRITION FOR INBORN ERRORS OF METABOLISM AFFECTING SKELETAL MUSCLE

The metabolic myopathies are inborn errors of metabolism that impair substrate metabolism in skeletal muscle and result in exercise intolerance (**Table 1**). Fatty acid oxidation defects (FAOD), glycogen storage disease (GSD), and mitochondrial cytopathies represent the three main groups of disorders. In general, the GSDs present with symptoms during higher intensity and anaerobic type of activities, whereas the FAODs and the mitochondrial cytopthies display symptoms during endurance type activity or under fasted or other metabolically stressful conditions, such as a super-imposed illness. The remainder of this article will consider how exercise training and dietary interventions can be manipulated for individuals with the aforementioned conditions as therapeutic strategies. For a summary of suggested treatments for metabolic myopathies (**Table 2**).

Glycogen Storage Disease

The glycogen storage diseases refer to a group of disorders characterized by inborn errors of metabolism in glycogen synthesis, glycogenolysis, or glycolysis. Although there are 13 main variants of GSDs with some subcategories, this article shall focus on GSD V (phosphorylase deficiency or McArdle's disease) and GSD VII (PFK deficiency or Tarui's disease), given that almost all of the exercise physiology work and dietary manipulation studies have been completed in these GSD subgroups.

Exercise intolerance results from the inability to breakdown glycogen (ie, phosphorylase deficiency) or flux through glycolysis (PFK deficiency) to provide energy via anaerobic or aerobic glycolysis. Although most patients are limited by the impairment

Table 1
Inborn errors of metabolism affecting skeletal muscle, major category examples

Major Category	Examples
Mitochondrial myopathy	MELAS, MERRF, CPEO, Kearn-Sayre Syndrome, complex I deficiency, cytochrome b mutations, cytochrome c oxidase mutations.
Fat oxidation defect	CPT I, CPT II, TFP, VLCAD, -deficiency; glutaric aciduria type II.
Glycogen storage disease	phosphorylase, PFK, acid maltase, phosphorylase b kinase, phosphoglycerate mutase, phosphoglycerate kinase -deficiency.

Abbreviations: CPEO, chronic progressive external ophthalmoplegia; CPT, carnitine palmitoyl transferase; MELAS, mitochondrial encephalomyopathy lactic acidosis and stroke-like episodes; MERRF, myoclonic epilepsy and ragged red fibers; TFP, trifunctional protein; VLCAD, very long acyl-COA dehydrogenase deficiency; other short-forms are given in the text.

in anaerobic glycolysis and manifest symptoms of muscle cramps and pain during the rest-to-exercise transition or with higher exercise intensities, most patients also have a low VO_2max.[216–219] The low VO_2max can be improved by the provision of carbohydrate in the case of McArdle's disease, but not PFK deficiency.[217,220] The improvement in exercise capacity and metabolic variables from the infusion of lactate in patients with PFK deficiency[221] further supports the concept that much of the exercise limitation in disorders of glycolysis and glycogenolysis are the result of a lower capacity to provide pyruvate to the tricarboxylic acid cycle via the PDH pathway. Both groups of patients have a hyperdynamic circulatory response to exercise with a rapid increase in heart rate and cardiac output.[216,219,222]

Because of the reduced flux through glycolysis, there is a marked attenuation of lactate production during ischemic and semi-ischemic work, and this forms the basis of the forearm exercise diagnostic test.[223] During exercise,[8] P magnetic resonance spectroscopy usually demonstrates a lack of acidosis,[224] with distal defects in glycolysis, such as PFK deficiency, also showing a characteristic increase in phosphomonoesters.[225] With the reduction in glycolytic flux, there is a compensatory increase in flux through the adenylate kinase greater than the myoadenylate deaminase

Table 2
Summary of suggested treatments for metabolic myopthies disease treatment

Disease	Treatment
Glycogen storage disease	Progressive exercise training Pre-exercise carbohydrates Creatine monohydrate Possible high protein diet, pyridoxine
Fat oxidation defect	High carbohydrate diet Avoid fasting and no exercise during illness Carbohydrate before and during exercise Possible medium chain triglyceride oil or riboflavin
Mitochondrial cytopathy	Progressive exercise training Avoid fasting and no exercise during illness High fat diet (complex I only, possibly short-term only) Antioxidants (vitamin C, E, alpha lipoic acid) Cofactors (coenzyme Q10) Alternative substrate (creatine monohydrate)

pathway, with the generation of excessive amounts of ammonia and ultimately uric acid,[219] termed "myogenic hyperuricemia."[226]

For patients with phosphorylase deficiency but not those with PFK deficiency, there is a process called the "second wind phenomenon," whereby the initial bout of exercise results in tachycardia and breathlessness and muscle cramps. But after a brief rest or a reduction in intensity, there is a reduced perception of effort and the ability to continue exercise at a lower intensity.[217,220] This phenomenon is caused by the delivery of blood-born substrates (primarily glucose) to the working muscle.[217,220] From a treatment perspective, most patients adjust their life-style by avoiding precipitating activities, such as brief bursts of high intensity activity. Interestingly, cautious but progressive aerobic conditioning improves functional capacity in patients with McArdle's disease,[27,28] occasionally to the lower levels of the healthy control range.[227] Furthermore, McArdle's disease patients who have a more active lifestyle have a reduced perception of daily muscle pain, and up to 17% can actually attain some level of competitive athletic endeavors.[227]

It is likely that the adaptations to endurance exercise training mentioned above for healthy individuals allows for more rapid substrate delivery and a greater proportion of lipid oxidation at any given exercise intensity. From a nutritional perspective, the consumption of sucrose or glucose 15 to 20 minutes before exercise can provide an exogenous source of glucose and improve exercise capacity in patients with McArdle's disease.[22,228] This latter effect is caused by the delivery of glucose to the muscle that can be taken up by GLUT-4 and provide flux through the glycolytic pathway, effectively bypassing the metabolic block.

In contrast, patients with PFK deficiency do worse with glucose ingestion, for it inhibits lipolysis and they cannot take advantage of the exogenous glucose because of the block in glycolysis. Pyridoxine (vitamin B_6) supplementation has been suggested for those with McArdle's disease because it is stored in conjunction with phosphorylase (which is absent) and vitamin B_6 is a cofactor in amino acid oxidation. However, the use of pyridoxine has not been evaluated by a rigorous clinical trial and high doses can cause peripheral neuropathy. High protein diets have also been suggested to up-regulate an alternative fuel pathway, given the intact pathway of amino acid oxidation; however, given that amino acid oxidation represents such a small fraction of total energy supply during exercise and can only be used under aerobic conditions, the clinical utility is questionable.

Along these lines, the acute ingestion of branched chain amino acids did not improve exercise capacity in patients with McArdle's disease.[229] Given the fact that both PFK and phosphorylase deficiency result in a massive reduction in anaerobic energy transduction, the only degrees of freedom for the cell are the adenylate kinase greater than the AMP deaminase pathway and the phosphocreatine hydrolysis pathway. Consequently, trials have looked at the potential for McArdle's disease patients to benefit from creatine monohydrate supplementation.[230,231] One randomized, double-blind trial found that low dose creatine monohydrate supplementation was of some clinical benefit (0.06 g/kg per day);[230] yet a higher dose (0.15 g/kg day) actually impaired exercise capacity.[231] A recent Cochrane review concluded that the only potential therapy for McArdle's disease was the low dose creatine intervention, with the pre-exercise sucrose being only useful for planned exercise and tending to cause weight gain if sustained regularly for a long period of time.[228]

Fatty Acid Oxidation Defects

The FAODs all result in some impairment of β-oxidation within the mitochondrial matrix. Given the importance of fat oxidation in long duration endurance activity and during periods of fasting (see the section above on fat metabolism and substrate selection during endurance exercise), patients with FAODs generally report symptoms during long-duration endurance activities or when repeated activity is completed in the fasted state or without adequate replacement of carbohydrates. The most commonly documented FAOD leading to rhabdomyolysis and exercise intolerance is CPT II deficiency; however, there are also a wide variety of other FAODs described, including carnitine transporter deficiency, defects of β-oxidation (ie, LCAD, MCAD, trifunctional protein or TFP deficiency), carnitine translocase deficiency, and glutaric aciduria type II (electron transport flavoprotein mutations). Many of these conditions can present in infancy or childhood with a primary liver or encephalopathic picture, while the adult onset forms are predominately myopathic and result in endurance exercise intolerance.

The main myopathic FAODs presenting in adulthood with exercise intolerance include CPT II, TFP, and very long chain acyl-CoA dehydrogenase deficiencies. Although most of the FAODs are autosomal-recessive in their inheritance, it has been reported that more men are diagnosed with CPT II deficiency. This may relate to the previously discussed sex differences in metabolism, where women have a greater ability to oxidize FFA as compared with men, and are somehow protected from the impairment in FFA transport across the mitochondrial membrane seen in CPT II deficiency. Further support for this sex difference in susceptibility to the metabolic effects of CPT II deficiency comes from murine studies showing that male peroxisome proliferator-activated receptor (PPARα$^{-/-}$) mice given a blocker of CPT (etomoxir) developed hypoglycemia and died, whereas the females did not.[232]

Many patients with myopathic FAODs are asymptomatic, without the superimposition of a metabolic stress. In contrast to those with glycogen storage disease, these individuals can often perform anaerobic activity for short periods of time without difficulty; however, with more prolonged exercise, patients develop symptoms of cramps, muscle discomfort, and inability to continue the activity. These clinical observations are consistent with metabolic tracer studies in patients with CPT II deficiency, where FFA oxidation is normal at rest and severely impaired during endurance exercise.[233] Standard exercise stress testing is often normal, although the VO$_2$max can be somewhat diminished;[233] still, this is neither sensitive nor specific. Occasionally, a high RER during low intensity exercise may indicate the increased reliance upon carbohydrates,[233] although, this finding cannot rule in or rule out an FAOD.

The avoidance of prolonged exercise or exercise during fasting or a superimposed infection is important in the management of those with FAODs. Patients can improve exercise capacity with intravenous glucose infusion, yet do not appear to get the same benefit from oral glucose ingestion.[23] Fortunately, the provision of a high carbohydrate diet (a forme fruste of carbohydrate loading) did lead to improved exercise capacity in those with CPT II deficiency.[24] Although riboflavin to enhance electron transport flavoprotein function, and medium chain triglyceride oil to bypass the carnitine carrier system have been advocated as potential therapies, their efficacy has not yet been demonstrated in a randomized, double blind trial or with metabolic tracers to evaluate the effect on metabolism during exercise. To date, no studies have systematically evaluated the potential benefit of aerobic training in patients with FAODs.

Mitochondrial Disorders

Mitochondrial disorders collectively represent a diverse group of conditions with a primary defect in electron transport chain function. The first mutations definitely linked to a mitochondrial disease were those for Leber's hereditary optic neuropathy (G11778A), chronic progressive external ophthalmoplegia (mitochondrial DNA deletions) and mitochondrial encepahlopmyopathy, lactic acidosis, and stroke-like episodes (MELAS, A3243G) in the late 1980s. Since then there have been many mitochondrial DNA point mutations described, and more recently a number of nuclear genes encoding for mitochondrial proteins have been discovered. Several reviews regarding mitochondrial medicine[234,235] and the role of exercise and nutrition[18,236] have been written recently, and the reader is referred to these for more details.

Many of the cellular consequences of mitochondrial dysfunction can be linked to a decrease in aerobic energy production. Because the mitochondria are the final common pathway for the oxidative metabolism of fats, proteins, and carbohydrates, it is understandable that mitochondrial dysfunction can be precipitated by superimposed metabolic stress, including exercise, infection, or prolonged fasting. Although there is extreme phenotypic and genotypic heterogeneity in the phenotype of the mitochondrial cytopathies, many adult patients will have exercise intolerance as a major feature. The impairment in aerobic energy transduction is reflected by low or very low VO_2max values.[19,21,29,237] In contrast with the fatty acid oxidation defects and glycogen storage diseases, it is not common for patients with mitochondrial cytopathies to have rhabdomyolysis or myoglobinuria; however, this can be seen in cytochrome b, cytochrome c oxidase, and MELAS A3260G mutations.

Exercise testing in mitochondrial cytopathies usually demonstrates a markedly reduced maximal aerobic capacity (VO_2max) or a high RER (early lactate production) with cycle ergometry testing (for review, see.)[18,235] Near infrared spectroscopy or direct venous blood gas measurements often show a lack of deoxygenation consequent to the low oxygen consumption by defective mitochondria.[238,239] Mitochondrial disorders are a true example of a situation in which the VO_2max is limited by peripheral extraction and not delivery. Patients with mitochondrial cytopathy show an increase in delivery of oxygen to the periphery,[31,239] similar to that seen in the glycogen storage diseases. Phosphorus magnetic resonance spectroscopy often reveals an increased reliance on phosphocreatine hydrolysis or a delay in the after-exercise phosphocreatine recovery.[29,31,224,240,241]

Therapeutic strategies for the mitochondrial cytopathies have focused on increasing aerobic energy transduction through the electron transport chain (cofactors and exercise training), reducing free radical production (antioxidants), bypassing metabolic defects (cofactors, high fat diet), and the provision of alternative energy stores (creatine). Dichloroacetate has been tried to reduce lactate levels by enhancing flux through the PDH pathway, and although lactate is lowered, there were no improvements in function seen in the largest trial to date.[242] Peripheral neuropathy has emerged as a significant side effect with long-term use.[243] The most common cofactor that has been studied is coenzyme Q10, and the balance of the evidence has shown that this compound is safe and has some benefits in surrogate clinical markers of efficacy (for a review of the studies see.[234–236,244,245]) Coenzyme Q10 has also been used as a therapy for the secondary mitochondrial dysfunction seen in Parkinson's disease, with some evidence of clinical efficacy and documented improvements in mitochondrial enzyme activity,[246–248] albeit at doses that were somewhat higher that those traditionally used in mitochondrial cytopathies.

Creatine monohydrate supplementation has been shown to be of some benefit in surrogate markers of strength and endurance and on some clinical features in some,[21,249–251] but not all,[252,253] studies. A recent Cochrane review on the use of creatine monohydrate supplementation did not find that there was a statistically significant improvement in surrogate markers of efficacy when all studies were combined.[254] However, the authors' finding of higher power output in repetitive high intensity contractions[21] is consistent with the literature in healthy men and women,[255,256] but of unclear clinical relevance at this point. The authors' group has found that a combination supplement of creatine monohydrate plus coenzyme Q10 plus α-lipoic acid lowered markers of oxidative stress and lactate in a cohort of subjects with mitochondrial cytopathy in a randomized, double-blind, cross-over study.[257] Given the clinical heterogeneity in the mitochondrial cytopathies and the relatively small numbers of identified patients at most institutions, there are some multicentered trials planned with coenzyme Q10 alone and in combination with creatine monohydrate.

Finally, a diet that is high in fat can theoretically increase the relative contribution of reducing equivalents to complex II of the electron transport chain, and a study has found improved exercise capacity in a cohort of subjects with complex I deficiency given a triglyceride infusion.[25] From a practical perspective, similar benefits were not seen in subjects with complex I deficiency on a high fat diet.[26] Studies have demonstrated improvement in exercise capacity and mitochondrial enzyme activity in subjects with mitochondrial cytopathy following an endurance exercise training program.[18,29–31,258] There was initial concern that endurance exercise may increase the mutational burden and ultimately lead to a worsening of the condition in the long run;[31] however, two subsequent studies did not find evidence for an increased mutational burden following endurance training.[30,259] Sporadic mitochondrial cytopathies do not result in the accumulation of mutations in the relatively quiescent satellite cells.[260,261] Consequently, their activation by direct toxin damage[260,261] and eccentric exercise[32] improves mitochondrial enzyme activity and lowers mutational burden through a process called mtDNA shifting.[32] Larger studies using weight lifting to induce mtDNA shifting will be difficult to complete because of the paucity of cases. However, there may be generic benefits of weight training for patients with mitochondrial disease related to muscle function, similar to those seen in older adults[33,34] who are known to also have mitochondrial dysfunction, that can be improved with weight training.[262–264]

REFERENCES

1. Friedlander A, Casazza G, Horning M, et al. Effects of exercise intensity and training on lipid metabolism in young women. Am J Physiol Endocrinol Metab 1998;275:E853.
2. Romijn JA, Coyle EF, Sidossis LS, et al. Regulation of endogenous fat and carbohydrate metabolism in relation to exercise intensity and duration. Am J Physiol 1993;256:E380.
3. Romijn JA, Coyle EF, Sidossis LS, et al. Substrate metabolism during different exercise intensities in endurance-trained women. J Appl Physiol 2000;88:1701.
4. Van Loon L, Greenhaff P, Constantin-Teodosiu D, et al. The effects of increasing exercise intensity on muscle fuel utilisation in humans. J Physiol 2001;536:295.
5. Venables MC, Achten J, Jeukendrup AE. Determinants of fat oxidation during exercise in healthy men and women: a cross-sectional study. J Appl Physiol 2005;98:160.
6. Bergman B, Brooks GA. Respiratory gas-exchange ratios during graded exercise in fed and fasted trained and untrained men. J Appl Physiol 1999;86:479.
7. Bergman B, Butterfield G, Wolfel E, et al. Muscle net glucose uptake and glucose kinetics after endurance training in men. Am J Physiol Endocrinol Metab 1999;277:E81.

8. Carter S, Rennie C, Tarnopolsky MA. Substrate utilization during endurance exercise in men and women after endurance training. Am J Physiol Endocrinol Metab 2001;280:E898–907.

9. Henriksson J. Training induced adaptation of skeletal muscle and metabolism during submaximal exercise. J Physiol 1977;270:661.

10. Holloszy J, Coyle EF. Adaptations of skeletal muscle to endurance exercise and their metabolic consequences. J Appl Physiol 1984;56:831.

11. Horowitz J, Leone T, Feng W, et al. Effect of endurance training on lipid metabolism in women: a potential role for PPARα in the metabolic response to training. Am J Physiol Endocrinol Metab 2000;279:E348.

12. Jansson E, Kaijser L. Substrate utilization and enzymes in skeletal muscle of extremely endurance-trained men. J Appl Physiol 1987;62:999.

13. Jeukendrup A, Mensink M, Saris W, et al. Exogenous glucose oxidation during exercise in endurance-trained and untrained subjects. J Appl Physiol 1997;82: 835–40.

14. Van Loon J, Jeukendrup A, Saris W, et al. Effect of training status on fuel selection during submaximal exercise with glucose ingestion. J Appl Physiol 1999;87: 1413.

15. Coyle EF, Jeukendrup AE, Oseto M, et al. Low-fat diet alters intramuscular substrate and reduces lipolysis and fat oxidation during exercise. Am J Physiol Endocrinol Metab 2001;280:E391.

16. Dyck D, Peters S, Wendling P, et al. Regulation of muscle glycogen phosphorylase activity during intense aerobic cycling with elevated FFA. Am J Physiol Endocrinol Metab 1996;270:E116–25.

17. Dyck D, Putman C, Heigenhauser G, et al. Regulation of fat-carbohydrate interaction in skeletal muscle during intense aerobic cycling. Am J Physiol Endocrinol Metab 1993;265:E852.

18. Taivassalo T, Haller RG. Exercise and training in mitochondrial myopathies. Med Sci Sports Exerc 2005;37:2094.

19. Taivassalo T, Jensen TD, Kennaway N, et al. The spectrum of exercise tolerance in mitochondrial myopathies: a study of 40 patients. Brain 2003;126:413.

20. Tarnopolsky MA. What can metabolic myopathies teach us about exercise physiology? Appl Physiol Nutr Metab 2006;31:21.

21. Tarnopolsky MA, Roy BD, MacDonald JR. A randomized, controlled trial of creatine monohydrate in patients with mitochondrial cytopathies. Muscle Nerve 1997;20:1502.

22. Vissing J, Haller RG. The effect of oral sucrose on exercise tolerance in patients with McArdle's disease. N Engl J Med 2003;349:2503.

23. Orngreen MC, Olsen DB, Vissing J. Exercise tolerance in carnitine palmitoyltransferase II deficiency with IV and oral glucose. Neurology 2002;59: 1046.

24. Orngreen MC, Ejstrup R, Vissing J. Effect of diet on exercise tolerance in carnitine palmitoyltransferase II deficiency. Neurology 2003;61:559.

25. Roef MJ, de Meer K, Reijngoud DJ, et al. Triacylglycerol infusion improves exercise endurance in patients with mitochondrial myopathy due to complex I deficiency. Am J Clin Nutr 2002;75:237.

26. de Meer K, Roef MJ, de Klerk JB, et al. Increasing fat in the diet does not improve muscle performance in patients with mitochondrial myopathy due to complex I deficiency. J Inherit Metab Dis 2005;28:95.

27. Haller RG, Wyrick P, Taivassalo T, et al. Aerobic conditioning: an effective therapy in McArdle's disease. Ann Neurol 2006;59:922.

28. Mate-Munoz JL, Moran M, Perez M, et al. Favorable responses to acute and chronic exercise in McArdle patients. Clin J Sport Med 2007;17:297.
29. Taivassalo T, De Stefano N, Argov Z, et al. Effects of aerobic training in patients with mitochondrial myopathies. Neurology 1998;50:1055.
30. Taivassalo T, Gardner JL, Taylor RW, et al. Endurance training and detraining in mitochondrial myopathies due to single large-scale mtDNA deletions. Brain 2006;129:3391.
31. Taivassalo T, Shoubridge EA, Chen J, et al. Aerobic conditioning in patients with mitochondrial myopathies: physiological, biochemical, and genetic effects. Ann Neurol 2001;50:133.
32. Taivassalo T, Fu K, Johns T, et al. Gene shifting: a novel therapy for mitochondrial myopathy. Hum Mol Genet 1999;8:1047.
33. Brose A, Parise G, Tarnopolsky MA. Creatine supplementation enhances isometric strength and body composition improvements following strength exercise training in older adults. J Gerontol A Biol Sci Med Sci 2003;58:11.
34. Fiatarone MA, Marks EC, Ryan ND, et al. High-intensity strength training in nonagenarians. Effects on skeletal muscle. JAMA 1990;263:3029.
35. Tseng BS, Marsh DR, Hamilton MT, et al. Strength and aerobic training attenuate muscle wasting and improve resistance to the development of disability with aging. J Gerontol A Biol Sci Med Sci 50 Spec No:113-119, 1995.
36. Spriet L, Watt M. Regulatory mechanisms in the interaction between carbohydrate and lipid oxidation during exercise. Acta Physiol Scand 2003;178:443.
37. Hermanse L, Hultman E, Saltin B. Muscle glycogen during prolonged severe exercise. Acta Physiol Scand 1967;71:129.
38. Stanley W, Connett R. Regulation of muscle carbohydrate metabolism during exercise. FASEB J 1991;5:2155.
39. Richter E, Derave W, Wojtaszewski J. Glucose, exercise and insulin: emerging concepts. J Physiol 2001;535:313.
40. Rose A, Richter E. Skeletal muscle glucose uptake during exercise: how is it regulated. Physiology 2005;20:260.
41. Ferrer J, Favre C, Gomis R, et al. Control of glycogen deposition. FEBS Lett 2003;546:172.
42. Roach P. Glycogen and its metabolism. Curr Mol Med 2002;2:101.
43. Lomako J, Lomako WM, Whelan WJ. The nature of the primer for glycogen synthesis in muscle. FEBS Lett 1990;268:8.
44. Lomako J, Lomako WM, Whelan WJ. Proglycogen: a low molecular-weight form of muscle glycogen. FEBS Lett 1993;279:223.
45. Lomako J, Lomako WM, Whelan WJ, et al. Glycogen synthesis in the astrocyte: from glycogenin to proglycogen to glycogen. FASEB J 1993;7:1386.
46. Jessen N, Goodyear L. Contraction signaling to glucose transport in skeletal muscle. J Appl Physiol 2005;99:330.
47. Ihlemann J, Galbo H, Ploug T. Calphostin C is an inhibitor of contraction, but not insulin-stimulated glucose transport, in skeletal muscle. Acta Physiol Scand 1999;167:69.
48. Lee A, Hansen P, Holloszy J. Wortmannin inhibits insulin-stimulated but not contraction-stimulated glucose transport activity in skeletal muscle. FEBS Lett 1995;361:51.
49. Lund S, Holman GD, Schmitz O, et al. Contraction stimulates translocation of glucose transporter GLUT4 in skeletal muscle through a mechanism distinct from that of insulin. Proc Natl Acad Sci USA 1995;92:5817.

50. Bergeron R, Russell RR, Young L, et al. Effect of AMPK activation on muscle glucose metabolism in conscious rats. Am J Physiol Endocrinol Metab 1999; 276:E938.

51. Hayashi T, Hirshman M, Kurth E, et al. Evidence for 5' AMP-activated protein kinase mediation of the effect of muscle contraction on glucose transport. Diabetes 1998;47:1369.

52. Henricksen E, Rodnibk K, Holloszy J. Activation of glucose transport in skeletal muscle by phospholipase C and phorbol ester. Evaluation of the regulatory roles of protein kinase C and calcium. J Biol Chem 1989;264:21535–43.

53. Coggan A, Raguso C, Williams B, et al. Glucose kinetics during high-intensity exercise in endurance-trained and untrained humans. J Appl Physiol 1995;78: 1203.

54. Zinker B, Lacy D, Bracy D, et al. Regulation of glucose uptake and metabolism by working muscle. An in vivo analysis. Diabetes 1993;42:956–65.

55. Wegener G, Krause U. Different modes of activating phosphofructokinase, a key regulatory enzyme of glycolysis, in working vertebrate muscle. Biochem Soc Trans 2002;30:264.

56. Sugden M, Holness M. Recent advances in mechanisms regulating glucose oxidation at the level of the pyruvate dehydrogenase complex by PDKs. Am J Physiol Endocrinol Metab 2003;284:E855.

57. Spriet L, Howlett R, Heigenhauser G. An enzymatic approach to lactate production in human skeletal muscle during exercise. Med Sci Sports Exerc 2000;32: 756.

58. De Stefano N, Matthews P, Ford B, et al. Short-term dichloroacetate treatment improves indices of cerebral metabolism in patients with mitochondrial disorders. Neurology 1995;45:1193.

59. Steensberg A, Vissing J, Pedersen B. Lack of IL-6 production during exercise in patients with mitochondrial myopathy. Eur J Appl Physiol 2001;84:155.

60. Helge JW, Watt PW, Richter EA, et al. Fat utilization during exercise: adaptation to a fat-rich diet increases utilization of plasma fatty acids and very low density lipoprotein-triacyclglycerol in humans. J Physiol 2001;537:1009.

61. Krssak M, Petersen K, Bergeron R, et al. Intramuscular glycogen and intramyocellular lipid utilization during prolonged exercise and recovery in man: a 13C and 1H nuclear magnetic resonance spectroscopy study. J Clin Endocrinol Metab 2000;85:748.

62. Roepstorff C, Donsmark M, Thiele M, et al. Sex differences in hormone-sensitive lipase expression, activity, and phosphorylation in skeletal muscle at rest and during exercise. Am J Physiol Endocrinol Metab 2006;291:1106.

63. Schrauwen-Hinderling V, van Loon L, Koopman R, et al. Intramyocellular lipid content is increased after exercise in nonexercising human skeletal muscle. J Appl Physiol 2003;95:2328.

64. White L, Ferguson M, McCoy S, et al. Intramyocellular lipid changes in men and women during aerobic exercise: a 1H-magnetic resonance spectroscopy study. J Clin Endocrinol Metab 2003;88:5638.

65. Zehnder M, Ith M, Kreis R, et al. Gender-specific usage of intramyocellular lipids and glycogen during exercise. Med Sci Sports Exerc 2005;37:1517.

66. Bergman B, Butterfield G, Wolfel E, et al. Evaluation of exercise and training on muscle lipid metabolism. Am J Physiol Endocrinol Metab 1999;276:E106–17.

67. Roepstorff C, Steffensen CH, Madsen M, et al. Gender differences in substrate utilization during submaximal exercise in endurance-trained subjects. Am J Physiol 2002;282:E435.

68. Steffensen CH, Roepstorff C, Madsen M, et al. Myocellular triacylglycerol breakdown in females but not in males during exercise. Am J Physiol Endocrinol Metab 2002;282:E634.
69. Guo Z. Triglyceride content in skeletal muscle: variability and the source. Anal Biochem 2000;298:1.
70. Guo Z, Burguera B, Jensen MD. Kinetics of intramuscular triglyceride fatty acids in exercising humans. J Appl Physiol 2000;89:2057.
71. Kiens B, Essen-Gustavsson B, Christensen N, et al. Skeletal muscle substrate utilization during submaximal exercise in man: effect of endurance training. J Physiol 1993;469:459.
72. Wendling P, Peters S, Heigenhauser G, et al. Variability of triacylglycerol content in human skeletal muscle biopsy samples. J Appl Physiol 1996;81:1150.
73. Martin W, Dalsky G, Hurley B, et al. Effect of endurance training on plasma free fatty acid turnover and oxidation during exercise. Am J Physiol 1993;265:E708.
74. Staron RS, Hikida R, Murray T, et al. Lipid depletion and repletion in skeletal muscle following a marathon. J Neurol Sci 1989;94:29.
75. Decombaz J, Schmitt B, Ith M, et al. Postexercise fat intake repletes intramyocellular lipids but no faster in trained than in sedentary subjects. Am J Physiol Regul Integr Comp Physiol 2001;281:R760.
76. Howald H, Boesch C, Kreis R, et al. Content of intramyocellular lipids derived by electron microscopy, biochemical assays, and 1H-MR spectroscopy. J Appl Physiol 2002;92:2264.
77. Ranallo R, Rhodes E. Lipid metabolism during exercise. Sports Med 1998;26:29.
78. Luiken J, Schaap F, van Nieuwenhoven F, et al. Cellular fatty acid transport in heart and skeletal muscle as facilitated by proteins. Lipids 1999;34:S169.
79. Glatz J, Schaap F, Binas BB, et al. Cytoplasmic fatty acid-binding protein facilitates fatty acid utilization by skeletal muscle. Acta Physiol Scand 2003;178:367.
80. Mittendorfer B, Horowitz JF, Klein S. Effect of gender on lipid kinetics during endurance exercise of moderate intensity in untrained subjects. Am J Physiol Endocrinol Metab 2002;283:E58.
81. Kiens B, Roepstorff C, Glatz J, et al. Lipid-binding proteins and lipoprotein lipase activity in human skeletal muscle: influence of physical activity and gender. J Appl Physiol 2004;97:1209.
82. Kjaer M, Howlett K, Langfort J, et al. Adrenaline and glycogenolysis in skeletal muscle during exercise: a study in adrenalectomised humans. J Physiol 2000; 528:371.
83. Watt M, Steinberg G, Chan S, et al. Beta-adrenergic stimulation of skeletal muscle HSL can be overridden by AMPK signaling. FASEB J 2004;18:1445.
84. Howlett R, Parolin M, Dyck D, et al. Regulation of skeletal muscle glycogen phophorylase and PDH at varying exercise power outputs. Am J Physiol Regul Intergr Comp Physiol 1998;275:R418.
85. Zammit V. Carnitine acyltransferases: functional significance of subcellular distribution and membrane topology. Prog Lipid Res 1999;38:199.
86. McGarry JM, SE, Long C, et al. Observations on the affinity for carnitine, and malonyl-CoA sensitivity, of carnitine palmitoyltransferase I in animal and human tissues. Demonstration of the presence of malonyl-CoA in non-hepatic tissues of the rat. Biochem J 1983;214:21.
87. Bruce C, Thrush A, Mertz V, et al. Endurance training in obese humans improves glucose tolerance and mitochondrial fatty acid oxidation and alters muscle lipid content. Am J Physiol Endocrinol Metab 2006;291:99.
88. Eaton S. Control of mitochondrial B-oxidation flux. Prog Lipid Res 2002;41:197.

89. El-Khoury A, Forslund A, Olsson R, et al. Moderate exercise at energy balance does not affect 24-h leucine oxidation or nitrogen retention in healthy men. Am J Physiol Endocrinol Metab 1997;273:E394.

90. Hamadeh MJ, Devries MC, Tarnopolsky MA. Estrogen supplementation reduces whole body leucine and carbohydrate oxidation and increases lipid oxidation in men during endurance exercise. J Clin Endocrinol Metab 2005;90:3592–9.

91. Lamont L, McCullough A, Kalhan S. B-adrenergic blockade heightens the exercise-induced increase in leucine oxidation. Am J Physiol Endocrinol Metab 1995;268:E910.

92. Phillips S, Atkinson SA, Tarnopolsky MA, et al. Gender differences in leucine kinetics and nitrogen balance in endurance athletes. J Appl Physiol 1993;75:2134.

93. Boyer B, Odessey R. Kinetic characterization of branched chain ketoacid dehydrogenase. Arch Biochem Biophys 1991;285:1.

94. Howarth K, Burgomaster K, Phillips S, et al. Exercise training increases branched-chain oxoacid dehydrogenase kinase content in human skeletal muscle. Am J Physiol Regul Integr Comp Physiol published online June 20th, 2007;293:R1335–41.

95. Shimomura Y, Fujii H, Suzuki M, et al. Branched-chain 2-oxo acid dehydrogenase complex activation by tetanic contractions in rat skeletal muscle. Biochim Biophys Acta 1993;1157:290.

96. Kasperek G. Regulation of branched-chain 2-oxo acid dehydrogenase activity during exercise. Am J Physiol Endocrinol Metab 1989;256:E186.

97. Murakami T, Matsuo M, Shimizu A, et al. Dissociation of branched-chain alpha-keto acid dehydrogenase kinase (BDK) from branched-chain alpha-keto acid dehydrogenase complex (BCKDC) by BDK inhibitors. J Nutr Sci Vitaminol (Toyko) 2005;51:48.

98. Chang T, Goldberg A. The metabolic fates of amino acids and the formation of glutamine in skeletal muscle. J Biol Chem 1978;253:3685.

99. Lamont L, McCullough A, Kalhan S. Gender differences in leucine, but not lysine, kinetics. J Appl Physiol 2001;91:357.

100. Achten J, Jeukendrup A. Optimizing fat oxidation through exercise and diet. Nutrition 2004;20:716.

101. Jeukendrup A. Modulation of carbohydrate and fat utilization by diet, exercise and environment. Biochem Soc Trans 2003;31:1270.

102. Hurley B, Nemeth P, Martin W III, et al. Muscle triglyceride utilization during exercise: effect of training. J Appl Physiol 1986;60:562.

103. Klein S, Coyle E, Wolfe R. Fat metabolism during low-intensity exercise in endurance-trained and untrained men. Am J Physiol 1994;267:E934.

104. McKenzie S, Phillips S, Carter SL, et al. Endurance exercise training attenuates leucine oxidation and BCOAD activation during exercise in humans. Am J Physiol Endocrinol Metab 2000;278:E580.

105. Phillips SM, Green HJ, Tarnopolsky MA, et al. Effects of training duration on substrate turnover and oxidation during exercise. J Appl Physiol 1996;81:2182.

106. Turcotte L, Swenberger J, Tucker M, et al. Training-induced elevation in FABP(PM) is associated with increased palmitate use in contracting muscle. J Appl Physiol 1999;87:285.

107. Turcotte L, Richter E, Kiens B. Increased plasma FFA uptake and oxidation during prolonged exercise in trained vs. untrained humans. Am J Physiol 1992;262:E791.

108. Phillips SM, Green HJ, Tarnopolsky MA, et al. Progressive effect of endurance training on metabolic adaptations in working skeletal muscle. Am J Physiol Endocrinol Metab 1996;270:E265.
109. Stallknecht B, Simonsen L, Bulow J, et al. Effect of training on epinephrinestimulated lipolysis determined by microdialysis in human adipose tissue. Am J Physiol 1995;269:E1059.
110. Gibala MJ, Little JP, van Essen M, et al. Short-term sprint interval versus traditional endurance training: Similar initial adaptations in human skeletal muscle and exercise performance. J Physiol 2006;575:901.
111. Goodpaster BH, He J, Watkins S, et al. Skeletal muscle lipid content and insulin resistance: evidence for a paradox in endurance-trained athletes. J Clin Endocrinol Metab 2001;86:5755.
112. Howald H, Hoppeler H, Classen H, et al. Influences of endurance training on the ultrastructural composition of the different muscle fibre types in humans. Pflugers Arch 1985;403:369.
113. Pruchnic R, Katsiaras A, He J, et al. Exercise training increases intramyocellular lipid and oxidative capacity in older adults. Am J Physiol Endocrinol Metab 2004;287:E857.
114. Schrauwen-Hinderling V, Schrauwen P, Hesselink M, et al. The increase in intramyocellular lipid content is a very early response to training. J Clin Endocrinol Metab 2003;88:1610.
115. Thamer C, Machann J, Bachmann O, et al. Intramyocellular lipids: anthropometric determinants and relationships with maximal aerobic capacity and insulin sensitivity. J Clin Endocrinol Metab 2003;88:1785.
116. van Loon J, Koopman R, Manders R, et al. Intramyocellular lipid content in type 2 diabetes patients compared with overweight sedentary men and highly trained endurance athletes. Am J Physiol Endocrinol Metab 2004;287:E558.
117. Carter S, Rennie C, Hamilton S, et al. Changes in skeletal muscle in males and females following endurance training. Can J Physiol Pharmacol 2001;79:386.
118. Kristiansen S, Gade J, Wojtaszewski J, et al. Glucose uptake is increased in trained vs. untrained muscle during heavy exercise. J Appl Physiol 2000;89:1151.
119. Terada S, Tabata I, Higuchi M. Effect of high-intensity intermittent swimming training on fatty acid oxidation enzyme activity in rat skeletal muscle. Jpn J Physiol 2004;54:47.
120. Tremblay A, Simoneau J, Bouchard C. Impact of exercise intensity on body fatness and skeletal muscle metabolism. Metabolism 1994;43:814.
121. Tikkanen H, Naveri H, Harkonen M. Alteration of regulatory enzyme activities in fast-twitch and slow-twitch muscles and muscle fibers in low-intensity endurance trained rats. Eur J Appl Physiol Occup Physiol 1995;70:281.
122. Bonen A, Dyck D, Ibrahimi A, et al. Muscle contractile activity increases fatty acid metabolism and transport and FAT/CD36. Am J Physiol Endocrinol Metab 1999;276:E642.
123. Host H, Hansen P, Nolte L, et al. Rapid reversal of adaptive increases in muscle GLUT-4 and glucose transport capacity after training cessation. J Appl Physiol 1998;84:798.
124. Dela F, Handberg A, Mikines K, et al. GLUT 4 and insulin receptor binding and kinase activity in trained human muscle. J Physiol 1993;469:615.
125. Greiwe J, Hickner R, Hansen P, et al. Effects of endurance exercise training on muscle glycogen accumulation in humans. J Appl Physiol 1999;87:222.

126. Putman CJ, NL, Hultman E, et al. Effects of short-term submaximal training in humans on muscle metabolism in exercise. Am J Physiol 1998;275:E132.
127. Richter E, Jensen P, Kiens B, et al. Sarcolemmal glucose transport and GLUT-4 translocation during exercise are diminished by endurance training. Am J Physiol Endocrinol Metab 1998;274:E89.
128. Hickner R, Fisher J, Hansen P, et al. Muscle glycogen accumulation after endurance exercise in trained and untrained individuals. J Appl Physiol 1997;83:897.
129. Nakatani A, Han DH, Hansen P, et al. Effect of endurance exercise training on muscle glycogen supercompensation in rats. J Appl Physiol 1997;82:711.
130. Friedman J, Sherman W, Reed M, et al. Exercise training increases glucose transporter protein GLUT-4 in skeletal muscle of obese Zucker (fa/fa) rats. FEBS Lett 1990;268:13.
131. Goodyear L, Hirshman M, Valyou P, et al. Glucose transporter number, function, and subcellular distribution in rat skeletal muscle after exercise training. Diabetes 1992;41:1091.
132. Gulve E, Spina R. Effect of 7–10 days of cycle ergometer exercise on skeletal muscle GLUT-4 protein content. J Appl Physiol 1995;79:1562.
133. Phillips A, Han X-X, Green H, et al. Increments in skeletal muscle GLUT-1 and GLUT-4 after endurance training in humans. Am J Physiol 1996;270:E456.
134. Hickner RC, Racette SB, Binder EF, et al. Effects of 10 days of endurance exercise training on the suppression of whole body and regional lipolysis by insulin. J Clin Endocrinol Metab 2000;85:1498.
135. Coggan A, Kohrt W, Spina R, et al. Endurance training decreases plasma glucose turnover and oxidation during moderate-intensity exercise in men. J Appl Physiol 1990;68:990.
136. Friedlander A, Casazza G, Horning M, et al. Endurance training increases fatty acid turnover, but not fat oxidation, in young men. J Appl Physiol 1999;86:2097.
137. Mendenhall L, Swanson S, Habash D, et al. Ten days of exercise training reduces glucose production and utilization during moderate-intensity exercise. Am J Physiol Endocrinol Metab 1994;266:E136.
138. Coggan A, Swanson S, Mendenhall L, et al. Effect of endurance training on hepatic glycogenolysis and gluconeogenesis during prolonged exercise in men. Am J Physiol 1995;268:E375.
139. Leblanc P, Howarth K, Gibala M, et al. Effects of 7 wk of endurance training on human skeletal muscle metabolism during submaximal exercise. J Appl Physiol 2004;97:2148.
140. Friedlander AL, Casazza GA, Horning MA, et al. Training-induced alterations of carbohydrate metabolism in women: women respond differently from men. J Appl Physiol 1998;85:1175.
141. Horton TJ, Pagliassotti MJ, Hobbs K, et al. Fuel metabolism in men and women during and after long-duration exercise. J Appl Physiol 1998;85:1823.
142. Tarnopolsky LJ, MacDougall JD, Atkinson SA, et al. Gender differences in substrate for endurance exercise. J Appl Physiol 1990;68:302.
143. Tarnopolsky MA, Atkinson SA, Phillips SM, et al. Carbohydrate loading and metabolism during exercise in men and women. J Appl Physiol 1995;78:1360.
144. Devries M, Hamadeh MJ, Phillips SA, et al. Menstrual cycle phase and sex influence muscle glycogen utilization and glucose turnover during moderate intensity endurance exercise. Am J Physiol Regul Integr Comp Physiol 2006;291:R1120.
145. Blatchford F, Knowlton R, Schneider D. Plasma FFA responses to prolonged walking in untrained men and women. Eur J Appl Physiol Occup Physiol 1985;53:343.

146. Bunt J. Metabolic actions of estradiol: significance for acute and chronic exercise responses. Med Sci Sports Exerc 1990;22:286.

147. Kendrick ZV, Steffen CA, Rumsey WL, et al. Effect of estradiol on tissue glycogen metabolism in exercise oophorectomized rats. J Appl Physiol 1987;63:492.

148. Burke L, Hawley J, Angus D, et al. Adaptations to short-term high-fat diet persist during exercise despite high carbohydrate availability. Med Sci Sports Exerc 2002;34:83.

149. Stellingwerff T, Spriet L, Watt M, et al. Decreased PDH activation and glycogenolysis during exercise following fat adaptation with carbohydrate metabolism. Am J Physiol Endocrinol Metab 2006;290:E380.

150. Stepto N, Carey A, Staudacher H, et al. Effect of short-term fat adaptation on high-intensity training. Med Sci Sports Exerc 2002;34:449.

151. Andrews J, Sedlock D, Flynn M, et al. Carbohydrate loading and supplementation in endurance-trained women runners. J Appl Physiol 2003;95:584.

152. Rauch L, Rodger I, Wilson G, et al. The effects of carbohydrate loading on muscle glycogen content and cycling performance. Int J Sport Nutr 1995;5:25.

153. Roepstorff C, Thiele M, Hillig T, et al. Higher skeletal muscle alpha-2-AMPK activation and lower energy charge and fat oxidation in men than in women during submaximal exercise. J Physiol 2006;574:125.

154. Speechly D, Taylor S, Rogers G. Differences in ultra-endurance exercise in performance-matched male and female runners. Med Sci Sports Exerc 1996;28:359.

155. Froberg K, Pedersen P. Sex differences in endurance capacity and metabolic response to prolonged, heavy exercise. Eur J Appl Physiol Occup Physiol 1984;52:446.

156. Melanson E, Sharp T, Seagle H, et al. Effect of exercise intensity on 24-h energy expenditure and nutrient oxidation. J Appl Physiol 2002;92:1045.

157. Tarnopolsky M, Bosman M, Macdonald J, et al. Postexercise proteincarbohydrate and carbohydrate supplements increase muscle glycogen in men and women. J Appl Physiol 1997;83:1877.

158. Horton T, Grunwald G, Lavely J, et al. Glucose kinetics differ between women and men, during and after exercise. J Appl Physiol 2006;100:1883.

159. Forsberg A, Nilsson E, Werneman J, et al. Muscle composition in relation to age and sex. Clin Sci 1991;81:549.

160. Tarnopolsky M, Rennie C, Robertshaw H, et al. The influence of endurance exercise training and sex on intramyocellular lipid and mitochondrial ultrastructure, substrate use, and mitochondrial enzyme activity. Am J Physiol Regul Integr Comp Physiol 2006;292:R1271.

161. Devries MC, Lowther SA, Glover AW, et al. IMCL area density, but not IMCL utilization, is higher in women during moderate-intensity endurance exercise, compared with men. Am J Physiol Regul Integr Comp Physiol 2007;293:R2336–42.

162. Burguera B, Proctor D, Dietz N, et al. Leg free fatty acid kinetics during exercise in men and women. Am J Physiol Endocrinol Metab 2000;278:E113.

163. Horton TJ, Commerford S, Pagliassotti MJ, et al. Postprandial leg uptake of triglyceride is greater in women than in men. Am J Physiol Endocrinol Metab 2002;283:E1192.

164. Campbell SE, Febbraio MA. Effect of the ovarian hormones on GLUT 4 expression and contraction-stimulated glucose uptake. Am J Physiol 2002;282:E1139.

165. Kendrick ZV, Ellis GS. Effect of estradiol on tissue glycogen metabolism and lipid availability in exercised male rats. J Appl Physiol 1991;71:1694.

166. Carter SL, McKenzie S, Mourtzakis M, et al. Short-term 17-beta-estradiol decreases glucose Ra but not whole body metabolism during endurance exercise. J Appl Physiol 2001;90:139.

167. Devries M, Hamadeh MJ, Graham TE, et al. 17-beta-estradiol supplementation decreases glucose Ra and Rd with no effect on muscle glycogen utilization during moderate intensity exercise in men. J Clin Endocrinol Metab 2005;90:6218–25.

168. Ruby BC, Robergs RA, Waters DL, et al. Effects of estradiol on substrate turnover during exercise in amenorrheic females. Med Sci Sports Exerc 1997;29:1160.

169. Tarnopolsky MA, Roy BD, MacDougall JD, et al. Short-term 17-beta-estradiol administration does not affect metabolism in young males. Int J Sports Med 2001;22:175.

170. Campbell SE, Angus DJ, Febbraio MA. Glucose kinetics and exercise performance during phases of the menstrual cycle: effect of glucose ingestion. Am J Physiol Endocrinol Metab 2001;281:E817.

171. Hackney AC. Influence of oestrogen on muscle glycogen utilization during exercise. Acta Physiol Scand 1999;167:273.

172. Zderic TW, Coggan AR, Ruby BC. Glucose kinetics and substrate oxidation during exercise in the follicular and luteal phases. J Appl Physiol 2001;90:447.

173. Casazza GA, Jacobs KA, Suh S-H, et al. Menstrual cycle phase and oral contraceptive effects on triglyceride mobilization during exercise. J Appl Physiol 2004;97:302.

174. Horton T, Miller E, Bourret K. No effect of menstrual cycle phase on glycerol or palmitate kinetics during 90 min of moderate exercise. J Appl Physiol 2006;100:917.

175. Horton T, Miller E, Glueck D, et al. No effect of menstrual cycle phase on glucose kinetics and fuel oxidation during moderate-intensity exercise. Am J Physiol Endocrinol Metab 2002;282:E752.

176. Nicklas BJ, Hackney AC, Sharp RL. The menstrual cycle and exercise: performance, muscle glycogen, and substrate responses. Int J Sports Med 1989;10:264.

177. Suh S, Casazza GA, Horning MA, et al. Luteal and follicular glucose fluxes during rest and exercise in 3-h postabsorptive women. J Appl Physiol 2002;93:42.

178. Bergstrom J, Hermansen L, Hultman E, et al. Diet, muscle glycogen and physical performance. Acta Physiol Scand 1967;71:140.

179. Bergstrom J, Hultman E. The effect of exercise on muscle glycogen and electrolytes in normals. Scand J Clin Lab Invest 1966;18:16.

180. Hultman E, Bergstrom J. Muscle glycogen synthesis in relation to diet studied in normal subjects. Acta Med Scand 1967;182:109.

181. Madsen K, Pedersen P, Rose P, et al. Carbohydrate supercompensation and muscle glycogen utilization during exhaustive running in highly trained athletes. Eur J Appl Physiol 1990;61:467.

182. Sherman W, Costill D, Fink W, et al. Effect of exercise-diet manipulation on muscle glycogen and its subsequent utilization during performance. Int J Sports Med 1981;2:114.

183. Bussau V, Fairchild T, Rao A, et al. Carbohydrate loading in human muscle: an improved 1 day protocol. Eur J Appl Physiol 2002;87:290.

184. Fairchild T, Fletcher S, Steele P, et al. Rapid carbohydrate loading after a short bout of near maximal-intensity exercise. Med Sci Sports Exerc 2002;34:980.

185. Hawley J, Palmer G, Noakes T. Effects of 3 days of carbohydrate supplementation on muscle glycogen content and utilization during a 1-h cycling performance. Eur J Appl Physiol 1997;75:407.
186. James A, Lorraine M, Cullen D, et al. Muscle glycogen supercompensation: absence of a gender-related difference. Eur J Appl Physiol 2001;85:533.
187. Tarnopolsky MA, Zawada C, Richmond L, et al. Gender differences in carbohydrate loading are related to energy intake. J Appl Physiol 2001;91:225–30.
188. Goforth H, Arnall DJ, Bennett B, et al. Persistence of supercompensated muscle glycogen in trained subjects after carbohydrate loading. J Appl Physiol 1997; 82:342.
189. Roberts K, Noble E, Hayden D, et al. Simple and complex carbohydrate-rich diets and muscle glycogen content of marathon runners. Eur J Appl Physiol 1988;57:70.
190. Walker J, Heigenhauser G, Hultman E, et al. Dietary carbohydrate, muscle glycogen content, and endurance performance in well-trained women. J Appl Physiol 2000;88:2151.
191. Karlsson J, Saltin B. Diet, muscle glycogen, and endurance performance. J Appl Physiol 1971;31:203.
192. Lynch N, Galloway S, Nimmo M. Effects of moderate dietary manipulation on intermittent exercise performance and metabolism in women. Eur J Appl Physiol 2000;81:197.
193. Derave W, Van Den Bosch L, Lemmens G, et al. Skeletal muscle properties in a transgenic mouse model for amyotrophic lateral sclerosis: effects of creatine treatment. Neurobiol Dis 2003;13:264.
194. Wallis G, Dawson R, Achten J, et al. Metabolic response to carbohydrate ingestion during exercise in males and females. Am J Physiol Endocrinol Metab 2006; 290:E708.
195. Riddell M, Partington S, Stupka N, et al. Substrate utilization during exercise performed with and without glucose ingestion in female and male endurance trained athletes. Int J Sports Med 2003;13:407.
196. Coggan A, Coyle E. Carbohydrate ingestion during prolonged exercise: effects on metabolism and performance. Exerc Sport Sci Rev 1991;19:1.
197. Jentjens R, Achten J, Jeukendrup A. High rates of exogenous carbohydrate oxidation from multiple transportable carbohydrates ingested during prolonged exercise. Med Sci Sports Exerc 2004;36:1551.
198. Jentjens R, Jeukendrup A. High exogenous carbohydrate oxidation rates from a mixture of glucose and fructose ingested during prolonged cycling exercise. Br J Nutr 2005;93:485.
199. Jentjens R, Moseley L, Waring R, et al. Oxidation of combined ingestion of glucose and fructose during exercise. J Appl Physiol 2004;96:1277.
200. Jentjens R, Shaw C, Birtles T, et al. Oxidation of combined ingestion of glucose and sucrose during exercise. Metabolism 2005;54:610.
201. Jentjens R, Venables M, Jeukendrup A. Oxidation of exogenous glucose, sucrose, and maltose during prolonged cycling exercise. J Appl Physiol 2004; 96:1285.
202. Wallis G, Rowlands D, Shaw C, et al. Oxidation of combined ingestion of maltodextrins and fructose during exercise. Med Sci Sports Exerc 2005;37:426.
203. Jeukendrup A, Brouns F, Wagenmakers A, et al. Carbohydrate-electrolyte feedings improve 1 h time trial cycling performance. Int J Sports Med 1997;18:125.
204. Sugiura K, Kobayashi K. Effect of carbohydrate ingestion on sprint performance following continuous and intermittent exercise. Med Sci Sports Exerc 1998;30: 1624.

205. Burke L, Angus D, Cox G, et al. Effect of fat adaptation and carbohydrate restoration on metabolism and performance during prolonged cycling. J Appl Physiol 2000;89:2413.
206. Fleming J, Sharman M, Avery N, et al. Endurance capacity and high-intensity exercise performance responses to a high fat diet. Int J Sport Nutr Exerc Metab 2003;13:466.
207. Goedecke J, Christie G, Wilson G, et al. Metabolic adaptations to a high-fat diet in endurance cyclists. Metabolism 1999;48:1509.
208. Havemann L, West S, Goedecke J, et al. Fat adaptation followed by carbohydrate loading compromises high-intensity sprint performance. J Appl Physiol 2006;100:194.
209. Helge J, Richter E, Kiens B. Interaction of training and diet on metabolism and endurance during exercise in man. J Physiol 1996;492:293.
210. Helge J, Wulff B, Kiens B. Impact of a fat-rich diet on endurance in man: role of the dietary period. Med Sci Sports Exerc 1998;30:456.
211. Lambert E, Goedecke J, Zyle C, et al. High-fat diet versus habitual diet prior to carbohydrate loading: effects of exercise metabolism and cycling performance. Int J Sport Nutr Exerc Metab 2001;11:209.
212. Lambert E, Speechly D, Dennis S, et al. Enhanced endurance in trained cyclists during moderate intensity exercise following 2 weeks adaptation to a high fat diet. Eur J Appl Physiol 1994;69:287.
213. Vogt M, Puntschart A, Howald H, et al. Effects of dietary fat on muscle substrates, metabolism, and performance in athletes. Med Sci Sports Exerc 2003;35:952.
214. Zehnder M, Christ E, Ith M, et al. Intramyocellular lipid stores increase markedly in athletes after 1.5 days lipid supplementation and are utilized during exercise in proportion to their content. Eur J Appl Physiol 2006;98:341.
215. Phinney S, Bistrian B, Evans W, et al. The human metabolic response to chronic ketosis without caloric restriction: preservation of submaximal exercise capacity with reduced carbohydrate oxidation. Metabolism 1983;32.
216. Haller RG, Lewis SF, Cook JD, et al. Myophosphorylase deficiency impairs muscle oxidative metabolism. Ann Neurol 1985;17:196.
217. Haller RG, Vissing J. Spontaneous "second wind" and glucose-induced second "second wind" in McArdle disease: oxidative mechanisms. Arch Neurol 2002;59:1395.
218. Riley M, Nicholls DP, Nugent AM, et al. Respiratory gas exchange and metabolic responses during exercise in McArdle's disease. J Appl Physiol 1993;75:745.
219. Sahlin K, Areskog NH, Haller RG, et al. Impaired oxidative metabolism increases adenine nucleotide breakdown in McArdle's disease. J Appl Physiol 1990;69:1231.
220. Haller RG, Vissing J. No spontaneous second wind in muscle phosphofructokinase deficiency. Neurology 2004;62:82.
221. Bertocci LA, Haller RG, Lewis SF. Muscle metabolism during lactate infusion in human phosphofructokinase deficiency. J Appl Physiol 1993;74:1342.
222. Chaussain M, Camus F, Defoligny C, et al. Exercise intolerance in patients with McArdle's disease or mitochondrial myopathies. Eur J Med 1992;1:457.
223. Tarnopolsky M, Stevens L, MacDonald JR, et al. Diagnostic utility of a modified forearm ischemic exercise test and technical issues relevant to exercise testing. Muscle Nerve 2003;27:359.
224. Argov Z, De Stefano N, Arnold DL. ADP recovery after a brief ischemic exercise in normal and diseased human muscle—a 31P MRS study. NMR Biomed 1996;9:165.

225. Grehl T, Muller K, Vorgerd M, et al. Impaired aerobic glycolysis in muscle phosphofructokinase deficiency results in biphasic post-exercise phosphocreatine recovery in 31P magnetic resonance spectroscopy. Neuromuscul Disord 1998;8:480.

226. Mineo I, Tarui S. Myogenic hyperuricemia: what can we learn from metabolic myopathies? Muscle Nerve 1995;3:S75.

227. Ollivier K, Hogrel JY, Gomez-Merino D, et al. Exercise tolerance and daily life in McArdle's disease. Muscle Nerve 2005;31:637.

228. Quinlivan R, Beynon RJ. Pharmacological and nutritional treatment for McArdle's disease (Glycogen Storage Disease type V). Cochrane Database Syst Rev 2004;(3):CD003458.

229. MacLean D, Vissing J, Vissing SF, et al. Oral branched-chain amino acids do not improve exercise capacity in McArdle disease. Neurology 1998;51:1456.

230. Vorgerd M, Grehl T, Jager M, et al. Creatine therapy in myophosphorylase deficiency (McArdle disease): a placebo-controlled crossover trial. Arch Neurol 2000;57:956.

231. Vorgerd M, Zange J, Kley R, et al. Effect of high-dose creatine therapy on symptoms of exercise intolerance in McArdle disease: double-blind, placebo-controlled crossover study. Arch Neurol 2002;59:97.

232. Djouadi F, Weinheimer CJ, Saffitz JE, et al. A gender-related defect in lipid metabolism and glucose homeostasis in peroxisome proliferator-activated receptor alpha-deficient mice. J Clin Invest 1998;102:1083.

233. Orngreen MC, Duno M, Ejstrup R, et al. Fuel utilization in subjects with carnitine palmitoyltransferase 2 gene mutations. Ann Neurol 2005;57:60.

234. DiMauro S, Hirano M, Schon EA. Approaches to the treatment of mitochondrial diseases. Muscle Nerve 2006;34:265.

235. Tarnopolsky MA, Raha S. Mitochondrial myopathies: diagnosis, exercise intolerance, and treatment options. Med Sci Sports Exerc 2005;37:2086.

236. Mahoney DJ, Parise G, Tarnopolsky MA. Nutritional and exercise-based therapies in the treatment of mitochondrial disease. Curr Opin Clin Nutr Metab Care 2002;5:619.

237. Tarnopolsky MA, Maguire J, Myint T, et al. Clinical, physiological, and histological features in a kindred with the T3271C MELAS mutation. Muscle Nerve 1998;21:25.

238. Grassi B, Marzorati M, Lanfranconi F, et al. Impaired oxygen extraction in metabolic myopathies: detection and quantification by near-infrared spectroscopy. Muscle Nerve 2007;35:510.

239. Taivassalo T, Abbott A, Wyrick P, et al. Venous oxygen levels during aerobic forearm exercise: an index of impaired oxidative metabolism in mitochondrial myopathy. Ann Neurol 2002;51:38.

240. Argov Z, Arnold DL. MR spectroscopy and imaging in metabolic myopathies. Neurol Clin 2000;18:35.

241. Argov Z, Lofberg M, Arnold DL. Insights into muscle diseases gained by phosphorus magnetic resonance spectroscopy. Muscle Nerve 2000;23:1316.

242. Stacpoole PW, Kerr DS, Barnes C, et al. Controlled clinical trial of dichloroacetate for treatment of congenital lactic acidosis in children. Pediatrics 2006;117:1519.

243. Kaufmann P, Engelstad K, Wei Y, et al. Dichloroacetate causes toxic neuropathy in MELAS: a randomized, controlled clinical trial. Neurology 2006;66:324.

244. Haas RH. The evidence basis for coenzyme Q therapy in oxidative phosphorylation disease. Mitochondrion 2007;(Suppl 7):S136–45.

245. Tarnopolsky MA, Beal MF. Potential for creatine and other therapies targeting cellular energy dysfunction in neurological disorders. Ann Neurol 2001;49:561.

246. Muller T, Buttner T, Gholipour AF, et al. Coenzyme Q10 supplementation provides mild symptomatic benefit in patients with Parkinson's disease. Neurosci Lett 2003;341:201.

247. Shults CW, Haas RH, Beal MF. A possible role of coenzyme Q10 in the etiology and treatment of Parkinson's disease. Biofactors 1999;9:267.

248. Shults CW, Oakes D, Kieburtz K, et al. Effects of coenzyme Q10 in early Parkinson disease: evidence of slowing of the functional decline. Arch Neurol 2002;59:1541.

249. Barisic N, Bernert G, Ipsiroglu O, et al. Effects of oral creatine supplementation in a patient with MELAS phenotype and associated nephropathy. Neuropediatrics 2002;33:157.

250. Komura K, Hobbiebrunken E, Wilichowski EK, et al. Effectiveness of creatine monohydrate in mitochondrial encephalomyopathies. Pediatr Neurol 2003;28:53.

251. Tarnopolsky MA, Simon D, Roy B, et al. Attenuation of free radical production and paracrystalline inclusions by creatine supplementation in a patient with a novel cytochrome b mutation. Muscle Nerve 2004;29:537.

252. Klopstock T, Querner V, Schmidt F, et al. A placebo-controlled crossover trial of creatine in mitochondrial diseases. Neurology 2000;55:1748.

253. Kornblum C, Schroder R, Muller K, et al. Creatine has no beneficial effect on skeletal muscle energy metabolism in patients with single mitochondrial DNA deletions: a placebo-controlled, double-blind 31P-MRS crossover study. Eur J Neurol 2005;12:300.

254. Kley RA, Vorgerd M, Tarnopolsky MA. Creatine for treating muscle disorders. Cochrane Database Syst Rev 2007;1:CD004760.

255. Tarnopolsky MA, MacLennan DP. Creatine monohydrate supplementation enhances high-intensity exercise performance in males and females. Int J Sport Nutr Exerc Metab 2000;10:452.

256. Terjung RL, Clarkson P, Eichner ER, et al. American College of Sports Medicine roundtable. The physiological and health effects of oral creatine supplementation. Med Sci Sports Exerc 2000;32:706.

257. Rodriguez MC, MacDonald JR, Mahoney DJ, et al. Beneficial effects of creatine, CoQ10, and lipoic acid in mitochondrial disorders. Muscle Nerve 2007;35:235.

258. Taivassalo T, Matthews PM, De Stefano N, et al. Combined aerobic training and dichloroacetate improve exercise capacity and indices of aerobic metabolism in muscle cytochrome oxidase deficiency. Neurology 1996;47:529.

259. Jeppesen TD, Schwartz M, Olsen DB, et al. Aerobic training is safe and improves exercise capacity in patients with mitochondrial myopathy. Brain 2006;129:3402.

260. Andrews RM, Griffiths PG, Chinnery PF, et al. Evaluation of bupivacaine-induced muscle regeneration in the treatment of ptosis in patients with chronic progressive external ophthalmoplegia and Kearns-Sayre syndrome. Eye 1999;13(Pt 6):769.

261. Clark KM, Bindoff LA, Lightowlers RN, et al. Reversal of a mitochondrial DNA defect in human skeletal muscle. Nat Genet 1997;16:222.

262. Melov S, Tarnopolsky MA, Beckman K, et al. Resistance exercise reverses aging in human skeletal muscle. PLoS ONE 2007;2:e465.

263. Parise G, Brose AN, Tarnopolsky MA. Resistance exercise training decreases oxidative damage to DNA and increases cytochrome oxidase activity in older adults. Exp Gerontol 2005;40:173.

264. Parise G, Phillips SM, Kaczor JJ, et al. Antioxidant enzyme activity is upregulated after unilateral resistance exercise training in older adults. Free Radic Biol Med 2005;39:289.

Section 3

Variables in Sport

Enhancement Drugs and the Athlete

Francesco Botrè[a,b,*], Antonio Pavan, MD[c]

KEYWORDS

- Enhancement drugs • Athletic competition
- Doping substances • Athletic regulations

PERFORMANCE-ENHANCING DRUGS: A (BRIEF) HISTORICAL OVERVIEW

The use of performance-enhancing drugs (PEDs) is perhaps as old as sport itself. The ingestion of plant and animal extracts to improve sport performance dates back to the origins of competitive sport, when Greek athletes competed in the ancient Olympics. Later, Roman gladiators had special potions prepared using a wide variety of natural products, including mushrooms, roots, and wines,[1,2] to attempt to supplement performance. The use of PEDs became more systematic, no longer based on sorcery and alchemy but instead biochemistry and pharmacology, during the twentieth century, when the Olympic Games were reinvented after the recovery and promotion of the Olympic spirit heralded by Baron Pierre de Coubertin.

To compare the lifespan of the ancient Olympics with that of the modern Olympic Games, the first ancient Olympic Games took place in 776 BC and the last one was held in 393 AD, when, although the Games already had degenerated, they officially were abolished by the Roman emperor Theodosius, who, as a Christian, was against the heathen spirit of the Games.[3,4] The modern Olympic Games, the first edition of which took place in Athens in 1896, celebrates their 112th anniversary in Beijing in August 2008. It follows that the history of the ancient Olympics, spanning more than 11 centuries, is approximately 10 times longer than that of the modern Olympic Games.

The history of PED use strictly follows the history of scientific development that took place at the time of the ancient and the modern Olympic Games; although the drugs

This article originally appeared in *Neurologic Clinics*, Volume 26, Issue 1.
This work was supported in part by Grants from the Italian Department of Health ("Commissione per la Vigilanza sul Doping e la Tutela Sanitaria delle Attività Sportive").
[a] Laboratorio Antidoping, Federazione Medico Sportiva Italiana, Largo Giulio Onesti 1, 00197 Rome RM, Italy
[b] Dipartimento per le Tecnologie, le Risorse e lo Sviluppo, "Sapienza" Università di Roma, Via del Castro Laurenziano 9, 00161 Rome RM, Italy
[c] Dipartimento di Medicina Sperimentale, "Sapienza" Università di Roma and Servizio di Immunoematologia e Medicina Trasfusionale, Azienda Ospedaliera Sant' Andrea, Via di Grottarossa, 1035–1039, 00189 Rome RM, Italy
* Corresponding author. Laboratorio Antidoping, Federazione Medico Sportiva Italiana, Largo Giulio Onesti 1, 00197 Rome RM, Italy.
E-mail address: francesco.botre@uniroma1.it (F. Botrè).

Phys Med Rehabil Clin N Am 20 (2009) 133–148
doi:10.1016/j.pmr.2008.10.010

used by athletes competing in the first ancient Olympic Games approximately were the same of those used 1 millennium later by their colleagues or by Roman gladiators, the illicit pharmacologic support to sport performance proceeded at a much faster pace in the twentieth century, with a further dramatic increase from the early 1960s to the present.

The problem of drug abuse in sport first was tackled by the international sport authorities, in the form of the International Olympic Committee (IOC), during the 1960s. An official definition of doping first was given by the IOC in 1964 and the first programs of antidoping tests were activated by the IOC and its newborn Medical Commission in 1967.[5–7] It was in the late 1960s when, in parallel to the official sport competitions, another race began and continues to the present: the race between testers and cheaters.

CLASSIFICATION OF PERFORMANCE-ENHANCING DRUGS: THE "PROHIBITED LIST"

The first official antidoping tests performed on the occasion of a multisport, international event took place at the Olympic Games of Mexico City in 1968. At that time, the only prohibited substances were those capable of producing a significant effect on sport performance only if administered, in sufficient amounts, right before or during the competition. Although short (compared with its current equivalent), that first list continuously was updated to include any new form of doping substance or method of administration. The periodic upgrades of the list were performed by the IOC Medical Commission until the constitution of the World Anti-Doping Agency (WADA) in 1999. Since then, as mandated by the World Anti-Doping Code,[8] the WADA has been responsible for the upgrade and publication of the list. In the framework of the World Anti-Doping Code, the list is an international standard identifying substances and methods, classified by categories, that are prohibited in competition, out of competition, and in particular sports. In the past 40 years, the "prohibited list" has expanded progressively (**Box 1**): it now reports hundreds of compounds, including so-called "related substances" (ie, substances with similar chemical structure or similar biologic effects to those of a banned prototype) and several prohibited methods, including blood transfusions and gene doping.[9]

The chronologic evolution of the "prohibited list" over the past 4 decades leads to identifying three main steps in the parallel expansion of the abuse of drugs in sport:

1. The first period, ranging from the origin of the modern Olympic Games to the early 1970s, coincides with the use of drugs whose efficacy, as discussed previously, is maximal if the administration takes place right before or even during the competition. This is the case with stimulants, narcotics, and some drugs of abuse (eg, cocaine).
2. In the second period, the PEDs also included those compounds—mainly AAS—requiring repeated administration over a prolonged period of time to be effective. It is with the use of synthetic AAS that doping substances start to be used off label (ie, with the aim of achieving one or more effects that are different from those for which a specific drug originally had been developed and authorized). This period also marks the transition from pinpoint, in-competition doping, to carefully planned, out-of-competition, systematic doping.
3. The third period follows the pharmaceutical industry development of routine techniques in protein chemistry, molecular biology, and genetic engineering, and led to the abuse of peptide hormones (including, but not limited to, erythropoietin, growth hormone, and gonadotropins). The use of PEDs belonging to the class of peptide and glycoproteic hormones led to the development of new analytic strategies for their detection, including the use of "indirect" methods based on the measurements of specific markers.

Box 1
World Anti-Doping Code: the 2008 "prohibited list"

Substances and methods prohibited at all times (in and out of competition)

Prohibited substances

S1. Anabolic agents

1. Anabolic androgenic steroids (AAS)

a. Exogenous AAS (eg, methyltestosterone, nandrolone, and stanozolol)

b. Endogenous AAS (eg, testosterone, androsteonedione, DHT, and DHEA)

2. Other anabolic agents (eg, clenbuterol and selective androgen receptor modulators)

S2. Hormones and related substances (eg, EPO, human growth hormone, insulin-like growth factors, gonadotropins, insulins)

S3. β_2-Agonists (eg, salbutamol, salmeterol, terbutaline, and formoterol)

S4. Hormone antagonists and modulators (eg, antiestrogens and myostatin inhibitors)

S5. Diuretics and other masking agents (eg, diuretics, epitestosterone, probenecid, α-reductase inhibitors, and plasma expanders)

Prohibited methods

M1. Enhancement of oxygen transfer (eg, blood transfusions and use of blood derivatives and analogs)

M2. Chemical and physical manipulation (eg, tampering and intravenous infusions)

M3. Gene doping

Substances and methods prohibited in competition

S6. Stimulants (eg, amphetamines, cocaine, strychnine, and ecstasy-like drugs)

S7. Narcotics (eg, morphine and opioids)

S8. Cannabinoids (eg, hashish and marijuana)

S9. Glucocorticosteroids

Substances prohibited in particular sports

P1. Alcohol

P2. β-Blockers

Abbreviations: DHEA, dehydroepiandrosterone; DHT, dihydrotestosterone; EPO, erythropoietin.
Data from The World Anti-Doping Code. The 2008 prohibited list international standard. World Anti-Doping Agency. Montreal (Canada); 2007. Available at: www.wada.ama.org. Accessed October 31, 2007.

A fourth period (the recourse to gene doping) is feared by many as the next step in the illicit search for the ultimate PEDs and methods. It is expected that gene doping will develop as soon as gene therapy is available practically.

Regardless of its complexity and length, the prohibited list stands as the fundamental reference document classifying all prohibited PEDs, prohibited methods, and masking agents. The fight against doping in sport has been based—and still continues to be based—on the capability of the antidoping laboratories to develop and apply analytic procedures for the most effective detection of all substances and methods included in the prohibited list.

THE ROLE OF THE WORLD ANTI-DOPING AGENCY–ACCREDITED ANTIDOPING LABORATORIES

There currently are 33 antidoping laboratories accredited by the WADA in the world (**Box 2**), performing more than 200,000 antidoping tests per year. A comprehensive report of the results of the analyses performed by the WADA laboratories worldwide is released yearly by WADA and made available for consultation through their website (www.wada-ama.org). In spite of the high number of tests, little information can be drawn simply on the basis of results of the antidoping analyses on the real toxic potential and the related mechanism of action of the many PEDs included in the WADA prohibited list. The antidoping analyses are forensic, but not diagnostic, tests. This means that the aim of the analysis is not to verify the "state of health or disease" of athletes but instead "to supply evidence"—based on the principle of strict liability—of the presence in the biologic sample of a substance (drug/metabolite/marker) included in the WADA prohibited list. It follows that the information supplied by the WADA-accredited antidoping laboratories refers to the identification of "markers of exposure," not of "markers of effect," of doping agents and methods.

The data supplied by the WADA-accredited antidoping laboratories also are of little epidemiologic value for the following reasons:

1. Despite the outstanding number of antidoping tests performed worldwide, the total number of positive samples is too limited to support any epidemiologic conclusions.
2. All samples analyzed by the laboratories are anonymous and, therefore, critical information necessary for the correct compilation of a reference database is not available (eg, ethnicity, age, height, weight, body mass index, genetic endowment, training level and regimen, and diet).
3. Samples are not collected as a part of a controlled study, and, therefore, it is impossible to carry out a real toxicity study correctly because of the potential influence of other confounding factors.
4. Finally, the WADA rules state clearly that the biologic samples collected in the framework of official antidoping tests cannot be used for purposes other than the antidoping test itself: this means that the activity of the laboratory has to be limited to the identification of specific compounds (drugs/metabolites/markers) whose

---

Box 2
Geographical distribution of the 33 antidoping laboratories accredited by the World Anti-Doping Agency

Africa: South Africa (Bloemfontein), Tunisia (Tunis)

Americas: Brazil (Rio de Janeiro), Canada (Montreal), Colombia (Bogota), Cuba (La Habana), United States (Los Angeles, Salt Lake City)

Asia: China (Beijing), Korea (Seoul), Japan (Tokyo), Malaysia (Penang), Thailand (Bangkok)

Europe: Austria (Seibersdorf), Belgium (Ghent), Czech Republic (Prague), Finland (Helsinki), France (Paris), Germany (Cologne, Kreischa), Greece (Athens), Italy (Rome), Norway (Oslo), Poland (Warsaw), Portugal (Lisbon), Russian Federation (Moscow), Spain (Barcelona, Madrid), Sweden (Stockholm), Switzerland (Lausanne), Turkey (Ankara), United Kingdom (London)

Oceania: Australia (Sydney)

presence (or whose concentration above a threshold value) is to be considered a proof of doping. No additional tests (including diagnostic tests) are allowed.

The same points hold true for the research activity performed within the network of the WADA-accredited laboratories via the World Association of Anti-Doping Scientists (WAADS), the international scientific society promoting the sharing of knowledge among the accredited laboratories and the basic and applied research in development of new analytic methods. Because the result of a positive test constitutes the basis for the possible sanctioning of an athlete, all efforts are not devoted to diagnosing the health risks consequent to the use of PEDs but instead to guaranteeing the maximum of solidity of the experimental results. The International Standard Organization 17025 accreditation has been imposed since 2000 as a further prerequisite of accredited antidoping laboratories, and criteria for reporting positive samples must be in compliance with the WADA rules.

It is self-evident that there is little or no room, at present, for toxicologic evaluations. The potential toxicologic risks for abuse of performance-enhancing substances and methods cannot be evaluated fully by a single measurement of urinary/blood concentration values of drugs, metabolites, or other representative indicators of administration. Therefore, no toxicokinetic information can be estimated.

A further step forward will be represented by the final implementation of longitudinal studies, also known as the "athlete passport:" the goal is to build a database for all athletes in which the main hematologic and hormonal parameters are recorded and monitored. Although these strategies are being developed with the main purpose of detecting, via the evaluation of indirect parameters, some forms of doping otherwise problematic to identify (eg, autologous blood transfusions), they also will contribute to shedding further light on the chronic effects of the abuse of PEDs. The implementation of novel diagnostic approaches, to be performed independently of the forensic antidoping tests, for the overall assessment of the toxicity of PEDs will remain mandatory to fully accomplish the requirements of an effective antidoping strategy.[10]

THE ADVERSE SIDE EFFECTS OF PERFORMANCE-ENHANCING DRUGS: WHAT IS KNOWN AND UNKNOWN

The possible health risks of doping substances and methods have been the subject of several review articles, monographs, and conference proceedings.[11–16] Mostly, these studies have been based on and supported by review of the scientific and medical literature, which have considered the results obtained in controlled, randomized clinical trials and the direct evidence obtained from clinical practice. It is impossible in this context to review, discuss, and outline the biochemical mechanisms of all the adverse effects of the PEDs described so far. To give an approximate idea of the variety of potential side effects of the different classes of substances included in the WADA-prohibited list (with the exception of alcohol, not a drug in the strict sense of the word), **Table 1** lists the most common potential direct and indirect effects and the corresponding side effects of PEDs. It is evident that the risks/benefits ratio is always unbalanced toward the risks. Also, it is virtually impossible for a single drug to produce all or none of the effects listed in **Table 1** in one subject.

To correctly assess the real toxicologic potential of PEDs (which easily can include additional effects not considered in **Table 1**) is not an easy task. Most of the side effects tend to be the same as those reported after the therapeutic use of the same drugs. It is even more difficult to evaluate the actual toxicity for athletes, because information supplied by the WADA-accredited antidoping laboratories is insufficient.

Table 1
Most common undesired side effects of the main classes of prohibited substances considered in the World Anti-Doping Agency list

Class of the World Anti-Doping Agency Prohibited List	Potential Direct/Indirect Effects Enhancing Sport Performance	Side Effects Reported Most Commonly
S1. Anabolic agents AAS (endogenous and exogenous)	Generic anabolic effect, produced with the aim of enhancing muscle growth and weight and increasing strength, power, speed, endurance, and aggressiveness. Recovery times also should be improved.	A broad variety of effects (exhaustively reviewed in Ref. [30]), including, but not limited, to the following: Cardiovascular: hypertension, elevated risk of brain hemorrhages, myocardiac damage Hepatic: abnormal liver functions, cholestasis, development of androgen-dependent adenomas, depletion of high-density lipoprotein production Skeletal: water retention Dermal: seborrhea (steroid acne), oily skin, folliculitis, furunculosis Behavioral: increase of aggressiveness (aggressive psychoses), change in the libido, mood swings (euphoria followed by depression), mental disorders, headaches, dependence, or addiction Specific effects for men: testicular atrophy, altered spermatogenesis, prostate hypertrophy, gynecomastia Specific effects for women: virilization, atrophy of the uterus, effects on the ovary (polycystic ovary syndrome, ovary inflammations), reduction of the breast gland, hirsutism, hypothyroidism, lowering of the voice, alteration of the menstrual cycle, alopecia, effects on the connective tissue (striae distensae)
Other anabolic agents	Same as previously.	For the side effects of clenbuterol, see "S3. β₂-Agonists" Side effects of selective androgen receptor modulators still are under evaluation (these drugs are not yet marketed)

S2. Hormones and related substances		Risk common to all peptide hormones: immunogenicity
Human growth hormone, insulin-like growth factors	Anabolic effect	Data on the effects of prolonged recombinant human growth hormone treatment in adults are limited
		Acute overdosing could lead to hyperglycemia.
		Long-term overdosing could result in signs and symptoms of gigantism or acromegaly consistent with the known effects of excess growth hormone
		Other reported effects are hypertension, cardiomyopathy, respiratory disease, diabetes, abnormal lipid metabolism, and osteoarthritis
		Increase risk for breast and colorectal cancer
Recombinant erythropoietins	Increased production of red blood cells and hemoglobin, resulting in an augmented efficacy of the transport of oxygen to the muscle	Hypertension, thromboses (thrombophlebitis, microvascular thrombosis, and thrombosis of the retinal artery, and temporal and renal veins), pulmonary embolism, cerebral embolism, seizures
		Other effects include pyrexia, headache, arthralgias, nausea, edema, fatigue, diarrhea, vomiting, chest pain, skin reaction (on the site of injection), asthenia, dizziness
Gonadotropins (human chorionic gonadotropin, luteinizing hormone, and follicle-stimulating hormone)	To stimulate the endogenous production of androgens, and to contrast the negative effects of testosterone doping	Prostate carcinoma or other androgen-dependent neoplasm
		Sudden ovarian enlargement resulting from ovarian hyperstimulation, ascites with or without pain, or pleural effusion, rupture of ovarian cysts with resultant hemoperitoneum
		Arterial thromboembolism, headache, irritability, restlessness, depression, fatigue, edema, precocious puberty, gynecomastia, pain at the site of injection
Insulin	To improve glucose transport to muscle	All adverse effects of hypoglycemia (including loss of consciousness, coma, and death)
		Respiratory adverse effects
		Chest pain, dry mouth, otitis media

(continued on next page)

Table 1
(Continued)

Class of the World Anti-Doping Agency Prohibited List	Potential Direct/Indirect Effects Enhancing Sport Performance	Side Effects Reported Most Commonly
S3. β₂-Agonists	To achieve stimulants and anabolic effects after systemic administration of high doses, significantly higher than those prescribed—by inhalation—for the treatment of asthma	Cardiac arrest and even death may be associated with the abuse of any sympathomimetic medications. Other cardiovascular effect include, but are not limited to, increased pulse rate and blood pressure, ECG changes, seizures, angina, hypertension or hypotension, tachycardia with rates up to 200 beats/minute, arrhythmias. Hypokalemia also may occur. Nervousness, headache, insomnia, tremor, dry mouth, palpitation, nausea, dizziness, fatigue, malaise, and sleeplessness
S4. Hormone antagonists and modulators Aromatase inhibitors (eg, anastrozole, letrozole, aminoglutethimide, exemestane, formestane, and testolactone)	To increase the production or decrease the biotransformation of endogenous AAS	At therapeutic doses: nonspecific toxic side effects, including (but not limited to) asthenia, headache, nausea, peripheral edema, fatigue, vomiting, and dyspepsia. Long-term endocrinologic side effects can be severe if administered in sequence or in combination with tamoxifen or selective estrogen receptor modulators
Selective estrogen receptor modulators (eg, raloxifene, tamoxifen, and toremifene)	Same as previously	Hot flashes, flu-like syndrome, joint pain, rhinitis. Blood clots, including deep vein thrombosis, and pulmonary embolus (rare)
Other antiestrogenic substances (eg, clomiphene, cyclofenil, and fulvestrant)	Same as previously	At high doses, nonspecific toxic side effects, including (but not limited to) nausea, vomiting, vasomotor flushes, visual blurring, spots or flashes, scotomata, ovarian enlargement with pelvic or abdominal pain
Agents modifying myostatin functions	To improve muscle growth by interfering with the action of myostatin.	Unknown: myostatin inhibitors never have been tested in human trials

S5. Diuretics and other masking agents Diuretics	1. To obtain a rapid and reversible reduction of the total body mass, an evident potential advantage in sports where weight categories are involved 2. To alter the normal urinary excretion of other PEDs or their metabolites (eg, by increasing the volume of urine and diluting them), making their detection by the antidoping laboratories more problematic	Hypotension Kidney dysfunction, dehydration (risk for central volume depletion), salt and water imbalance, electrolyte dispairement (eg, hyperosmolality, hyponatremia, hypokalemia, hypomagnesemia, hypocalcemia), muscle cramps Dizziness or lightheadedness, gastric effects, rash, impotence, secondary gout
Probenecid	To interfere with the normal excretion of other PEDs, especially AAS	Metabolic effects: precipitation of acute gouty arthritis Central nervous system: headache, dizziness Gastrointestinal: hepatic necrosis, nausea, anorexia, sore gums, vomiting Genitourinary: nephritic syndrome, uric acid stones with or without hematuria, renal colic, costovertebral pain, urinary frequency Hematologic: aplastic anemia, leucopenia, hemolytic anemia Integumental: dermatitis, alopecia, flushing (Rarely) severe allergic reactions and anaphylaxis
Epitestosterone	To adjust the value of the ratio of testosterone to epitestosterone	Unknown (epitestosterone is not a registered drug), even if likely overlapping to many of the side effects of the AAS
α-Reductase inhibitors (eg, finasteride and dutasteride)	Alteration of the endogenous steroid profile, interfering with the quantitation of some AAS and with the correct evaluation of longitudinal data	Alteration of the sexual function (impotence, decreased libido, decreased volume of ejaculate and other ejaculation disorders, breast enlargement, breast tenderness)
Plasma volume expanders (eg, dextran, hydroxyethylstarch and other modified polysaccharides)	To mask the effects of blood doping by blood dilution	Febrile response, infection at the site of injection, venous thrombosis or phlebitis extending from the site of injection, extravasation, hypervolemia
S6. Stimulants	Increased alertness	Increased alertness
Including, but not limited to	Improvement in coordination	Insomnia, anxiety

(continued on next page)

Table 1
(Continued)

Class of the World Anti-Doping Agency Prohibited List	Potential Direct/Indirect Effects Enhancing Sport Performance	Side Effects Reported Most Commonly
Central nervous system stimulants	Increased strength and endurance, as a consequence of a decreased perception of pain and fatigue	Inhibited judgment
Respiratory stimulants Cardiovascular stimulants Appetite suppressants	Glycogen sparing effect in muscle	Increased competitiveness, aggressiveness, and hostility Reduced fatigue (risks for muscle and cardiac overload) Tremor Effect on the cardiovascular systems (increased heart rate and blood pressure) Increased risk for stroke, heart attack, or sudden death Effects on the skeletal muscle (rhabdomyolysis).
S7. Narcotics	Increased tolerance to pain and fatigue Transient reduction of tremor in precision events	Addiction (also as gateway to other drugs), tolerance, physical and psychologic dependence Increased pain threshold Euphoria Excitement, psychologic stimulation Incorrect perception of danger Loss of coordination/equilibrium Reduced capacity of concentration Nausea, vomiting, constipation Depression Reduced breath capacity Reduced cardiac frequency/output Overdosing can lead to respiratory depression and death Effects on the skeletal muscle (rhabdomyolysis)
S8. Cannabinoids	To relieve precompetition tension Social drugs: motivation for their use or abuse may be different from the illicit enhancement of sport performance	Drug dependence Psychomotor changes Antimotivational syndrome (loss of ambition)

S9. Glucocorticosteroids	Effect on glucose metabolism (stimulation of de novo synthesis of glucose, conversion of amino acids into glucose, release of glucose from glycogen storage, and activation of the lipolysis in fat cells) Anti-inflammatory and analgesic properties, accompanied by euphoria Effects on the immune system	Acute: Hyperglycemia Fluid retention Mood alteration Chronic: Immunosuppression Suppression of the hypothalamic-pituitary-adrenal axis Musculoskeletal problems, also due to alteration of calcium metabolism and bone homeostasis Nonspecific effects (cataracts, diabetes mellitus, hypertension, peptic ulcer disease, weight gain, skin thinning, ecchymoses, striae, acne, hirsutism, fat redistribution, and various psychiatric disorders)
P2. β-Blockers	To reduce tremor, which gives a competitive advantage in specific sports/disciplines (eg, shooting, archery, curling, gymnastics)	Cardiovascular effects: bradycardia, cold extremities, postural hypotension, leg pain Central nervous system/neuromuscular effects: reversible mental depression progressing to catatonia, emotional lability, dizziness, vertigo, tiredness, fatigue, lethargy, drowsiness, depression, insomnia Hematologic effects: agranulocytosis Allergic: fever, sore throat, laryngospasm, respiratory distress Gastrointestinal: mesenteric arterial thrombosis, ischemic colitis, diarrhea, nausea Respiratory effects: wheeziness, dyspnea Other effects: impotency, hypoglycemia

Also, administration of a drug for the enhancement of sport performance clearly is different from rules regulating the administration of the same drug when used within correctly planned therapeutic schemes in patients. The range of side effects can be wider than expected and intensity more severe (discussed later).

Use of Off-Label Drugs

With the noteworthy exception of designer steroids (discussed later), all drugs administered for nonphysiologic enhancement of sport performance are well known drugs; but when they are administered within the framework of a doping strategy, they are used off label (ie, out of the range of therapeutic application for their original intent). In most cases, athletes understand that a drug is being used beyond its indicated uses. Under these circumstances, it could be difficult to extrapolate the theoretic side effects and compare with those observed in routine medical practice to obtain a representative picture of the actual risks for athletes.

Overdosing (Acute or Chronic)

Doping agents generally are used at doses higher than therapeutic doses. Therefore, it is reasonable to think that adverse effects could be more severe as the administered dose increases. Although good pharmacologic practice recommends minimizing administered doses and duration of use, this situation is reversed when the desired effect instead is improvement of sport performance.

Drug-Drug Interaction

PEDs seldom are administered alone. Many are used in association with other drugs (banned or allowed) and with a wide variety of nutritional supplements. Drugs may be combined to reach different goals, such as maximizing overall efficacy of the doping treatment, reducing risks for undesired side effects, and complicating their detection by accredited laboratories. Because the range of desired effects is broad, it is reasonable to expect that most of the corresponding drug-drug interactions never have been considered. No therapeutic scheme has been considered for the parallel administration (again, to a healthy person) of combined "therapeutic" schemes, which may include (1) erythropoietin, (2) anticoagulant agents, (3) anabolic steroids, (4) branched-chain amino acids, (5) glucocorticosteroids, and (6) diuretics.[17] It is evident that in such conditions the range of undesired side effects cannot be foreseen adequately.

Physical Activity

The overall evaluation of PED side effects has to consider that active principles are administered during intense physical exercise in competition or out of competition (ie, during the training sessions). It is not unlikely to expect the range of undesired effects are more broad than those that listed in **Table 1** or their intensity much more pronounced, given their use at the time of concurrent intense training.

THE RISKS OF THE UNKNOWN: THE DARK SIDE OF DESIGNER STEROIDS

Although used off label, many PEDs officially are approved drugs and have undergone a full toxicologic premarketing evaluation. A series of antidoping investigations performed recently have revealed that that new families of drugs, previously unknown to more mainstream pharmacology methodologies, have been developed to be used by athletes seeking enhancement of sport performance. Most of these drugs have been designed to obtain completely new substances, with only some minor modifications in their molecular structure from known synthetic AAS—these are called "designer steroids." These previously unknown compounds have been synthesized illicitly by clandestine laboratories, operating out of the channel of the pharmaceutical industry. These steroids were supposed to be undetectable, because the practice of the antidoping laboratories is based on the availability of certified reference materials for all target substances: the final proof of the presence of a target within a biologic sample requires the comparison of the analytic signal with that obtained on a certified positive reference sample. There is no reference material available for detection of many of the designer steroids. Furthermore, no pharmacokinetic data are available regarding the metabolism and the excretion profile of the designer steroids. Therefore, it has been nearly impossible for laboratory-mediated selection of suitable urinary markers to detect designer steroids. Consequently, designer steroids have been referred to as the perfect anabolic agents: effective and invisible.

The discovery of the first designer steroid was in 2002, when a previously unknown synthetic AAS, norbolethone, was identified by the WADA-accredited antidoping laboratory of Los Angeles.[18] The discovery of norbolethone was followed by detection of other designer AAS, including tetrahydrogestrinone and desoxy-methyl testosterone (or madol).[19–21] The antidoping laboratories reacted immediately to face this new analytic challenge by making available suitable reference materials (most of them through the WAADS network) and developing a new series of analytic procedures for the detection of designer steroids and related substances. This task has been made possible by the development of a new generation of scientific instruments that provides additional tools for the early detection of designer steroids. A particularly promising approach couples a liquid chromatographer to a time-of-flight mass spectrometer.[22] The unique feature of time-of-flight mass spectrometer is its ability to record a broad amount of information from a single assay, giving the ability to return to a previously stored electronic data file and reassess for the possible presence of substances unknown at the time of initial analysis. Other analytic strategies, based on the use of simpler instrumentation, are those based on the use of triple quadrupole liquid chromatography coupled to mass spectrometry with sequential fragmentations (LC/MS-MS) operating in precursor ion scan acquisition mode, a technique that allows identification of compounds derived from a prototype molecular structure based on class-specific fragmentation patterns. This process can be applied to the screening not only of AAS but also other classes of structurally related compounds.[23,24] Although designer steroids no longer may be invisible to antidoping laboratories, their toxicologic profiles remain unknown. Designer steroids add a further item to the list of substances sought after, but because they are not "known" drugs, there have not been any official toxicologic studies performed on them.[25]

The process by which the effectiveness and toxicity of a newly developed drug are determined with human volunteers can be structured into three stages (phases) after a drug is designed, synthesized, and preliminarily tested in vitro and in animal models.

1. In phase I clinical trials, a new drug or treatment is tested for the first time in a small group of people (20–80) to evaluate its activity, determine a safe dosage range, and identify the most evident side effects.
2. In phase II clinical trials, a study drug or treatment is administered to a larger group of people (100–300) to verify efficacy and further evaluate safety.
3. In phase III studies, a study drug or treatment is given to large groups of people (1000–3000) to confirm evidence obtained in phases I and II, to monitor the potential side effects further, to compare features to those of reference drugs and treatments, and to collect as much clinical information as possible to a the drug or treatment to be used safely in routine medical practice.

None of these steps ever has been performed or considered for designer steroids. For this reason, designer steroids represent perhaps the most dangerous threat to the health of athletes, and the administration of these drugs or any illicitly produced drug should be discouraged.

THE HIDDEN RISKS OF NUTRITIONAL SUPPLEMENTS AND THE PARALLEL MARKET

A final aspect that has to be considered is the massive use by athletes of nonpharmaceutical products, especially nutritional supplements. These products (originally containing only amino acids, vitamins, and mineral salts) readily are available, actively marketed, and massively used by athletes. Because nutritional supplements are not drugs and generally seen as "performance-allowing" rather than "performance-enhancing" substances (and, as such, not included in the WADA-prohibited list), they are not actively included in many studies. If used correctly, nutritional supplements generally are believed safe, with the only known health risks consequent to intolerance or overdosing.[26,27] There are some cases in which the situation is not that simple: for instance, when a product contains one or more substances (or their precursors) included in the WADA list, especially when an athlete is not aware of their presence.[28] This is the case for (1) herbal products, in which the active principles may be indicated with different names (eg, ma huang instead of ephedrine); (2) prohormones, in which the active principles, correctly indicated in the label, are metabolic precursors of endogenous steroid hormones (such as androstenedione and norandrostenedione, precursors of testosterone and nandrolone, respectively); and (3) contaminated or mislabeled products, in which an athlete may be unaware of the presence of a forbidden substance. In the last case, presence of the illicit substance can be the result of accidental contamination or fraud. This problem was identified first by WADA-accredited laboratories. The Cologne Laboratory performed a thorough investigation of the products available on the international market (including those marketed via the Internet), identifying a high percentage of contaminated products.[29] Even in those products in which the concentration of nonlabeled ingredients is low (less than 0.01%), the risks for accumulation cannot be neglected, as many athletes regularly ingest considerable doses of nutritional supplements for long durations of time.

These observations also apply to the broad variety of pseudopharmaceutical products that increasingly are available via the Internet: in these cases, the lack of any pharmaceutical-grade quality control during their productive process could add further risks to those described for "pure" substances. The basic recommendation (as stated by the IOC Medical Commission in 2001) is to limit the use of nutritional supplements to certified products. Any other product should be evaluated carefully and possibly tested by specialized laboratories before being used.

SOME CONCLUSIONS AND PERSPECTIVES: TOWARD A COMPREHENSIVE TOXICOLOGY OF PERFORMANCE-ENHANCING DRUGS

The study of the adverse side effects of PEDs is far from complete. Stimulation of the development of novel investigative tools could complement (1) the toxicologic studies performed as a part of the development of any new drug; (2) the statistic data supplied by the WADA-accredited antidoping laboratories (also considering the forthcoming activation of specific protocols for the longitudinal follow-up of athletes); (3) the indirect evidence obtained by studies performed on animal models; and (4) the anecdotic information circulated within athletes' environments. A complete assessment of the overall toxicologic profile of the many different PEDs likely will result from such thorough investigations.

The authors also believe that a decisive contribution could originate from the results of ad hoc in vitro studies, which could simulate conditions in which PEDs are used. It is ethically unacceptable to design toxicity studies on humans to reproduce the effects of a real doping protocol; at the same time, the simple extrapolation of results obtained from animal models likely are overly simplistic. The toxic effects of a drug likely are different in patients or healthy volunteers versus intensively training athletes, who are exposed to acidosis, hypoxemia, and tachycardia; toxicodynamic and toxicokinetics can be altered in those conditions. A further result of such an integrated approach would be to shift the interest in use of PEDs from a forensic to a clinical context, allowing not only the identification of markers of exposure to but also of markers of effects of doping substances and methods.

REFERENCES

1. Zerbini M. Alle Fonti del Doping. Fortune e prospettive di un tema storico-religioso. Roma (Italy): "L'Erma" di Bretschneider; 2001 [in Italian].
2. Christopoulos GA, editor. The Olympic games in ancient Greece. Athens (Greece): Ekdotike Hellados S.A.; 2003.
3. Yalouris N. Origin and history of the games. In: Christopoulos GA, editor. The Olympic games in ancient Greece. Athens (Greece): Ekdotike Hellados S.A.; 2003. p. 88–93.
4. Kyrkos B. The development of sport in Hellenistic and Roman Periods. In: Christopoulos GA, editor. The Olympic games in Ancient Greece. Athens (Greece): Ekdotike Hellados S.A.; 2003. p. 289–300.
5. Wagner JC. Enhancement of athletic performance with drugs. An overview. Sports Med 1991;12:250–65.
6. Le Mondenard JP. Dopage aux jeux olympiques. Condé-Sur-Noireau (France): Editions Amphora SA; 1996 [in French].
7. Guezennec CY. Doping: effectiveness, consequences, prevention. Ann Endocrinol (Paris) 2001;62:33–41.
8. The World Anti-Doping Code. World anti-doping agency. Montreal (Canada). 2003. Available at: www.wada-ama.org. Accessed October 31, 2007.
9. The World Anti-Doping Code. The 2008 prohibited list international standard. World Anti-doping Agency. Montreal (Canada); 2007. Available at: www.wada-ama.org. Accessed October 31, 2007.
10. Botrè F. Drugs of abuse and abuse of drugs in sportsmen: the role of in vitro methods to study effect and mechanism. Toxicol In Vitro 2003;17:509–13.
11. Donohoe T, Johnson N. Foul play? Drug abuse in sport. Oxford (United Kingdom): Blackwell; 1986.
12. Wadler GI, Hainline B. Drugs and the athlete. Philadelphia: FA Davis Company; 1989.
13. Cowan DA, Kicman AT. Doping in sport: misuse, analytical tests, and legal aspects. Clin Chem 1997;43:1110–3.
14. Segura J. Sports. In: Karch SB, editor. Drug abuse handbook. Boca Raton (USA): CRC Press; 1998. p. 641–726.
15. Peters C, Schulz T, Michna H, editors. Biochemical side effects of doping. Köln (Germany): Sport & Büch Strauss; 2001.
16. Botrè F. Classi di sostanze e metodi doping. Schede riassuntive. In: Il CONI contro il doping. 2nd edition. Rome (Italy): National Italian Olympic Committee; 2001. p. 19–37 [in Italian].
17. Menthéour E, Blanchard C. Secret Défonce. Ma vérité sur le dopage. Paris: J-C Lattès; 1999 [in French].

18. Catlin DH, Ahrens BD, Kucherova Y. Detection of norbolethone, an anabolic steroid never marketed, in athletes' urine. Rapid Commun Mass Spectrom 2002;16:1273–5.

19. Catlin DH, Sekera MH, Ahrens BD, et al. Tetrahydrogestrinone: discovery, synthesis, and detection in urine. Rapid Commun Mass Spectrom 2004;18:1245–9.

20. Sekera MH, Ahrens BD, Chang YC, et al. Another designer steroid: discovery, synthesis, and detection of 'madol' in urine. Rapid Commun Mass Spectrom 2005;19:781–4.

21. Malvey TC, Armsey TD II. Tetrahydrogestrinone: the discovery of a designer steroid. Curr Sports Med Rep 2005;4:227–30.

22. Georgakopoulos C, Vonaparti A, Stamou M, et al. Preventive doping control analysis: liquid and gas chromatography time-of-flight mass spectrometry for detection of designer steroids. Rapid Commun Mass Spectrom 2007;21:2439–46.

23. Thevis M, Geyer H, Mareck U, et al. Screening for unknown synthetic steroids in human urine by liquid chromatography-tandem mass spectrometry. J Mass Spectrom 2005;40:955–62.

24. Mazzarino M, Turi S, Botrè F. A screening method for the detection of synthetic glucocorticoids in human urine by liquid chromatography—mass spectrometry based on class characteristic fragmentation pathways. Anal Bioanal Chem, in press.

25. Botrè F. I controlli antidoping nel terzo millennio: mai più sostanze 'invisibili'? Med Sport 2007;60:119–31 [in Italian].

26. Botrè F, Tranquilli C. Uso e diffusione degli integratori in Italia: opinioni a confronto. Med Sport 2001;54:263–74 [in Italian].

27. Caprino L, Braganò MC, Botrè F. Gli integratori fitoterapici nello sport: uso ed abuso. Ann Ist Super Sanita 2005;41:35–8 [in Italian].

28. Pipe A, Ayotte C. Nutritional supplements and doping. Clin J Sport Med 2002;12:245–9.

29. Geyer H, Parr MK, Mareck U, et al. Analysis of non-hormonal nutritional supplements for anabolic-androgenic steroids—results of an international study. Int J Sports Med 2004;25:124–9.

30. Spitzer G. Doping with children. In: Peters C, Schulz T, Michna H, editors. Biochemical side effects of doping. Köln (Germany): Sport & Büch Strauss; 2001. p. 127–39.

Sleep, Recovery, and Performance: The New Frontier in High-Performance Athletics

Charles Samuels, MD, CCFP, DABSM[a,b,*]

KEYWORDS

• Sleep • Fatigue • Sleep deprivation • Sleep quality

The relationship between sleep and post-exercise recovery (PER) and performance in elite athletes has become a topic of great interest because of the growing body of scientific evidence confirming a link between critical sleep factors, cognitive processes, and metabolic function. Although a complete understanding of the function of sleep in humans remains unknown and contested on many fronts, certain indisputable facts remain: sleep restriction (sleep deprivation) is linked causally to cognitive impairment;[1] there is interindividual variability in the response to sleep deprivation with respect to the degree of cognitive impairment;[2] and critical metabolic, immunologic and restorative physiologic processes are negatively affected by sleep restriction, sleep disturbance, and forced desynchrony of the human circadian sleep/wake phase.[3]

Sleep has been identified by elite athletes, coaches, and trainers as an important aspect of the PER process, and is thought to be critical for optimal performance,[4] even though there is little scientific evidence supporting this observation. The first comprehensive review of sleep and sport[5] concluded that

1) Little is known about the relationship between sleep to PER and performance in elite athletes.
2) Current interventions are based largely on clinical experience and evidence derived from research in other fields, far removed from elite athletics.
3) More sophisticated research methodology is required.

This article originally appeared in *Neurologic Clinics*, Volume 26, Issue 1.

[a] Centre for Sleep and Human Performance, #106, 51 Sunpark Drive SE, Calgary, Alberta, Canada T2X 3V4

[b] Department of Family Medicine, Faculty of Medicine, University of Calgary Health Sciences Centre, 3330 Hospital Drive NW, Calgary, Canada AB T2N 4N1

* Centre for Sleep and Human Performance, #106, 51 Sunpark Drive SE, Calgary, Alberta, Canada T2X 3V4.

E-mail address: chuck@centreforsleep.com

Phys Med Rehabil Clin N Am 20 (2009) 149–159

doi:10.1016/j.pmr.2008.10.009

Previous research in the fields of aviation, transportation, and the military has established that sleep is an active physiologic state, during which critical metabolic, immunologic, and cognitive/memory processes occur.[6] Sleep-deprivation studies have demonstrated a significant effect on glucose metabolism, appetite, and fat deposition.[1] Cognitive performance (psychomotor vigilance) has been shown to be directly affected by sleep deprivation, with a distinct interindividual variability in the response to various doses of sleep deprivation.[2] The impact of sleep disturbance on learning and neural plasticity has also been established. The positive or mitigating effect of recovery sleep (strategic napping) has been established as well in sleep-deprivation studies.[3]

Current research performed to explore the relationship between sleep and PER and performance in athletes has been of questionable value because of the multiple variables affecting sleep in athletes, the limitations of the research methodology, and the small sample sizes. To establish an effective research plan, the first step is to identify the key sleep factors of interest (primary outcomes) and to identify valid, reliable measures for subjective capture of these data. With these tools, the relationship of sleep to PER and performance can be explored in a structured fashion. Sleep length (total sleep requirement: hours/night), sleep quality (sleep disturbance or fragmentation), and sleep phase (circadian timing of sleep) are the key factors affecting the overall recuperative outcome of the sleep state.[7] Valid, reliable, subjective and objective measures of these factors can be used to explore the relationship of sleep to PER and performance in athletes. This article describes the theoretic concepts, discusses the results of pilot study data and proposes future research directions.

THEORETICAL CONCEPTS
Sleep Requirement (Total Sleep Time)

There is great interest and debate over the optimum amount of sleep (sleep length) required for humans to recuperate and function normally. Van Dongen and colleagues[2] have shown a dose-response relationship between hours of sleep deprivation and decline in cognitive function using the psychomotor vigilance task. Although a research subject's performance was relatively stable over the course of the experiment, there were significant differences among subjects in their responses to the negative effects of sleep deprivation.[2] In other words, different subjects respond differently to the same amount of sleep deprivation. Walker and Stickgold[3] have summarized the relationship of sleep to consolidation of skill memory and performance enhancement, concluding that sleep restriction poses a risk to sleep-dependent memory consolidation and neural plasticity. Thus a causal relationship exists among sleep, memory, and performance. These results substantiate the importance of adequate sleep (amount and quality) for athletes to ensure optimal performance when cognitive tasks and psychomotor vigilance is required. Human sleep deprivation studies support the assumption that sleep restriction (sleep debt) has a negative effect on neuroendocrine and immune function.[8] Critical metabolic and immune processes are known to occur during specific stages of sleep. Therefore, a critical relationship exists between physiologic recovery during the sleep state and an athlete's ability to train at maximum capacity with optimal results. Overtraining syndrome or chronic training fatigue is a common phenomenon that negatively affects athletes, and is believed to be predominantly the result of immunologic,[9] neuroendocrinological,[10] and musculoskeltal[11] factors. Therefore, determination of an athlete's total sleep need and ongoing sleep debt is likely a critical factor affecting PER, performance and susceptibility to overtraining syndrome.

Sleep Quality (Sleep Disturance)

Nonrestorative sleep is the descriptor used to account for the fact that some people get enough sleep (achieve their total sleep need) on a nightly basis, but the quality of the sleep is inadequate. Sleep quality is disturbed by sleep fragmentation as a result of recurrent arousal throughout the sleep period, without full awakening, or light sleep as a result of a hyperaroused state, with recurrent awakening throughout the sleep period.[12] Brief arousal and full awakening during the sleep period are associated with a sympathoadrenal response that negatively impacts sleep quality. Athletes who suffer with nonrestorative sleep may be tired from training as well as from not achieving the full restorative benefit of their sleep. Therefore, determining the athlete's sleep quality is another sleep factor that could be a critical determinant of PER, performance, and prevention of overtraining.

Timing of Sleep (Circadian Phase)

The circadian timing of sleep directly affects sleep length and sleep quality. The circadian phase is both genetically and environmentally determined in humans.[13,14] Each athlete has a preferred sleep schedule that suits his or her circadian phase; however, training, school, and work commitments can have a substantial impact on the athlete's ability to match the circadian phase to the sleep schedule. If the circadian preference and sleep schedule are not matched and are out of phase, this will affect the amount and quality of the sleep. For example, night owls who prefer to go to bed later and sleep in (1 AM–9 AM) and who then have to wake up at 5 AM to train at 6 AM will curtail their sleep by 2 to 4 hours per night, missing critical periods of rapid eye movement (REM) sleep and slow wave sleep.

THE CLINICAL SIGNIFICANCE OF SLEEP, RECOVERY, AND PERFORMANCE
Case 1

A 19-year-old male university swimmer presented with a 3-year history of increasing fatigue and inability to tolerate standard training volume and intensity, following a prolonged viral illness. The sleep history was significant for a lifetime of light nonrestorative sleep and intermittent violent myoclonic jerking in sleep. Teammates would not share a room with him because of his habit of banging the wall throughout the night. His mother reported an occasion when the athlete was sleeping in the passenger seat of a car and he struck her while she was driving. The provisional diagnosis was periodic limb movement disorder and nonrestorative sleep. The hypnogram of sleep (**Fig. 1**) revealed an absolutely normal night of sleep with appropriate sleep staging. The sleep electroencephalograph (EEG) revealed a pattern, referred to as alpha-delta intrusion, consistent with that seen in patients who describe "nonrestorative sleep." The synchronized digital video revealed normal myoclonic jerking in sleep. The key clinical factor in this case is the fact that this athlete is being chronically sleep restricted by 1 to 2 hours per day when morning training begins at 6 AM. The chronic sleep restriction deprives the athlete of a long period of REM sleep in the morning. The combination of chronic sleep restriction and REM sleep deprivation contributes to ongoing fatigue; impaired memory, cognition, and learning; and finally impaired immunologic function. This could account for the prolonged recovery from the viral insult.

Case 2

A 17-year-old female ice hockey goalie presented with initial insomnia and situational anxiety. She was diagnosed with a delayed sleep phase, with a preferred sleep

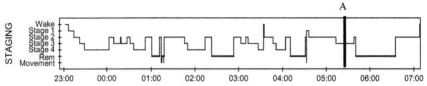

Fig. 1. Hypnogram: Progression of Sleep Staging through the night based on the sleep EEG. Nineteen-year-old national team swimmer sleep hypnogram from nocturnal polysomnography. Sleep staging on the X-axis descends from wake through stages 1 and 2 light non-REM sleep to stages 3 and 4 deep slow wave sleep to REM sleep (indicated by heavy black lines). The Y-axis indicates time 11:00 PM bed time and 7:00 AM wake time. The hypnogram represents a perfectly normal descent into sleep for a 19-year-old with slow wave sleep dominating the first third of the sleep period and a progressive increase in REM density and frequency toward morning intermixed with light stages 1 and 2. The key factor in the hypnogram is to note that rising at 5:30 AM (A) for early morning training clearly eliminates a large REM period on a daily basis and restricts the sleep chronically by 1–2 hours per day.

schedule of 1 AM to 9 AM. Attempts at going to sleep earlier than 11 PM resulted in a 2-hour sleep onset latency, causing anxiety over not being able to fall asleep. This was inadequately treated with a sedative/hypnotic (7.5 mg of zopiclone nightly at bedtime). She was waking early for training at 6 AM and having trouble with her training regimen. Once the delayed sleep phase was treated with a seasonal affective disorder (SAD) light,[15] which advances the sleep phase by adjusting melatonin secretion, she was able to adjust her training schedule. She was then able to fall asleep earlier and wake spontaneously at 7 to 8 AM. She began going to the gym later, at 9 AM, and experienced major positive benefits in her training, including weight gain, improved strength, and better performance. The sedative medication was no longer needed once the sleep phase was advanced. Delayed sleep phase syndrome is a circadian rhythm disorder that is best treated with chronotherapy (SAD light and/or melatonin) and not a sedative/hypnotic. This case illustrates the importance of a comprehensive sleep assessment for determination of the cause of initial insomnia. Additionally, adjustment of the sleep phase improved the training regimen and response.

Case 3

A 20-year-old female university swimmer who had a 6-year history of chronic daytime fatigue and recurrent upper respiratory tract infections followed by a bout of mononucleosis was referred for a sleep assessment. The sleep history revealed a preference for a delayed sleep phase, predisposition to initial insomnia, and according to the parents, loud, disruptive snoring. She was referred for ongoing fatigue and possible sleep disorder. The medical workup for fatigue was negative. She was being treated for depression with 20 mg of citalopram every morning, and her mood was stable. Sleep history was unremarkable except for the snoring. A sleep apnea screening study was performed, and she had evidence of high upper airway resistance associated with the snoring.[16] This is a well-described phenomenon that is known to cause recurrent arousals throughout the night, similar to sleep apnea, as a result of partial closure of the airway, increased resistance to airflow, and increased respiratory effort. A therapeutic trial of an autotitrating positive airway pressure (autoPAP) device was done for 2 weeks, followed by 2 weeks off therapy. The patient noted a substantial improvement in her daytime fatigue with therapy. This case points to the importance of careful exploration of the sleep history in order to determine if any primary sleep disorders could be disturbing the quality of the sleep on a chronic basis.

These clinical cases exemplify the importance of determining the athlete's total sleep requirement, the presence of sleep disturbance/fragmentation, and the athlete's preferred circadian sleep phase. Evaluating these sleep factors may explain an athlete's ongoing problems with nonrestorative sleep and chronic training fatigue. More importantly, optimizing these sleep factors for the athlete may have a substantial impact on training, PER, and performance.

A PILOT STUDY OF SLEEP QUALITY AND CIRCADIAN SLEEP PHASE IN COMPETITIVE ATHLETES

In an effort to determine the prevalence of poor sleep quality, circadian sleep phase preference, and possible sleep disorders in a spectrum of competitive athletes, a pilot survey of two groups of athletes was performed. The preliminary results of this pilot project are discussed below.

National Sport School

The National Sport School (NSS) is a special school within the Calgary Board of Education for junior athletes in grades 9 through 12 (**Table 1**) that accommodates tier travel, training, and competition schedules. Forty-six athletes attended the 2-hour educational program. Each athlete/student anonymously completed the Pittsburgh Sleep Quality Index (PSQI)[17] and Athlete Morningness/Eveningness Scale (AMES).[18] All athletes were offered a consultation with the sleep physician.

Pittsburgh sleep quality index

The PSQI is a validated, adult, self-report questionnaire providing a global score of sleep quality. The questionnaire is composed of 19 questions divided into seven component scores: (1) sleep quality, (2) sleep latency, (3) sleep duration, (4) habitual sleep efficiency, (5) sleep disturbance, (6) use of sleep medication, and (7) daytime dysfunction. There is no validated psychometric tool for the assessment of sleep quality in adolescents. The PSQI does provide some indication of sleep quality based on the above parameters, and has face validity for this pilot study. A global score of 5 or higher is considered to indicate poor sleep quality, although a more conservative score of 8 or higher is occasionally used. These cutoffs are based on the assumption that a total sleep time of 7 hours per night is adequate for an adult. However it is well-known and advocated by the National Sleep Foundation that adolescents require 8 to 10 hours of sleep per day.[19] Therefore, a PSQI global score cutoff of 5 or higher in this adolescent population likely underestimates the prevalence of poor sleep quality based on the parameter of total sleep time alone.

Students achieved global scores ranging from 2 to 16 (**Fig. 2**). Eighty-five percent of the athletes scored greater than or equal to 5, and 21% of the athletes scored greater

Table 1 National Sport School Demographics				
(N[a] = 46)	n[b]	Percent (%)	Mean	Range
Age (yrs)	46		15.58	14–18
Gender				
Male	25/44[c]	56.8		
Female	19/44[c]	43.18		

[a] Total Sample Size.
[b] Group Sample Size.
[c] Two did not indicate gender.

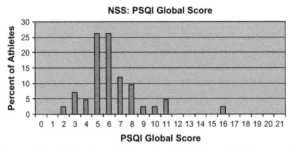

Fig. 2. National Sport School Pittsburgh Sleep Quality Index global score distribution. Approximately 85% of athletes surveyed scored greater than or equal to 5 on the PSQI, indicating a substantial prevalence of poor sleep quality in this pilot population of adolescent athletes.

than or equal to 8 (**Table 2**). Clearly there is a wide range of sleep qualities, with a preponderance of poor sleep quality in this population. In fact, most of these athletes were found to be getting less than 8 hours of sleep per night, and this would not be detected as abnormal using the adult scoring system. Therefore it is likely that a higher percentage of the athletes would have been found to be abnormal if the total sleep time was adjusted for age.

The athlete morningness/eveningness scale

The AMES is a four-item, self-report questionnaire designed to classify the respondent's chronotype in terms of preferred sleep/wake phase and preferred competition and training time. The questionnaire has not been validated, but is the only chronotype questionnaire specifically designed for athletes. The AMES provides a global score within a numeric range of 10 (extreme evening type) to 31 (extreme morning type). Score categories break down in ranges as follows: extreme evening type (10–12), moderate evening type (13–17), mid-range type (18–23), moderate morning type (24–28) and extreme morning type (29–31).

The assumption in this adolescent population of athletes was that there would be a preponderance of moderate and extreme evening types, because of the normal tendency for the sleep phase to delay in adolescence. This would be a significant factor affecting total sleep time and scheduled morning training sessions in athletes whose sleep phase was delayed. The consequences are expressed as difficulty waking for morning training (common in swimmers) and chronically restricting the total sleep time because of difficulty falling asleep at night (initial insomnia). The author

Table 2					
National Sport School Pittsburgh Sleep Quality Index: Global Score Distribution					
(N[a] = 42/46[b])	n[c]	Percent (%)	Mean	SD[d]	Range
PSQI Global Score			6.28	2.49	2–16
≥ 5	36	85.71			
≥ 8	9	21.43			

[a] Total Sample Size.
[b] Four were invalid.
[c] Group Sample Size.
[d] Standard Deviation.

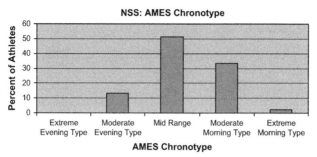

Fig. 3. National Sport School Athlete Morningness/Eveningness chronotype distribution. Only 13% of these adolescent athletes were classified as "Moderate Evening Type". The remainder of the athletes were classified as "Mid Range" or "Morning Type," which is contrary to what would be expected in this population. This finding may reflect the impact of environmental factors such as forced early awakening for training and school.

speculates that the origin of chronic training fatigue in elite adult athletes is related to inadequate time for recovery during critical adolescent years as a result of long-term chronic sleep restriction.

Interestingly and contrary to hypothesis, the results of the AMES indicate that most athletes (>85%) are mid-range to morning types (**Fig. 3**; **Table 3**). Only 13% of the athletes are moderate evening types, and there were no extreme evening types (see **Fig. 3**; **Table 3**). Although the natural tendency toward a delayed sleep phase in adolescence may not be highly relevant, this tendency still occurs in more than 10% of such athletes, and should be evaluated and addressed in individual cases in order to improve sleep-related training and performance issues.

Bobsleigh Canada Skeleton

Bobsleigh Canada Skelton (BCS) incorporated a sleep education component into its 2007 summer training camp, consisting of four sessions, each 2 to 3 hours long, addressing the basic science of sleep, sleep disorders, and travel fatigue. Athletes who attended the sessions (**Table 4**) were asked to anonymously fill out the PSQI and AMES. All athletes were offered a consultation with the sleep physician.

Table 3
National Sport School Athlete Morningness/Eveningness Chronotype Distribution

(N[a] = 45[b]/46)	n[c]	Percent (%)
AMES Chronotype		
Extreme Evening Type	0	–
Moderate Evening Type	6	13.33
Mid Range	23	51.11
Moderate Morning Type	15	33.33
Extreme Morning Type	1	2.22

[a] Total Sample Size.
[b] One was invalid.
[c] Group Sample Size.

Table 4
Bobsleigh Canada Skeleton Demographics

(N[a] = 24)	n[b]	Percent (%)	Mean	Range
Age (yrs)			27	21–36
Gender				
Male	10	41.67		
Female	14	58.33		

[a] Total Sample Size.
[b] Group Sample Size.

Pilot Survey Results

The results of the PSQI for the BCS athletes were similar to the NSS results. Approximately 78% of the athletes had a global PSQI score of 5 or higher and 26% had a score of 8 or higher (**Table 5; Fig. 4**). Therefore, even with a conservative cutoff for poor sleep quality of 5, a substantial number of athletes suffer from poor sleep quality and would benefit from further clinical evaluation. More importantly in the BCS group more than 10% of the athletes have global scores above 10 which clearly indicates a significant sleep problem that requires further evaluation. The distribution of the global scores for both the NSS and BCS can be seen in **Fig. 5** and reveals a similar distribution with a peak in the moderately abnormal range of 5–7 which displays the magnitude of the problem.

AMES results are more consistent with what would be expected in an adult population. More than 85% of the BCS athletes were in the mid-range to extreme morning type and there were no extreme evening types and only 14% were moderate evening types (see **Fig. 6; Table 6**).

SUMMARY

A pilot study of sleep quality and circadian sleep phase in two groups of competitive athletes spanning the lifecycle of a typical athlete, from adolescence to adulthood, suggests that the prevalence of poor sleep quality is substantial. The author's hypothesis that a delayed sleep phase (evening type), a common phenomenon in adolescence, would be prevalent in this population was not upheld. Improved sleep screening and case detection is necessary to address the concerns of athletes, parents, coaches, and trainers regarding sleep issues. Future research should focus on the validation of a sleep screening tool, and the determination of prevalence and

Table 5
Bobsleigh Canada Skeleton Pittsburgh Sleep Quality Index: Global Score Distribution

(N[a] = 23[b]/24)	n[c]	Percent (%)	Mean	SD[d]	Range
PSQI Global Score			6.304	0.672	2–13
≥5	18	78.26			
≥8	6	26.08			

[a] Total Sample Size.
[b] One was invalid.
[c] Group Sample Size.
[d] Standard Deviation.

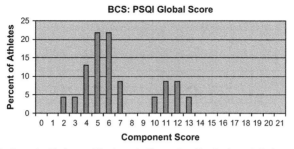

Fig. 4. Bobsleigh Canada Skeleton Pittsburgh Sleep Quality Index global score distribution. Approximately 78% of athletes surveyed scored greater than or equal to 5, indicating a substantial prevalence of poor sleep quality in this pilot population of adult athletes.

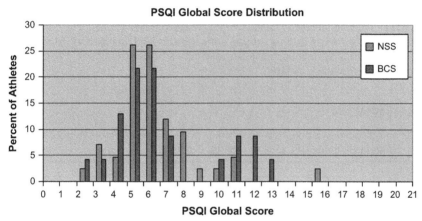

Fig. 5. PSQI Global Score Distribution National Sport School and Bobsleigh Canada Skeleton. The prevalence and distribution of abnormal PSQI global scores are similar in both groups of athletes, which suggests that sleep problems are common and occur throughout the life-cycle of an elite athlete.

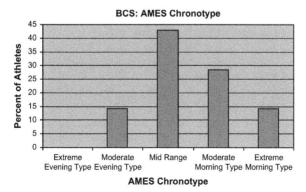

Fig. 6. Bobsleigh Canada Skeleton Athlete Morningness/Eveningess Chronotype Distribution. The distribution of chronotype in the adult athletes is in keeping with what would be expected in this age range.

Table 6
Bobsleigh Canada Skeleton Athlete Morningness/Eveningness Chronotype

(N^a = 21^b/24)	n^c	Percent (%)
AMES Chronotype		
Extreme Evening Type	–	–
Moderate Evening Type	3	14.28
Mid Range	9	42.85
Moderate Morning Type	6	28.57
Extreme Morning Type	3	14.28

[a] Total Sample Size.
[b] Three were invalid.
[c] Group Sample Size.

incidence of sleep problems in athletes. Finally, well-designed and appropriately powered studies investigating the relationship of sleep to training, PER, and performance need to be performed in order to address the fundamental question: do sleep restriction, circadian sleep phase, and sleep quality affect training response, PER, and performance in competitive athletes?

ACKNOWLEDGMENTS

The author acknowledges the assistance of the National Sport School and Bobsleigh Canada Skeleton of Calgary, Alberta, Canada.

REFERENCES

1. Spiegel K, Leproult R, Van Cauter E. Impact of sleep debt on metabolic and endocrine function. Lancet 1999;254(October 23):1435–9.
2. Van Dongen HPA, Baynard MD, Maislin G, et al. Systematic interindividual differences in neurobehavioral impairment from sleep loss: evidence of trait-like differential vulnerability. Sleep 2004;27(3):423–33.
3. Walker MP, Stickgold R. It's practice, with sleep, that makes perfect: implications of sleep-dependent learning and plasticity for skill performance. In: Postolache T, editor. Sports chronobiology. Clinics sports medicine, vol. 24(2). Philadelphia: W.B Saunders Company; 2005. p. 301–18.
4. O'Toole M. Overreaching and overtraining in endurance athletes. In: Postolache T, editor. Sports chronobiology. Clinics sports medicine, vol. 24(2). Philadelphia: W.B Saunders Company; 2005. p. 3–17.
5. Postolache T. Sports chronobiology. Clinics sports medicine, vol. 24(2). Philadelphia: W.B Saunders Company; 2005.
6. Parmeggiani PL. Physiologic regulation in sleep. In: Kryger MH, Roth T, Dement WC, editors. Principles and practice of sleep medicine. 4th edition. Philadelphia: Elsevier Saunders; 2005. p. 185–91.
7. Roehrs T. Normal sleep and its variations. In: Kryger MH, Roth T, Dement WC, editors. Principles and practice of sleep medicine. 4th edition. Philadelphia: Elsevier Saunders; 2005. p. 1–100.
8. Basta M, Chrousos GP, Vela-Bueno A, et al. Chronic insomnia and the stress system. Sleep Medicine Clinics 2007;2(2):279–91.

9. Mackinnon LT. Effects of overreaching and overtraining on immune function. In: Kreider RB, Fry AC, O'Toole ML, editors. Overtraining in sport. Windsor (Ontario): Human Kinetics Publishers, Inc; 1998. p. 219–42.

10. Keizer HA. Neuroendocrine aspects of overtraining. In: Kreider RB, Fry AC, O'Toole ML, editors. Overtraining in sport. Windsor (Ontario): Human Kinetics Publishers, Inc; 1998. p. 145–68.

11. Kibler WB, Chandler TJ. Musculoskeletal and orthopedic considerations. In: Kreider RB, Fry AC, O'Toole ML, editors. Overtraining in sport. Windsor (Ontario): Human Kinetics Publishers, Inc; 1998. p. 169–92.

12. Vgontzas AN. Understanding insomnia in the primary care setting: a new model. Insomnia Series 2004;9(2):1–7.

13. Vitaterna MH, Pinto LH, Turek FW. Molecular genetic basis for mammalian circadian rhythms. In: Kryger MH, Roth T, Dement WC, editors. Principles and practice of sleep medicine. 4th edition. Philadelphia: Elsevier Saunders; 2005. p. 363–74.

14. Viola AU, Archer SN, James LM, et al. PER3 polymorphism predicts sleep structure and waking performance. Curr Biol 2007;17:613–8.

15. Chesson AL, Littner M, Davilla D, et al. Practice parameters for the use of light therapy in the treatment of sleep disorders. Sleep 1999;22(5):641–60.

16. Velamuri K. Upper airway resistance syndrome. Sleep Medicine Clinics 2006;1: 475–82.

17. Buysse DJ, Reynolds CF, Monk TH, et al. The Pittsburgh Sleep Quality Index: a new instrument for psychiatric practice and research. Psychiatry Res 1989; 28(2):193–213.

18. Postolache T, Hung T-M, Rosenthal RN, et al. Sport chronobiolgoy consultation: from the lab to the arena. Sports chronobiology. Clinics sports medicine 2005; 24(2):415–56.

19. National Sleep Foundation 2006 Sleep in America Poll. National Sleep Foundation. Available at: http://www.sleepfoundation.org/atf/cf/{F6BF2668-A1B4-4FE8-8D1A-A5D39340D9CB}/2006_summary_of_findings.pdf. Accessed August 20, 2007.

Neuromuscular Fatigue in Racquet Sports

Olivier Girard, PhD[a],*, Grégoire P. Millet, PhD[b]

KEY WORDS

- Fatigue • Muscular fatigue • Tennis • Racquetball
- Table tennis • Squash

This article describes the physiologic and neural mechanisms that cause neuromuscular fatigue in racquet sports; table tennis, tennis, squash and badminton. In these intermittent and dual activities, performance may be limited as a match progresses because of a reduced central activation, linked to changes in neurotransmitters concentration or in response to afferent sensory feedback. Alternatively, modulation of spinal loop properties may occur because of changes in metabolic or mechanical properties within the muscle. Finally, increased fatigue manifested by mistimed strokes, lower speed, and altered on-court movements may be caused by ionic disturbances and impairments in excitation-contraction coupling properties. These alterations in neuromuscular function contribute to decrease in racquet sports performance observed under fatigue.

TECHNICAL CHARACTERISTICS AND PHYSIOLOGIC DEMANDS OF RACQUET SPORTS

Badminton, squash, and table tennis are among the most popular racquet sports, even if tennis is probably the most widely practiced. Before discussing the potential mechanisms that limit performance, the technical characteristics of these sports and the physiologic strain imposed on the players have to be described. In racquet sports, the activity pattern is intermittent; that is, characterized by repetitions of fast starts and stops and alternating brief periods of exercise at maximal or near maximal intensity, and longer periods of lower intensity.[1,2] Performance arises from complex interaction between technical, tactical, physiologic, and psychologic skills that often have to be sustained in hostile environmental conditions. To successfully endure tournament competition, racquet sports players must accelerate, decelerate, change direction, move quickly, maintain balance, and repeatedly generate optimum stroke production. This physiologic strain is influenced by hydration and nutritional status.[1–4] The duration of competition in racquet sports can vary from 30 to 60 minutes

This article originally appeared in *Neurologic Clinics*, Volume 26, Issue 1.
[a] EA 2991—Motor Efficiency and Deficiency Lab, Faculty of Sport Sciences, University of Montpellier 1, 700, avenue du Pic St Loup, Montpellier 34090, France
[b] ASPIRE—Academy for Sports Excellence, P.O. Box 22287, Doha, Qatar
* Corresponding author.
E-mail address: oliv.girard@gmail.com (O. Girard).

in squash and badminton to more than 5 hours in tennis, but average durations of 30 to 90 minutes are common in all racquet sports.[2] In most high-level matches, the rallies last on average between 2 and 15 seconds and the work-to-rest ratio varies between 1.1 and 1.5. Nevertheless, match activity varies widely across racquet sports. In tennis, the mean durations of rally and resting periods are approximately 4 to 8 seconds and 15 to 20 seconds, respectively.[1] The average effective playing time ranges usually between 10% and 30% of the game duration. In squash, the point duration is longer (10–20 seconds) and the resting period is shorter (7–8 seconds); so the effective playing time is 50% to 70% of game duration.[5,6] A summary of the results of several notational analyses of racquet sports is presented in **Table 1**.[1,2,5–7]

Research on the physiologic demands of racquet sports indicate that these sports place considerable demands on both aerobic and anaerobic pathways, but their relative contributions are controversial.[1,2,5] Estimates of exercise intensity (oxygen uptake, heart rate, or blood lactate concentrations) are described in **Table 2**.[1,2,5–7] In racquet sports, the physiologic demand may vary to a large extent, and is influenced by a multitude of factors such as the style of the player, gender, the level and style of the opponent, the surface, the equipment (ie, missile and racquet characteristics), and environmental factors (ie, temperature and humidity).[1,2]

Cardiorespiratory fitness has been traditionally measured by maximal oxygen uptake. Racquet sports players possess moderate (table tennis: $\sim$50 mL.min^{-1}.kg^{-1}; tennis: $\sim$50–55 mL.min^{-1}.kg^{-1}) to high (badminton: $\sim$55 mL.min^{-1}.kg^{-1}; squash: >60 mL.min^{-1}.kg^{-1}) aerobic capabilities, similar to those of team-sports players but obviously lower than those of endurance athletes.[2] However, an elevated cardiovascular endurance is a prerequisite attribute to compete at the elite level (ie, fast recovery between points) in all racquet sports but table tennis. Flexibility, muscular endurance, strength, and power, as well as more specific factors such as acceleration, agility, balance, and response time have also been described as important physical factors in racquet sports. At the elite level, effective stroke production requires rapid on-court movements, explosive force, and the capacity to generate explosive bursts of power. As a consequence, success in the decisive rallies at the end of a long and demanding match can be determined by the ability to repeatedly perform sprints and generate effective powerful strokes. Therefore an important issue is to describe and understand how fatigue limits performance in racquet sports.

MANIFESTATION OF FATIGUE

A close inspection of the literature reveals that the effects of fatigue on performance in squash, badminton, or table tennis players have received little documentation.[2] During the last decades, several studies have provided scientific evidence to support the

Table 1
Notational analysis in racquet sports

Activity	PD (s)	RD (s)	W:R ratio	EPT (%)	References
Table tennis	3–4	8	1:3	35	2
Tennis	5–12	15–20	1:4	20–30	1–3
Badminton	4–8	10–16	1:2	40–50	2,7
Squash	15–20	8–10	1:1	50–70	2,5,6

Abbreviations: EPT, Effective playing time; PD, point duration; RD, recovery duration; W:R ratio, work-to-rest ratio.

Table 2				
Typical physiologic strain experienced in racquet sports				
Activity	%VO$_{2max}$	%HR$_{max}$	[La] (mmol.l^{-1})	References
Table tennis	–	80–85	2	2
Tennis	60–80	70–85	2–4	1–3
Badminton	75–85	75–90	3–6	2,7
Squash	80–85	85–92	6–10	2,5,6

Abbreviations: %HR$_{max}$, percentage of maximal heart rate; [La], lactate concentration; %VO$_{2max}$, percentage of maximal oxygen uptake.

observations made by coaches that fatigue impairs performance, as shown by mistimed shots (ie, power and precision) and altered on-court movements (ie, speed, positioning to the ball). In tennis, physiologic perturbations during training and simulated matches and their combined effects on a number of performance variables have been reviewed.[3] Fatigue-inducing protocols have been recently developed to determine the effects of fatigue on stroke production in specific conditions close to those of competition.[8,9] These studies have reported conflicting results regarding change in stroke velocity and accuracy. For example, Davey and colleagues[8] observed a large decrease in the accuracy of shots played (~69% and 30% for ground stroke and serve, respectively) during an exhausting tennis simulation test, whereas accuracy was only slightly reduced (ground stroke) or unchanged (serve) after a 2-hour, on-court strenuous training session.[9] However, the lack of sensitivity and the large variability in selected variables limit considerably the generalization of these findings. Another shortcoming is that fatigue levels experienced by players failed to reflect those recorded in match play (ie, format of the protocol, using a ball machine to administer pre- and post-fatigue on-court skill assessment; Ref. [8]). For example, it is questionable how an intermittent test leading to volitional exhaustion in approximately 35 minutes could induce a degree of physiologic strain comparable to that of actual competition. These limitations have guided investigators to evaluate the effects of fatigue on performance during simulated match conditions. For example, Mitchell and colleagues[10] have reported that fatigue after a 3-hour tennis match is manifested by a decreased velocity of the serve and longer time to complete tennis pattern shuttle-runs. Using a similar approach, Girard and colleagues[11] recently reported progressive reductions in maximal voluntary strength (~10%–13% in quadriceps) and leg stiffness highly correlated with increases in perceived exertion and muscle soreness throughout a 3-hour tennis match, whereas explosive strength was maintained and decreased only after the exercise. As recently outlined by Hornery and colleagues,[3] these studies are also limited by a lack of knowledge regarding mechanisms underlying potential fatigue. Finally, it is important to keep in mind that several factors, including the environmental conditions (hot/humid), dehydration status, and intake of carbohydrate and caffeine, have been shown to affect racquet sports performance and therefore the extent of muscle fatigue experienced by players.[3,4]

DEFINING AND QUANTIFYING NEUROMUSCULAR FATIGUE

Fatigue is a complex phenomenon and has been a major research topic for exercise scientists for the last half century. Neuromuscular fatigue refers to a transient reduction in the maximal force capacity of the muscle, and is measured objectively by an acute reduction of performance during exercise.[12] The inability to produce and maintain the required force can be attributed to several potential mechanisms occurring within cortical regions to muscular contractile elements, with each of these stages as a possible limiting factor.[13] Traditionally, studies of neuromuscular fatigue during exercise have focused on alteration in the recruitment of motor units or muscles themselves.[12] In reality, it is best to use the concepts of central fatigue (ie, an exercise-induced decrease of muscle force caused by a reduction in recruitment) and peripheral fatigue (ie, decrease in force caused by a decrease in muscle fiber contractility induced predominantly by metabolic events within the muscle). However, it is not within the scope of this article to describe in detail the central and peripheral aspects of fatigue. The reader is referred to the excellent reviews of Gandevia[14] and Fitts.[15]

Reliable assessment of neuromuscular fatigue can be studied in humans using percutaneous stimulation of nerve or muscle, although this method sometimes causes discomfort.[12,16,17] This method usually associates electromyography (EMG) and measurements of voluntary and evoked forces. It is possible to superimpose an electrical or magnetic stimulation on the motor nerve (ie, tibial nerve for the soleus muscle) or to perform transcranial magnetic stimulations to evaluate the level of central fatigue of a subject.[12] In short, the twitch superimposed to a maximal voluntary contraction (MVC) is compared with the twitch evoked on the relaxed muscle in order to calculate the level of voluntary activation (twitch interpolation technique Ref.[18]). If the electrical stimulus elicits an increase in force greater than MVC, then there is reduced motor drive and central fatigue has occurred. Electrical or magnetic stimulation can also be evoked on the relaxed muscle to explore peripheral fatigue (ie, amplitude of the mechanical response). By analyzing the changes in the integrated electromyographic signal (iEMG), or root mean square (RMS), and the compound action potential (M-wave) during voluntary and evoked contractions, respectively, EMG can also be considered as an acceptable noninvasive method of measuring neuromuscular fatigue.[12] With such indices it is possible to clarify whether a decrease in MVC force is completely attributable to the loss of muscle contractile properties, or whether central drive may contribute to this decrease. This method has been applied to isometric contractions more frequently than to dynamic ones of muscles groups of both upper and lower limbs.[14] In addition, peak MVC force is commonly assessed in humans to characterize fatigue, probably because it is an easily measurable variable under relatively standardized conditions, which ultimately allow valuable comparisons between studies.[17] In racquet sports, one issue to be resolved when assessing functional impairment of fatigued muscles is that the dynamic parameters such as the rate of force development, usually analyzed in other sports, does not reflect the specific fatigue that is induced by repeated accelerations-decelerations of brief durations in order to reach maximum velocity. Therefore one may underestimate the functional muscle impairment (ie, ability to generate fast movements) by analyzing force parameters only. Furthermore, the large variability in the contraction types, the muscle groups tested, and the testing protocols (ie, nature of the exercise, ergometers, fatigue variables) complicate the interpretation of mechanisms underlying neuromuscular fatigue for a given task.[17] However, a good reliability of measurements used for characterizing central (ie, voluntary activation level or EMG) and peripheral (ie, M-wave properties or peak twitch and peak doublet torques) fatigue was recently described by Place and colleagues.[19]

It is well-established that the magnitude and the etiology of fatigue depend on the exercise (task-dependency).[20] During racquet play, fatigue develops as the duration and intensity of physical exertion increase. Transient episodes of muscular fatigue generally occur after several consecutive intense rallies. As a result of this combination of repeated sprints and the prolonged pattern of exercise, the ability to maintain exercise intensity in racquet sports represents a unique challenge. During real competitions the changes in the sequence of movement are complex and unpredictable, and are widely affected by the level and game of the opponent,[1] so this variability imposes unique physiologic demands. Therefore, it is likely that the mechanisms underlying fatigue are different among the different racquet games.

The neuromuscular adaptation to fatigue has been widely studied in conditions of voluntary isometric muscle actions (ie, Duchateau and colleagues[21]) and electrical stimulation (ie, Boerio and colleagues[22]). Much less is known, however, about the effects of real exercise such as racquet games on the neuromuscular function. This lack of direct scientific information on racquet games-specific fatigue is only partly compensated for by interpretation of data from laboratory studies or of other intermittent activities (ie, team sports). The objective of the next two sections is to carry out an integrative review of the available literature on possible causes (peripheral and central) limiting muscular performance during racquet sports competitions.

PERIPHERAL FATIGUE
Muscle Activity

At the peripheral level, surface EMG recordings during evoked contractions have been used to indirectly explore neuromuscular fatigue.[12] In human experiments, the M-wave is commonly used as an index of neuromuscular transmission and action potential propagation in muscle fibers.[23] During intense short-term activities, reductions in ionic (Na+ and K+) trans-membrane gradients may occur, resulting in a decreased M-wave amplitude.[24] Briefly, the increased intracellular Na+ and reduced intracellular K+ could be attributed to insufficient activation of the Na+/K+ muscle pumps.[24,25] After prolonged continuous exercises,[26] changes in M-wave characteristics (ie, decreased amplitude, increased duration) are rather modest, suggesting that sarcolemmal excitability does not play a fundamental role in limiting performance in these activities. In accordance with these findings, no significant change in M-wave of both vastii has been observed during a 3-hour tennis match play.[27] Rather, fatigue related to Na+-K+ disruptions might be a transient phenomenon, which would explain the temporary loss of performance (ie, incapacity to repeat powerful movements) associated with periods of repeated intense exercise bouts with incomplete recovery periods, as typically observed in racquet sports. Correspondingly, Mohr and colleagues[28] have recently postulated that temporary fatigue during an intense soccer match could be linked to an accumulation of K+ in the muscle interstitium.

Excitation-Contraction Coupling

The excitation-contraction (E-C) coupling process is the sequence of movement that starts with release of acetylcholine at the neuromuscular junction and ends with the release of Ca^{2+} from the sarcoplasmic reticulum (SR).[29] Despite the influence of stiffness alteration of the muscle-tendon complex on the evoked twitch mechanical response, it has been proposed to study the changes in the shape of this parameter to determine whether impaired intracellular Ca^{2+} regulation by the SR is implicated in the fatigue process.[25] In examining modifications of single twitches (quadriceps, Ref.[27]; soleus, Ref.[30]) during a 3-hour tennis match play, a reduced peak twitch torque has been found to occur, suggesting a failure of the E-C coupling. Although early research focused on acidosis as the most likely cause of muscular fatigue, recent evidence provides substantial support for an increase in inorganic phosphate (Pi) having a key role.[31] Pi appears to interfere with muscle function because its entry into the SR induces a Ca^{2+}-Pi precipitation, and hence decreases the Ca^{2+} available for release.

This would in turn attenuate the binding of Ca^{2+} to troponin C. Fewer cross-bridges would be formed between actin and myosin molecules, and hence a lower force or power would be generated. Low-frequency fatigue shown by a large decrease of force following stimulation at low frequency (ie, 20 Hz) concomitant with small or no change in force evoked by a stimulation at high frequency (ie, 80 Hz) has been shown to be related to a reduction in Ca^{2+} release, and is generally considered to reflect E-C coupling failure.[32] Muscular damage following exertion and low-frequency fatigue are connected. Low-frequency fatigue has been observed after prolonged tennis playing.[27] This is not surprising considering the amount of stretch-shortening cycle movements (ie, serves, jumps, or changes of direction) and eccentric contractions (ie, flexions or breakages), which may induce some structural myofibrillar impairment.

Metabolic Energy Supply

Several factors including decreased phosphocreatine (PCr) availability, increased muscle acidity, decreased muscle carbohydrate (glycogen) stores, or a low blood glucose level have also been suggested as causes of fatigue at the muscle level. These are beyond the scope of this article, but they are presented briefly here because they may also contribute to fatigue.

Phosphocreatine availability

After a bout of intense/maximal work, a decrease in PCr stores occurs, and the complete replenishment can last between 3 and 5 minutes.[33] The recovery time between two consecutive efforts in racquets games is largely smaller (see **Table 1**), and thus PCr stores are only partially restored between rallies, leading to a progressive depletion during a match. In soccer, decreased muscle PCr was significantly correlated with impairment in sprint ability.[28] Conversely, performance in intense intermittent exercise was improved after a period of creatine supplementation.[28] It is doubtful, however, that the PCr depletion is a predominant factor of fatigue, because muscle ATP rarely falls below 60% of pre-exercise levels during exhaustive exercise.[34]

Acidosis

There are some strong correlations between muscle (skinned fibers) fatigue (ie, reduced isometric force and shortening velocity), and the presence of high lactate ([La]) or low pH concentrations;[35,36] however, recent studies have challenged the role of acidosis as a direct cause of muscle fatigue.[31] Generally, [La] levels (see **Table 2**) and hence muscle acidity are thought to remain low (table tennis, tennis) to moderate (badminton, squash) in racquet sports competitions[2] and to contribute little to fatigue. Temporary fatigue during a game (ie, a series of consecutive intense rallies), however, may be related to high [La] or muscle acidosis. Nevertheless, it is noteworthy that [La] measured infrequently can only reflect the exercise intensity immediately before sampling. In addition, results linking acidosis and performance in racquet sports are sometimes conflicting. For example, it has been reported that performance in repeated-sprints can be maintained despite increased muscle acidity.[37] Taken together, these findings suggest that acidosis is probably not the most important cause of neuromuscular fatigue in intermittent activities. However, further studies are required to determine the role of acidosis in racquet games.

Muscle glycogen

The close association between fatigue and glycogen depletion during prolonged continuous exercise is well-documented.[38] Although conflicting results have been reported (ie,[37]), there is good evidence that low muscular and hepatic glycogen concentrations play an important role in limiting performance during long-term high-intensity intermittent exercises. For example, soccer players who have low pre-match muscle glycogen spent more time walking and less time sprinting than their counterparts who had a higher muscle glycogen content.[38] However, there is little direct information concerning the rate and extent of muscle glycogen depletion during racquet sports. Carbohydrate intake has been found to improve explosive strength (Sargent jump) after 2 hours of tennis.[39] These findings suggest an unexplored relationship between low muscle glycogen levels and fatigue during prolonged racquet sports matches. In addition, it is known that glycogen concentrations directly influence the metabolism of neurotransmitters involved in the central component of fatigue.[40]

Glucose
In tennis, blood glucose concentration does not decrease significantly,[10] and in most cases actually increases.[41,42] Hypoglycemia (ie, low blood glucose) per se is therefore unlikely to be a factor in fatigue during tennis and probably more generally in the other racquet sports.

CENTRAL FATIGUE
Evidence of Central Activation Failure

There is a growing body of literature to support a predominant association between fatigue in racquet sports and reduced neural drive to muscle.[27,30,43] The role of central fatigue in neuromuscular perturbations can be studied using the twitch inter-polation technique, the ratio of the EMG signal during MVC normalized to the M-wave amplitude or the comparison of torques achieved with maximal voluntary and electrically-induced contractions.[12,26] Using a combination of these different methods on two lower limb muscle groups (ie, quadriceps and soleus muscles), it has been shown that central activation deficit occurs progressively during a 3-hour tennis match.[27,30] Such central activation failure has been observed by several au-thors during the latest stages of prolonged running and cycling exercises performed at a fixed intensity,[26] and more recently after repeated cycling sprints.[44] If different types of exercise (intense versus prolonged) produce acute changes in muscular per-formance, however, the magnitude of these changes differs according to the type of contraction involved, the muscle groups involved, and the exercise duration and in-tensity; a phenomenon termed "task-dependency".[20] Thus, it is likely that the mech-anisms underlying fatigue in the different racquet games are different. Future experimentation should therefore be designed to investigate the role of fatigue in the impairment of performance in badminton, table tennis, or squash. Based on their central governor model, St Clair Gibson and Noakes[45] proposed that during self-paced, continuous exercise, the central nervous system continuously modifies the pace as part of a complex, nonlinear dynamic system. This model predicts that the ultimate control of exercise performance resides in the brain's ability to vary the work rate and the metabolic demand by altering the number of skeletal muscle motor units recruited during exercise, with the end point of the exercise acting as the reference point. In the study by Girard and colleagues,[27] the progressive reduc-tion in normalized EMG and muscle activation level as the exercise progressed could be interpreted as a protective mechanism of the neuromuscular system.[14] However, "pacing" does not make sense in racquet sports because the games are not predict-able and are influenced by numerous factors, including the level and style of the op-ponents.[1] Collectively, these results indicate that a reduced number of motor units are voluntarily recruited by the subjects, or that the maximal discharge rate from ac-tive motor units is not attained[46] in the latter stages of an exhausting tennis match.[27,30] Nevertheless, the ability to identify central and peripheral fatigue is complicated by the facts that both supraspinal and spinal mechanisms are involved, and that spinal fatigue involves both positive and negative influences of afferent sensory feedbacks.

Supraspinal Fatigue

Changes in neurotransmitter concentrations and flux have been suggested to be involved in central fatigue (ie, supraspinal fatigue). Increase in serotonin, dopamine, and acetylcholine concentrations in the brain may reduce the rate of central neural drive, which negatively influences the excitement and recruitment of skeletal muscles.[47] It has been also clearly shown that an increase in the ratio of free tryptophan:-branched chain amino acids (BCAA) in the circulation could affect prolonged performance via an increased concentration of free tryptophan (the serotonin precursor) in the brain.[48] Struder and colleagues[43] have postulated that the fatigue-induced reduction in performance in racquet sports players has a supraspinal origin: indeed, 4 hours of singles tennis increased the free tryptophan:BCAA ratio more than 2.5-fold. In addition, it is thought that these changes in neurotransmitters concentration have an important effect on arousal, lethargy, sleepiness, and mood state,[48] which in turn may influence the cognitive and sensorial variables (ie, perception of effort, stress management, tactical choices) during decisive rallies. Interestingly, it has been suggested that nutritional status (especially the carbohydrate metabolism) affects neurotransmitter metabolism, such as with an increase in carbohydrate intake attenuating fatigue-related increases in serotonin.[40] In short, carbohydrate supplementation before or during exercise aims to limit depletion of muscle glycogen stores by attenuating the rise in free fatty acids, which in turn contributes to limiting the augmentation of some precursors of central fatigue (ie, plasma-free tryptophan:BCAA ratio). Thus, it is not surprising that carbohydrate supplementation is an efficient strategy to reduce fatigue after several hours of tennis play, even if performance variables (ie, ground stroke accuracy, number of games won and lost per match) remained unaffected by the treatment.[40] More recently, measuring handgrip force (ie, a muscle not involved in the fatiguing exercise) has also been proposed as a method of further exploration of the potential existence of supraspinal fatigue after prolonged exercise involving lower limbs.[26] However, no changes were observed in grip strength of the nondominant arm during a 3-hour tennis match suggesting that loss of cortical excitability per se is probably not the only cause of central fatigue.[30]

Spinal Fatigue

As previously stated, it is well-established that racquet sport performance may be associated with peripheral perturbations (ie, increase in metabolites, acidosis, lesser energy supply). Despite the direct effects that selected metabolites might have on muscle contractility,[15] it is also believed that neural-mediated afferent feedbacks from the muscle (ie, fusimotor system disfacilitation and presynaptic inhibition) play a role in the inhibition of motoneuron excitability.[49] Two major hypotheses have been proposed to explain the mechanisms responsible for the reduced neural drive to the muscle. The first hypothesis involves the decreased facilitation of the α-motoneuron pool concomitant to a progressive withdrawal of spinal-mediated fusimotor support.[50] The second hypothesis speculates that reduced neural activation depends on the reflex response from the contracting muscle itself to metabolic or mechanical changes.[51] An increased inhibitory drive to the α-motoneuron pool, probably mediated by small-diameter Group III and IV muscle afferents, contributes to the reduction in voluntary drive (at both spinal and supraspinal levels). Regarding racquet sports performance, this latter hypothesis is supported by a recent study[30] examining the excitability of spinal reflex loops by using combined measurements of evoked Hoffmann (H) reflex (at rest) and first volitional (V) wave (during contraction; ie, an electrophysiological variant of the H-reflex) responses during the course (each 30 minutes) of a 3-hour tennis match play. These reflexes reflect the efficiency (ie, estimate of α-motoneuron excitability) of the transmission in Ia afferent-α-motoneuron synapses (principally H-reflex) and the level of efferent and descending neural drive (mostly V-wave), and these evoked potentials are both

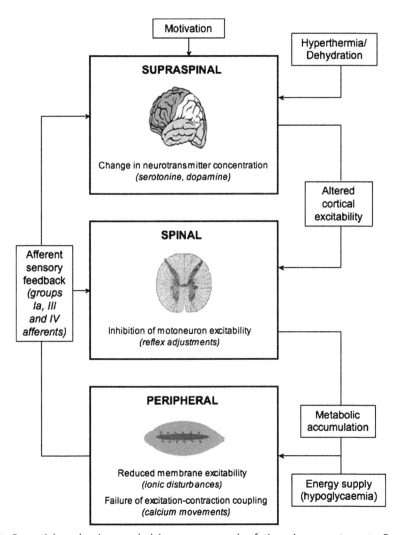

Fig. 1. Potential mechanisms underlying neuromuscular fatigue in racquet sports. Exercise performance may be limited (as match progresses) because of a reduced central activation, linked to changes in neurotransmitter metabolism or in response to afferent sensory feedbacks. Alternatively, modulation of spinal loop properties (ie, inhibition of motoneuron excitability) may occur because of changes in metabolic or mechanical properties within the muscle. Finally, the temporary fatigue observed after a series of consecutive intense rallies may be caused predominantly by a reduction in sarcolemmal excitability because of ionic disturbances and alterations in excitation contraction coupling (low-frequency fatigue).

influenced by reciprocal inhibition and recurrent inhibitions.[52] Significant reductions in H- and V-wave responses (normalized to the M-wave) were observed as the tennis match progressed, suggesting an inhibition of the spinal motoneurons (ie, modulation of spinal loop properties) during this prolonged intermittent exercise.[30] Similarly, in the other racquet sports a decrease in motoneuron excitability in response to metabolic disruptions remains a potential fatigue factor affecting the ability to fully activate the synergistic musculature (ie, ability to generate explosive power within a few seconds) (see **Table 2**). Nevertheless, future studies are needed to quantify the relative importance of the possible reflex adjustments in the neural origin of performance decrease in all racquet sports. Overall, these findings emphasize the possible role of the peripheral reflex pathways as a probable origin of the reduction in central efferent neural command in racquet sports. In addition, this suggests that the reflex may act as a protective mechanism to preserve force-generating capabilities and possibly avoid irreversible cellular damages (**Fig. 1**).[45]

SUMMARY

Fatigue impairs racquet sports performance, and can be manifested as mistimed shots, altered on-court movements, and incorrect cognitive (ie, tactical) choices. The etiology of muscle fatigue in racquet sports is a complex phenomenon that may involve impairment in both neural and contractile processes (see **Fig. 1**). Temporary fatigue observed after a series of consecutive intense rallies may be caused predominantly by a reduction in sarcolemmal excitability because of ionic disturbances and alterations in excitation contraction coupling (low-frequency fatigue). Future research should investigate if electromyostimulation[53] and resistance training[54] can improve racquet sports-related variables and delay central fatigue. Over time, research into fatigue-related mechanisms in athletes should be expanded to include other forms of sport.

REFERENCES

1. Fernandez J, Mendez-Villanueva A, Pluim B. Intensity of tennis match play. Br J Sports Med 2006;40(5):387–91.
2. Lees A. Science and the major racket sports: a review. J Sports Sci 2003;21(9): 707–32.
3. Hornery D, Farrow D, Mujika I, et al. Fatigue in tennis. Mechanisms of fatigue and effect on performance. Sports Med 2007;37(3):199–212.
4. Kovacs MS. Hydratation and temperature in tennis—a practical review. J Sci Med Sport 2006;5:1–9.
5. Girard O, Chevalier R, Habrard M, et al. Game analysis and energy requirements of elite squash. J Strength Cond Res 2007;21(3):909–14.
6. Montpetit RR. Applied physiology of squash. Sports Med 1990;10(1):31–41.
7. Cabello Manrique D, Gonzalez-Badillo JJ. Analysis of the characteristics of competitive badminton. Br J Sports Med 2003;37(1):62–6.
8. Davey PR, Thorpe RD, Williams C. Fatigue decreases skilled tennis performance. J Sports Sci 2002;20(4):311–8.
9. Vergauwen L, Spaepen AJ, Lefevre J, et al. Evaluation of stroke performance in tennis. Med Sci Sports Exerc 1998;30(8):1281–8.
10. Mitchell JB, Cole KJ, Grandjean PW, et al. The effect of a carbohydrate beverage on tennis performance and fluid balance during prolonged tennis play. Journal of Applied Sport Science Research 1992;6(2):174–80.

11. Girard O, Lattier G, Micallef J-P, et al. Changes in exercise characteristics, maximal voluntary contraction and explosive strength during prolonged tennis playing. Br J Sports Med 2006;40(6):521–6.
12. Vøllestad NK. Measurement of human muscle fatigue. J Neurosci Methods 1997; 74(2):219–27.
13. Enoka R. Muscle fatigue. In: Enoka R, editor. Neuromechanics of human movement. Champaign, Illinois: Human Kinetics; 2002. p. 374–96.
14. Gandevia SC. Spinal and supraspinal factors in human muscle fatigue. Physiol Rev 2001;81(4):1725–89.
15. Fitts RH. Cellular mechanisms of muscle fatigue. Physiol Rev 1994;74(1):49–94.
16. Allen GM, Gandevia SC, McKenzie DK. Reliability of measurements of muscle strength and voluntary activation using twitch interpolation. Muscle Nerve 1995; 18(6):593–600.
17. Cairns SP, Knicker AJ, Thompson MW, et al. Evaluation of models used to study neuromuscular fatigue. Exerc Sport Sci Rev 2005;33(1):9–16.
18. Merton PA. Voluntary strength and fatigue. J Physiol 1954;123(3):553–64.
19. Place N, Maffiuletti N, Martin A, et al. Assessment of the reliability of central and peripheral fatigue after sustained maximal voluntary contraction of the quadriceps muscle. Muscle Nerve 2007;35(4):486–95.
20. Enoka RM, Stuart DG. Neurobiology of muscle fatigue. J Appl Physiol 1992;72(5): 1631–48.
21. Duchateau J, Balestra C, Carpentier A, et al. Reflex regulation during sustained and intermittent submaximal contractions in humans. J Physiol 2002;541(3): 959–67.
22. Boerio D, Jubeau M, Zory R, et al. Central and peripheral fatigue after electrostimulation-induced resistance exercise. Med Sci Sports Exerc 2005;37(6):973–8.
23. Hicks A, McComas AJ. Increased sodium pump activity following repetitive stimulation of rat soleus muscles. J Physiol 1989;414(7):337–49.
24. Fowles JR, Green HJ, Tupling R, et al. Human neuromuscular fatigue is associated with altered Na+-K+-ATPase activity following isometric exercise. J Appl Physiol 2002;92(4):1585–93.
25. Green HJ. Mechanisms of muscle fatigue in intense exercise. J Sports Sci 1997; 15(3):247–56.
26. Millet GY, Lepers R. Alterations of neuromuscular function after prolonged running, cycling and skiing exercises. Sports Med 2004;34(2):105–16.
27. Girard O, Lattier G, Maffiuletti NA, et al. Neuromuscular fatigue during a prolonged intermittent exercise: application to tennis. J Electromyogr Kinesiol, in press.
28. Mohr M, Krustrup P, Bangsbo J. Fatigue in soccer: a brief review. J Sports Sci 2005;23(6):593–9.
29. Warren GL, Ingalls CP, Lowe DA, et al. Excitation-contraction uncoupling: major role in contraction-induced muscle injury. Exerc Sport Sci Rev 2001;29(2):82–7.
30. Girard O, Racinais S, Micallef JP, et al. Changes in motoneuron pool excitability during prolonged tennis playing. Med Sci Sports Exerc 2007;39(5):S434.
31. Westerblad H, Allen DG, Lannergren J. Muscle fatigue: lactic acid or inorganic phosphate the major cause? News Physiol Sci 2002;17(2):17–21.
32. Jones DA. High- and low-frequency fatigue revisited. Acta Physiol Scand 1996; 156(3):265–70.
33. Glaister M. Multiple sprint work: physiological responses, mechanisms of fatigue and the influence of aerobic fitness. Sports Med 2005;35(9):757–77.

34. Bangsbo J, Graham TE, Kiens B, et al. Elevated muscle glycogen and anaerobic energy production during exhaustive exercise in man. J Physiol 1992;451: 205–27.

35. Metzger JM, Moss RL. Greater hydrogen ion-induced depression of tension and velocity in skinned single fibres of rat fast than slow muscles. J Physiol 1987; 393(12):727–42.

36. Westerblad H, Lee JA, Lannergren J, et al. Cellular mechanisms of fatigue in skeletal muscle. Am J Physiol 1991;261(8):C195–209.

37. Krustrup P, Mohr M, Amstrup P, et al. The yo-yo intermittent recovery test: physiological response, reliability, and validity. Med Sci Sports Exerc 2003;35(4): 697–705.

38. Saltin B. Metabolic fundamentals in exercise. Med Sci Sports 1973;5(3):137–46.

39. Burke ER, Ekblom B. Influence of fluid ingestion and dehydratation on precision and endurance performance in tennis. In: Bachl N, Prokop L, Suckert R, editors. Current topics in sports medicine. Vienna (Austria): Urban & Schwarzenberg; 1984. p. 379–88.

40. Struder HK, Ferrauti A, Gotzmann A, et al. Effect of carbohydrates and caffeine on plasma amino acids, neuroendocrine responses and performance in tennis. Nutr Neurosci 1999;1:419–26.

41. Therminarias A, Dansou P, Chirpaz-Oddou MF, et al. Hormonal and metabolic changes during a strenuous tennis match. Effect of aging. Int J Sports Med 1991;12(1):10–6.

42. Bergeron MF, Maresh CM, Kraemer WJ, et al. Tennis: a physiological profile during match play. Int J Sports Med 1991;12(1):474–9.

43. Struder HK, Hollmann W, Duperly J, et al. Amino acid metabolism in tennis and its possible influence on the neuroendocrine system. Br J Sports Med 1995;29(1): 28–30.

44. Racinais S, Bishop D, Denis R, et al. Muscle deoxygenation and neural drive to the muscle during repeated sprint cycling. Med Sci Sports Exerc 2007;39(2): 268–74.

45. St Clair Gibson A, Noakes TD. Evidence for complex system integration and dynamic neural regulation of skeletal muscle recruitment during exercise in humans. Br J Sports Med 2004;38(6):797–806.

46. Kent-Braun JA, Le Blanc R. Quantification of central activation failure during maximal voluntary contractions in humans. Muscle Nerve 1996;19(7): 861–9.

47. Meeusen R, Watson P, Hasegawa H, et al. Central fatigue: the serotonine hypothesis and beyond. Sports Med 2006;36(10):881–909.

48. Davis JM, Bailey SP. Possible mechanisms of central nervous system fatigue during exercise. Med Sci Sports Exerc 1997;29(1):45–57.

49. Nicol C, Avela J, Komi PV. The stretch-shortening cycle: a model to study naturally occurring neuromuscular fatigue. Sports Med 2006;36(11):977–99.

50. Garland SJ. Role of small diameter afferents in reflex inhibsition during human muscle fatigue. J Physiol 1991;435(4):547–58.

51. Kniffki KD, Mense S, Schmidt RF. Responses of Group IV afferent units from skeletal muscle to stretch, contraction and chemical stimulation. Exp Brain Res 1978; 31(4):511–22.

52. Zehr PE. Considerations for use of the Hoffmann reflex in exercise studies. Eur J Appl Physiol 2002;86(6):455–68.

53. Gondin J, Duclay J, Martin A. Soleus- and gastrocnemii-evoked V-wave responses increase after neuromuscular electrical stimulation training. J Neurophysiol 2006;95(6):3328–35.
54. Aagaard P, Simonsen EB, Andersen JL, et al. Neural adaptation to resistance training: changes in evoked V-wave and H-reflex responses. J Appl Physiol 2002;92(6):2309–18.

Section 4

Neurologic Injuries in Team Sports

Peripheral Nerve Injuries in Baseball Players

Craig A. Cummins, MD*, David S. Schneider, DO

KEYWORDS

- Baseball • Peripheral nerve injury
- Nerve entrapment • Suprascapular nerve

Baseball is a sport requiring speed, coordination, strength and timing that is enjoyed by millions of people around the world. From a biomechanical perspective, the throwing motion, and in particular the pitching motion, places extreme stress on the throwing arm. Baseball pitchers are required to throw frequently, complicating the trauma placed across the pitcher's throwing arm. This combination of high stress placed on the shoulder and elbow during the throwing motion, coupled with the cumulative microtrauma caused from repetitive overuse, places baseball pitchers at increased risk for peripheral nerve injuries in the upper extremity. Neuropathies of the shoulder comprise less than 2% of all causes of pain and weakness for patients in this region.[1] Because of its uncommon nature, it is not unusual for the diagnosis of a neuropathy of the shoulder to be delayed. Signs and symptoms of a neuropathy typically overlap with more common causes of shoulder pain or weakness, further complicating diagnosis. Affected baseball players often have coexisting shoulder diagnoses such as rotator cuff pathology, labral tears, instability, and internal impingement, which may be the more dominant clinical finding. For example, patients who have suprascapular neuropathy may present with a more dominant impingement syndrome caused by to the weakness in the rotator cuff muscles as a result of the peripheral nerve injury. Baseball players are susceptible to nerve injuries seen in other sports (cervical radiculopathy, lumbar radiculopathy, "burners" or "stinger," carpal tunnel syndrome). The focus of this article is on reviewing forms of peripheral neuropathies more common to baseball players and resulting from their unique throwing motion.

BIOMECHANICS

The overhand throwing motion in baseball, initially described as occurring in three phases, has subsequently been subdivided to occur in six distinct phases (**Fig. 1**).[2,3] The initial phase of the throwing motion, stage 1, is the windup. The windup

This article originally appeared in *Neurologic Clinics*, volume 26, issue 1.

Lake Cook Orthopedic Associates, 27401 West Highway 22, #125, Barrington, IL 60010, USA

* Corresponding author.

E-mail address: ccummins@lakecookorthopedics.org (C.A. Cummins).

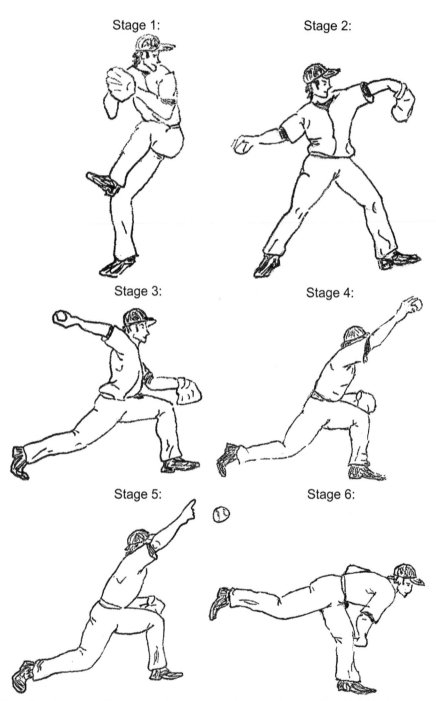

Fig. 1. The six phases of the baseball pitch: stage 1 (windup), stage 2 (early cocking), stage 3 (late cocking), stage 4 (acceleration), stage 5 (deceleration), and stage 6 (follow-through).

involves individualize body mechanics; however, it begins with the stride foot coiling backward, away from home plate, and the arms swinging overhead, imparting little stress to the upper extremity. The next portion of the throwing motion is broken up into the early cocking phase (stage 2) and the late cocking phase (stage 3). The early cocking phase begins when the ball leaves the nondominant gloved hand and ends when the forward foot comes in contact with the ground. The late cocking phase begins with the planting of the striding leg and ends with the shoulder in a position of maximum external rotation, which can be as much as 170° to 180°. In the terminal portion of the late cocking phase, the torso begins to open up and a shear force of 400 N is generated across the anterior shoulder, with the firing of the rotator cuff muscles generating a compressive force of 650 N.[4] During this phase the elbow is flexed between 90° and 120°, with forearm pronation increasing to 90°. Stage 4, the acceleration phase, rotates the shoulder internally at velocities of 7000 deg/sec, and ends with ball release. The acceleration phase occurs rapidly over a time period of approximately 0.05 seconds. During this phase the elbow accelerates as much as 3000 degrees/sec, with tremendous valgus stresses generated about the medial aspect of the elbow estimated as high as 64 N·m. The anterior bundle of the ulnar collateral ligament (UCL) complex bears the principal portion of these forces, with the secondary supporting structures being the flexor-pronator musculature.[4] Most elbow injuries occur during this acceleration phase of throwing. Stage 5, the deceleration phase, begins with ball release and ends with the cessation of humeral rotation. It is during the deceleration phase that the energy generated through the first four phases is dissipated and the upper extremity decelerates at a rate of almost 6180 deg/sec over a time span of only 50 msec.[5] During the deceleration phase a violent contraction of all muscle groups occurs, with eccentric contraction of the muscles required to slow down arm rotation.[6,7] Stage 6, the follow-through, is the final stage of the overhead throwing motion. This is the rebalancing phase where the body moves forward with the arm until motion stops. The entire throwing motion takes less than 2 seconds.[5]

PATHOPHYSIOLOGY

Peripheral nerves are highly susceptible to injury from stretch and compression. Both mechanisms of injury result in nerve ischemia, edema, microenvironmental changes, and conduction impairment. These changes are proportional to the magnitude and duration of the insult, and can lead to irreversible damage.[8–10] In a rabbit tibial nerve model, a stretch that increased in situ length as little as 6% resulted in conduction abnormalities.[8] In this same model, a stretch of 15% leads to irreversible neural functional deficits. Intraneural vascular supply to a rabbit tibial nerve was compromised when the nerve was elongated by 8%, with total occlusion at 15%.[9] Similar changes have been reported to occur with compression. The unique stresses and arm positions occurring during the baseball throwing motion likely place the peripheral nerves of the thrower's dominant upper extremity at risk for similar and significant mechanical insults. If these nerve injuries are recognized early, cessation of throwing and an appropriate rehabilitation program may be of benefit and preventative of more permanent injury.

SUPRASCAPULAR NEUROPATHY
Anatomy

The suprascapular nerve is a mixed motor and sensory nerve that arises from the upper trunk of the brachial plexus (C5 and C6 nerve roots) and supplies motor innervations to the supraspinatus and infraspinatus muscles, and sensory innervations to the coracohumeral and coracoacromial ligaments, subacromial bursa, and acromioclavicular and glenohumeral joint (**Fig. 2**). Although most anatomic studies have not identified any cutaneous innervation, cutaneous innervations of the proximal-lateral arm has been reported.[11]

After the suprascapular nerve originates from the brachial plexus, it initially courses through the posterior triangle of the neck before traveling deep to the trapezius muscle, underneath the clavicle, toward the suprascapular notch. The suprascapular nerve next crosses the suprascapular notch, passing beneath the transverse scapular ligament, with the suprascapular artery and vein traveling above the ligament. After the suprascapular nerve traverses the suprascapular notch, it typically sends two motor branches to the supraspinatus muscle, as well as sensory branches to the coracoclavicular and coracohumeral ligaments, the acromioclavicular joint, and the subacromial bursa. After passing through the suprascapular notch, the main branch of the suprascapular nerve travels inferiorly to the infraspinatus muscle, while providing a sensory branch to the posterior aspect of the glenohumeral joint.[12-14] Before reaching the infraspinatus muscle, the suprascapular nerve courses sharply around the spine of the scapular through a fibro-osseous tunnel formed by the spinoglenoid ligament and the spine of the scapula. The prevalence of the spinoglenoid ligament has been debated in the literature; however, more recent anatomic studies have identified the ligament in the majority of shoulder specimens examined.[15,16] Finally, the suprascapular nerve terminates in two to four branches innervating the infraspinatus muscle.

Etiology

The suprascapular nerve may be injured by direct trauma, including surgery, traction, clavicle fractures or dislocations.[17-19] Baseball players, however, typically sustain

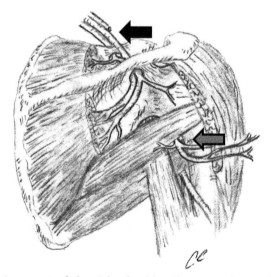

Fig. 2. The posterior aspect of the right shoulder. The supraspinatus, infraspinatus, and deltoid muscles have been partially removed. The suprascapular nerve (*black arrow*) can be identified passing under the superior transverse scapular ligament and around the spinoglenoid notch. The axillary nerve (*gray arrow*) can be identified exiting through the quadrilateral space.

injury to the suprascapular nerve because of the frequent and significant stresses place on their arms during the throwing motion. Various hypotheses have been proposed to explain suprascapular nerve injuries, including traction, compression, and vascular compromise; however, there is no consensus on which cause, if any, is dominant. A common location of injury is where the suprascapular nerve passes through the suprascapular notch underneath the superior transverse scapular ligament.[20] Injury at this location results in denervation, affecting both supraspinatus and infraspinatus muscles. Typically patients who have a suprascapular nerve injury at this location will present with posterior shoulder pain in addition to shoulder weakness.

Overhead throwing athletes seem to be particularly susceptible to distal injury to the suprascapular nerve at the spinoglenoid notch.[21–27] Patients who have injury to the suprascapular nerve at the spinoglenoid notch often present with isolated infraspinatus muscle atrophy. Because this location of nerve injury is distal to the sensory fibers from the suprascapular nerve, there may be no history of shoulder pain.[21,26] The incidence of distal suprascapular nerve injuries in overhead throwing athletes is likely significantly higher than in the general population. Not limited to baseball, asymptomatic atrophy of the infraspinatus muscle was identified in 12 of 96 top-level volleyball players.[26] Similar findings were observed in major league professional baseball players, with isolated infraspinatus muscle atrophy present in 4% of major league pitchers.[21] Infraspinatus muscle atrophy was more common among starting pitchers, more experienced pitchers, and pitchers who had thrown for more innings at the major league level, so amount of throwing appears to play a significant role.[21]

An additional cause of suprascapular nerve injury is compression by a ganglion cyst.[28,29] Baseball players can develop superior and posterior labral tears as a result of the stresses placed on the shoulder during the throwing motion. Ganglion cysts may develop because of labral tear acting as a one-way valve, permitting joint fluid to escape into the cyst cavity but not allowing the return of the synovial fluid back into the joint. The most common location for labral tears is the superior posterior labrum, which is probably why the most common location for a shoulder ganglion cyst is the spinoglenoid notch. This location of a ganglion cyst can result in compression to the suprascapular nerve once the ganglion cyst has reached sufficient size, leading to isolated denervation of the infraspinatus muscle.

Clinical Evaluation

History and examination

Patient presentation of suprascapular nerve injuries varies depending on the location of the nerve injury and the presence of additional shoulder pathology. Patients who have proximal lesions affecting the supra and infraspinatus muscles often present with posterior shoulder pain, atrophy of the involved muscles, and weakness of shoulder abduction and external rotation (**Fig. 3**). A similar presentation can be seen in patients who have chronic rotator cuff tears; however, patients who have large rotator cuff tears are typically older than the overhead throwing athlete who has a suprascapular nerve injury. Patients who have a more distal suprascapular nerve injury are often asymptomatic, and the nerve injury presentation may result from casual observation of the scapular muscle atrophy only. A small percentage of patients who have a distal suprascapular nerve injury may have posterior shoulder pain, however. This pain may be caused by dysfunction in the relationship of the posterior capsules sensory branch to the spinoglenoid ligament. Finally, it is common for a patient's initial presentation to be the result of other shoulder pathology. An example is patients who have a suprascapular nerve injury caused by a ganglion cyst, in which the labral tear associated with the ganglion cyst causes the shoulder pain leading to clinical attention.

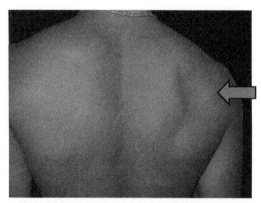

Fig. 3. Photograph of the posterior aspect of the right shoulder of an overhead athlete. Atrophy can be observed in the right infraspinatus muscle (*gray arrow*) located inferior to the right scapular spine.

Diagnostic studies

Patients who have a suspected suprascapular nerve injury should be evaluated with MRI, which not only aids in the diagnosis of suprascapular nerve injuries but also helps in the differentiation of proximal nerve injuries from more distal nerve injuries. In one investigation, Kullmer and colleagues[30] performed experimental denervation of the supraspinatus and infraspinatus muscles in rats by segmental excision of the suprascapular nerve. Identifiable muscle atrophy and increased signal intensity on T2-weighted MRI images appeared within 3 weeks of injury. MRI has the added advantage of being able to detect intra-articular lesions and ganglion cysts (**Fig. 4**). Increased sensitivity and specificity for the diagnosis of labral tears can be obtained

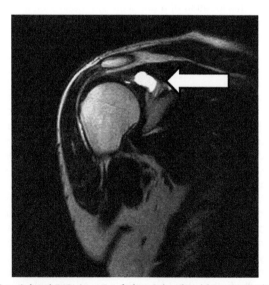

Fig. 4. Coronal T2-weighted MRI image of the right shoulder. A ganglion cyst is located superior to the glenoid fossa (*white arrow*), with extension into the spinoglenoid notch. Ganglion cysts present at this location can result in compression of the suprascapular nerve.

with the addition of intra-articular gadolinium contrast. MRI arthrography has been found to have a sensitivity of 91% and specificity of 93% for the diagnosis of labral lesions.[31]

Electrodiagnositic studies are also important in confirming the diagnosis of a suprascapular nerve injury, localizing the site of the nerve injury, and by excluding other etiologies in the differential diagnosis, such as cervical radiculopathy and brachial plexopathy. An increased latency when performing the suprascapular compound motor action potentials (CMAP) indicates demyelination or a conduction block. Although there are sensory innervations from the suprascapular nerve, there are no cutaneous nerve branches capable of generating a sensory nerve action potential (SNAP). Electromyography (EMG) is also a useful method for evaluating axonal loss from a suprascapular nerve injury by the demonstration of increased involuntary spontaneous activity with fibrillations and positive sharp waves. These changes tend to occur 2 to 3 weeks after the injury. Disadvantages of these electrodiagnositic studies include their invasiveness and user dependence; however, EMG has a high sensitivity and specificity for diagnosing the suprascapular neuropathy, and may have prognostic value. For example, identification of polyphasic potentials with large-amplitude and long-duration motor unit action potentials (MUAPS) with disappearance of involuntary activity indicates collateral sprouting, reinnervation, and the absence of ongoing denervation.

Treatment

Nonoperative

Nonoperative treatment of suprascapular nerve injuries should be considered as the initial treatment option, unless nerve compression is caused by a mass lesion. Nonoperative treatment includes the avoidance of activities felt to be causative, obviously including cessation of throwing. This treatment should be combined with a rehabilitation program. The initial focus of a rehabilitation program is on shoulder flexibility, with particular attention given to improving internal rotation contractures, postural training, and strengthening of the periscapular and deltoid muscles. Strengthening of the rotator cuff muscles can be started once symptoms of nerve impingement have subsided. The advancement of the rehabilitation program should be monitored closely to avoid reinjury to the nerve while it is healing. In general, success rates with nonoperative treatment are less satisfactory when the nerve injury results from a mass lesion such as a ganglion cyst. One concern with nonoperative treatment is that a delay in decompression of the suprascapular nerve may result in incomplete restoration of muscle function. It has been demonstrated that fatty atrophy in the rotator cuff muscle is not reversible following repair of large rotator cuff tears.[32] A similar situation likely occurs when portions of rotator cuff muscles (supraspinatus and infraspinatus) are denervated following nerve injury.

Operative treatment

The operative treatment of suprascapular nerve injuries depends on the etiology and location of the nerve lesion. When planning the surgical procedure it is important to understand the nerve injury location and the presence or absence of a ganglion cyst.

Surgical treatment of a suprascapular nerve injury when not related to a ganglion cyst is generally through a posterior surgical incision. When the nerve injury is located at the suprascapular notch, surgical management involves resection of the superior transverse scapular ligament, with or without deepening the suprascapular notch.[33] When the nerve injury is located at the spinoglenoid notch, surgical decompression involves the release of the spinoglenoid ligament, which is present in the majority of patients.[15,16] Additionally, some authors advocate deepening the spine of the scapula;[27,34] however, if the spine of the scapular is deepened more than 1 cm, the acromion is at risk of fracture. Surgical decompression, whether performed for a proximal or distal nerve injury, typically leads to resolution of patient's pain and a substantial increase in muscle strength; however, the return of muscle bulk is less predictable and requires many months to occur.[22,25,27,33–35] Reports of arthroscopic decompression of the suprascapular nerve have been described recently, but these techniques remain new and investigational.[36,37]

A different scenario exists when a ganglion cyst is compressing the suprascapular nerve; a shoulder arthroscopy should be performed to assess for a coexisting labral tear. The ganglion cyst can be drained using arthroscopic techniques at the site of the labral tear, following which the labral tear should be repaired.[38–40] Ganglion cysts can also be excised through an open incision; however, shoulder arthroscopy should be performed in this scenerio to address any underlying labral pathology[29] It is possible for ganglion cyst to recur following an open cyst excision when a labral tear has not been addressed. In one case report of a failed excision of a ganglion cyst, at a subsequent operation, arthroscopy identified a labral tear, which after correction led to no further recurrence of the ganglion cyst.[38]

AXILLARY NEUROPATHY
Anatomy

The axillary nerve supplies motor function to the deltoid and teres minor muscles, as well as providing sensation over the lateral shoulder. The axillary nerve is the terminal branch of the posterior cord of the brachial plexus, which arises from the C5 and C6 nerve roots. The nerve travels along the subscapularis muscle obliquely, and then courses under the axillary recess of the glenohumeral joint. The nerve subsequently exits posteriorly, accompanied by the posterior humeral circumflex artery, passing through the quadrilateral space, which is bound by the teres minor superiorly, the teres major inferiorly, the long head of the triceps medially, and the humeral shaft laterally (see **Fig. 2**). The axillary nerve divides into two major trunks after exiting the quadrilateral space. The posterior trunk provides motor innervations to the posterior deltoid muscle and the teres minor muscle before terminating as the superior lateral brachial cutaneous nerve supplying sensation to the lateral aspect of the shoulder. The anterior truck of the axillary continues anteriorly to the undersurface of the deltoid muscle, coursing around the humeral shaft to supply the middle and anterior deltoid muscle.

Etiology

Axillary nerve injuries are uncommon and represent less than 1% of all nerve injuries.[41] Injury to the axillary nerve in baseball players can occur as a result of a direct trauma or as the result of quadrilateral space syndrome. Direct trauma to the nerve can result from a traction injury, as can be seen with shoulder dislocations or fractures. The risk of injury to the nerve with shoulder dislocations increases with patient's age, severity of the trauma, and with the length of time that a shoulder is left unreduced.[42–44] Additionally, a direct blow to the outer aspect of the shoulder can injure the axillary nerve by compressing it against the proximal humerus. Another etiology for axillary nerve injuries is the quadrilateral space syndrome, an uncommonly reported syndrome identified in overhead throwing athletes in which the axillary nerve is compressed within the quadrilateral space. The most frequent reported cause of quadrilateral space syndrome is a fibrous band within the quadrilateral space.[45] The nerve may also be compressed because of a space-occupying lesion (ie, ganglion cyst).[46] Repetitive microtrauma may also play a causative role. Intermittent compression of the axillary nerve occurs when the shoulder is a position abduction and external rotation. This shoulder position occurs during the late cocking phase of pitching, and results in closing of the quadrilateral space by contraction of teres minor and teres major.

Clinical Evaluation

History and physical examination
Patients who have an axillary nerve injury following a direct trauma to the shoulder often provide a history of the shoulder trauma followed by decreased sensation over the lateral aspect of their upper arm. Patients may also report a history of weakness or fatigue of the arm with overhead activity or heavy lifting. Patients who have quadrilateral space syndrome generally do not report a history of trauma. It is not uncommon for the diagnosis to be delayed, and the condition may only be identified after failed treatment for other shoulder diagnoses. Pain is described as a dull ache or burning located over the posterior aspect of the shoulder. Asymmetry of the deltoid muscle or "squaring off" of the affected shoulder may be noted as a result of the deltoid atrophy. On physical examination, patients typically have tenderness over the region of the quadrilateral space, which may lessen with a diagnostic injection of local anesthetic. Although a positive FABER test (shoulder forward elevation, abduction, and external rotation held for more than 1 minute) may be suggestive of this diagnosis by leading to shoulder pain, this nonspecific finding may also occur in more common shoulder diagnoses such as internal impingement or impingement syndrome. Shoulder strength tests should be performed because the teres minor accounts for 45% of external rotation strength and the deltoid muscle provides the majority of strength in shoulder flexion, abduction, and extension.[47] If the posterior deltoid muscle and teres minor muscles are not affected, then an axillary nerve injury may have occurred distal to the quadrilateral space. During the history and physical examination it is important to evaluate for other more common neurologic etiologies within the differential diagnosis, including cervical pathology, thoracic outlet syndrome, or brachial plexus pathology. Additionally, clinical evaluation should also assess for intrinsic shoulder pathology such as adhesive capsulitis, osteoarthritis, and rotator cuff tears.

Diagnostic studies
Plain radiographs are important imaging studies to obtain, particularly when there is a history of trauma. In acute trauma, an EMG/nerve conduction velocity (NCV) should be obtained 3 weeks after the shoulder injury in order to confirm the diagnosis and aid in evaluating the severity of the nerve injury. As with assessment of the suprascapular nerve, EMG evaluation of other muscles will assist in ruling out a nerve root, brachial plexus, or other peripheral nerve injury. Like the suprascapular nerve, CMAP is obtainable and there is no readily obtainable SNAP. In patients who have quadrilateral space syndrome, EMG/NCV is not as sensitive, and may not become useful until later in the disease process. MRI will often be helpful in evaluating these patients (**Fig. 5**) through detection of changes of denervation in affected muscles as well as detection of ganglion cysts or other mass lesions compressing the axillary nerve. Additionally, MRI aids in evaluating for other causes of shoulder pain and dysfunction. It is not uncommon for the diagnosis of quadrilateral space syndrome to be suggested by an MRI performed to examine for other causes. In a prospective investigation, isolated teres minor atrophy was identified in 12 out of 217 patients (5.5%) who underwent consecutive shoulder MRI examinations over a 3-month period of time.[48] Subclavian

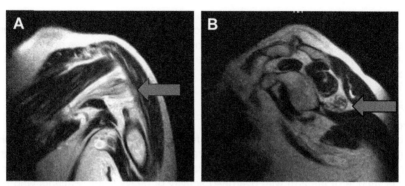

Fig. 5. T1-weighted MRI image of a left shoulder demonstrating signal changes in the teres minor muscle (*gray arrow*). (*A*) Coronal image. (*B*) Sagittal image.

arteriography can evaluate for compression of the axillary nerve by an arterial structure, such as with the posterior humeral circumflex artery as it passes through the quadrilateral space. Typically, the angiogram does not show reduced blood flow through the posterior humeral circumflex artery when the patients arm is held in adduction. With abduction and external rotation of the shoulder, however, the blood flow in the artery is attenuated. A concern with this test is the low specificity for making the diagnosis of quadrilateral space syndrome. One investigation using MR angiography demonstrated that 80% of asymptomatic patients had occlusion of arterial flow in the posterior humeral circumflex artery when the arm was placed in abduction and external rotation.[49]

Treatment

Nonoperative

In discussing the treatment options of axillary nerve injuries it is important to differentiate traumatic patients from those who have quadrilateral space syndrome. When the axillary nerve is injured from a fracture, dislocation, or contusion, the prognosis for nerve function and return to sport is good. Nonoperative treatment includes reassurance to the patient, relative rest, ice, and symptomatic management. As the acute pain subsides, physical therapy should be started to maintain shoulder mobility while awaiting nerve function to return. Additionally, electrical stimulation may be beneficial in reducing deltoid atrophy while nerve function recovers.[50,51]

The initial management of quadrilateral space syndrome, in the absence of a space-occupying lesion, is nonoperative treatment. It has been suggested that only 30% of symptomatic patients who have quadrilateral space syndrome require surgical intervention;[52] however, most of the literature on quadrilateral space syndrome is based on case reports or small case series. Nonoperative treatment consists of relative rest, and in the case of a baseball pitcher, refraining from throwing while symptomatic. Additionally, symptomatic treatment includes the use of anti-inflammatory medications and local corticosteroid injections into the quadrilateral space. A rehabilitation program is also essential in a baseball player's recovery and return to throwing, including a stretching program with particular emphasis on the posterior shoulder capsule and teres minor. As symptoms subside, and as the deltoid function returns to normal, an interval throwing program should be initiated in which the throwing arm is subjected to gradually increasing stresses based on the velocity and distance of throwing.

Additionally, it is important to assess the affected player for proper throwing mechanics.

Operative treatment

Surgical indications for treating an axillary nerve injury include surgically derived iatrogenic injuries, penetrating trauma, and a symptomatic patient who has no clinical or EMG/NCV evidence of nerve recovery by 3 to 6 months. The best surgical results are seen when surgery is performed within 6 months from the injury; however, functional improvement can still occur when surgery is performed up to 1 year after the injury occurred.[53–55] Surgical techniques involved include such procedures as neurolysis, neurorrhaphy, nerve grafting, nerve transfer, and neurotization. In general, these operations can be performed through both an anterior and posterior incision.

Surgical intervention for quadrilateral space syndrome should be considered when a space-occupying lesion is present, and when symptoms have persisted despite nonoperative interventions for a 3- to 6-month period of time.

Surgery for quadrilateral space syndrome can be performed through a muscle-sparing technique or with detachment of the deltoid muscle from the acromion. The axillary nerve and its branches should be identified as they exit the quadrilateral space, and any fibrous bands or space-occupying lesions that are compressing the nerve should be excised. Confirmation of an adequate decompression may involve placing the arm in an abducted and externally rotated position and palpating a pulse in the posterior humeral circumflex artery. Information regarding patient outcomes following surgical decompression of the axillary nerve at the quadrilateral space is limited, because most of the data are derived from small case series.[45,46,52,56–59] Of 23 patients reported in one study, 10 patients had dramatic relief of symptoms, 11 had improvement of symptoms, and 2 patients had no improvement.[59]

ULNAR NEUROPATHY
Anatomy

The ulnar nerve is a mixed sensorimotor nerve derived from the medial cord of the brachial plexus (C8 and T1). The motor innervations from the ulnar nerve are to the majority of the intrinsic muscles of the hand, the flexor carpi ulnaris muscle, and medial aspect of the flexor digitorum profundus. The sensory innervations are the dorsal and palmar surfaces of the fourth and fifth fingers and the ulnar border of the hand.

The ulnar nerve travels down the upper arm through the anterior compartment adjacent to the brachial artery. No significant branches of the ulnar nerve are present in the upper arm; however, occasionally there is a variant supracondylar motor branch to the flexor carpi ulnaris. In the middle third of the upper arm, the nerve pierces the medial intermuscular septum as it courses from the anterior to the posterior compartment, passing through the arcade of Struthers, a musculofascial band located approximately 8 cm proximal to the medial epicondyle. The ulnar nerve subsequently travels behind the medial epicondyle in a fibro-osseous groove that is bound by the medial epicondyle anteriorly, the olecranon and ulnohumeral ligament laterally, and a fibroaponeurotic band medially. Laxity of the fibroaponeurotic band can result in subluxation or dislocation of the ulnar nerve out of the epicondylar groove. This occurs during elbow flexion, with reduction during elbow extension. Asymptomatic hypermobility of the nerve is found in approximately 16% of the population, and is often bilateral.[60] Next the nerve passes between the two heads of the flexor carpi ulnaris, under a fascial band called Osborne's ligament. Elbow flexion causes stretching of Osborne's ligament, resulting in the cross-sectional shape of the tunnel changing from an oval to a flattened ellipse.[61] The ulnar collateral ligament relaxes and bulges medially, further narrowing the space available for the ulnar nerve. During elbow flexion, pressure within the tunnel increases sevenfold, and can increase more than 20-fold with contraction of the flexor carpi ulnaris.[62]

The diagnosis and treatment of ulnar nerve injuries in baseball players requires an understanding of the relationship between the unique anatomy of the elbow and the stresses placed across those structures during the throwing motion. The stability of the elbow joint is primarily supplied by the bony anatomy when the elbow is within 20° of extension or flexed beyond 120°. The primary provider of elbow stability between 20° and 120° of motion is the surrounding soft tissue.[63–65] In particular, during the throwing motion the anterior bundle of the ulnar collateral ligament is the primary restraint to valgus forces. This ligament encounters repetitive near-failure tensile stresses during the pitching motion.[4,64,66–69] The pathophysiology behind most elbow injuries in baseball players has been termed the "valgus extension overload syndrome."[48] The combination of large valgus forces and rapid extension of the elbow places tensile stress as high as 64 Nm along the medial side of the elbow.[4] Structures affected by these forces include the ulnar nerve, ulnar collateral ligament, flexor-pronator mass, and medial epicondyle apophysis in adolescents.

Etiology

Ulnar neuropathy at the elbow is the second most common compression neuropathy after carpal tunnel syndrome. The ulnar nerve travels in a superficial location behind the medial epicondyle, and can be injured as a result of a direct insult. More commonly, the ulnar nerve is injured because of compression or traction where it travels in the cubital tunnel between the upper arm and forearm. Injury to the nerve can occur at several locations within the cubital tunnel, including at the intermuscular septum, the arcade of Struthers, the fibro-osseous groove at the medial epicondyle, and between the two heads of the flexor carpi ulnaris origin. Baseball players are particularly prone to ulnar neuropathy because of the repetitive valgus stresses placed on the nerve during the throwing motion. Symptoms involving the ulnar nerve are very common in throwing athletes, and occur in more than 40% of athletes who have valgus instability and 60% of throwers who have medial epicondylitis.[70,71] The pressure within the ulnar nerve in the flexed elbow and extended wrist has been shown to be elevated more than three times the resting level.[72] When this elbow position is combined with shoulder abduction, the intraneural pressure may be elevated as much as six times the resting level. This is the arm position that occurs during the acceleration phase of throwing. As a result of the valgus extension overload syndrome, other changes occur in throwers' elbows, resulting in tethering of the ulnar nerve and increased intraneural pressures, such as with degenerative changes and osteophyte formation impinging on the ulnar groove. Other potential factors affecting the ulnar nerve include loose bodies, traction spurs, hypertrophy of the triceps and anconeus epitrochlearis muscles, synovitis, thickened retinaculum, scar tissue, and calcification of the UCL.

Clinical Evaluation

History and physical examination

Ulnar neuropathy is a diagnosis that is typically made via history and physical examination. Baseball pitchers typically present with a history of medial elbow pain, with or without radiation to the hand. The player may also report clumsiness of the hand and parasthesias in the little and ring fingers. These symptoms initially occur during times of throwing and subside with rest; however, as the disease progresses, symptoms may also occur at rest. Motor symptoms affecting the intrinsic hand muscles and extrinsic forearm muscles are often not observed in the initial stages, when most players present.

Physical examination is important in making the diagnosis of ulnar neuropathy and excluding other potential sources of the patient's neurologic symptoms. Evaluation for a cervical radiculopathy, brachial plexus injury, or coexisting nerve compression should be performed. In evaluating the patient who has ulnar nerve symptoms, the physician needs to assess for compression at more than one site.[73] Examination of the elbow should assess for areas of tenderness, range of motion, strength, and stability. Tenderness over the flexor pronator tendon origin reproduced with resisted wrist flexion and forearm pronation suggests a diagnosis of medial epicondylitis. Pain over the UCL reproduced with a valgus stress to the elbow is consistent with an injury to the UCL. The ulnar nerve should be evaluated for subluxation during elbow flexion. Pain over the ulnar nerve, a positive Tinel's sign posterior to the medial epicondyle, and a positive elbow flexion test all may suggest involvement of the ulnar nerve. As with the Phalen's test, the elbow flexion test is more sensitive than specific, with false-positive results reported in 10% of normal individuals. When motor weakness develops, involvement of the intrinsic muscles of the hand occurs before that of extrinsic forearm muscles, likely because of to a more superficial location of these nerve fascicles at the elbow.[74] One of the first signs of intrinsic motor weakness is an inability to adduct the little finger (Wartenberg's sign). When intrinsic weakness is severe and associated with muscle wasting, a claw hand deformity may be seen as a flexion of the fourth and fifth proximal and distal interphalyngeal joints, with extension of the fourth and fifth metacarpal phalyngeal joints.

Diagnostic studies

Radiographic imaging of the elbow is important when patients present with a history of trauma. Radiographic views should include an anterior posterior, lateral, and cubital tunnel view. If there is concern of elbow instability, then stress radiographs can also be obtained. Medial joint opening greater than 3 mm is consistent with instability.[65,75] MRI will allow assessment of soft tissue masses, but is not essential for diagnosis or planning appropriate treatment in most patients. If the patient's history and physical examination suggest an injury to the ulnar collateral ligament, however, then an MRI may be useful for evaluating for ligament avulsions, partial and complete ulnar collateral ligament tears, and for assessing the flexor pronator tendon origin.[75,76]

Electrodiagnositic studies can be an important adjunct in confirming the diagnosis of ulnar neuropathy and assessing the severity of the nerve injury when the diagnosis is not obvious based on clinical evaluation.[77] False-negatives can occur if the electrodiagnositic testing is performed too early in the disease process. In focal ulnar nerve compression, sensory fibers are affected before motor fibers. It is important to obtain the dorsal ulnar cutaneous SNAP because an absent response may indicate a moderate to severe lesion of the ulnar nerve at the elbow.[78] The most common technique for assessing proximal ulnar nerve function is evaluating the ulnar CMAP below and above the elbow. A nerve conduction velocity of less than 49 m/sec across the elbow[79] or a difference of 10 m/sec or greater between the arm and above the elbow to below elbow segment is considered abnormal.[80] When using this technique, it is important to perform the test with the elbow fully flexed, otherwise the true length of the nerve can be underestimated, leading to false slowing of conduction times.[79] The segment across the elbow should be greater than 10 cm to increase sensitivity. When conduction velocity is slowed, it is occasionally accompanied by a drop in CMAP amplitude of 20% to 30% at the site of the lesion at the elbow. An alternative method of finding a focal lesion at the elbow is to perform multiple short segmental stimulations of 1 cm, both proximal and distal to the medial epicondyle,[81] called an "inching technique." An increase in the latency of 0.4 msec or more is considered significant, and identifies a focal lesion at that segment.[82] EMG is helpful in confirming denervation in ulnar-innervated muscles as well as evaluating other forms of nerve injuries such as a C8/T1 radiculopathy or lower trunk/medial cord plexopathy.

Treatment

Nonoperative
Nonoperative management of ulnar nerve injuries at the elbow involves rest, avoidance of aggravating activities, and nonsteroidal anti-inflammatory medication. Local corticosteroid injections are not recommended. If the patient's symptoms occur at night or are more severe, splinting with the arm in slight flexion can be helpful. This can be particularly beneficial in patients who have ulnar nerve subluxation or dislocation. Players whose symptoms occur predominantly during throwing should not be allowed to throw until they are asymptomatic. Once the elbow is asymptomatic, the player should be started on a strengthening program focusing on the dynamic stabilizers of the elbow. The final stage of rehabilitation includes an interval throwing program, with the goal of having the player return to competitive throwing. Unfortunately, unlike the general population, athletes who have valgus instability of the elbow often have recurrence of their ulnar nerve symptoms with resumption of throwing.

Operative treatment
Indications for surgical intervention include failed nonoperative treatment or coexisting elbow pathology that requires surgical treatment. Additionally, patients who have more severe compression of the ulnar nerve, to include those patients who have axonal loss, profound sensory deficits, and motor weakness, may be considered for earlier surgical intervention. Surgical procedures include simple decompression, medial epicondylectomy, anterior subcutaneous transposition, and submuscular transposition. Simple decompression of the ulnar nerve and medial epicondylectomy in the throwing athlete are contraindicated. Both anterior subcutaneous transposition and submuscular transposition have demonstrated favorable outcomes in the overhead throwing athlete.[70,83–88] When this procedure is compared with submuscular transpositions, it has the advantage of less surgical dissection and faster rehabilitation. Potential disadvantages include the nerve being in a more superficial location and therefore vulnerable to direct trauma. Additionally, the ulnar nerve follows a less direct course, and can be iatrogenically compressed by the subcutaneous fascial-dermal sling. Submuscular transposition protects the transposed nerve from both direct and indirect trauma by placing the nerve deep to the flexor muscle mass.[85] Disadvantages of the submuscular transposition include increased surgical dissection, the need for temporary immobilization and protection of the repaired flexor tendon, and a longer rehabilitation period. There are surgical advocates for both procedures; however, there are no prospective randomized controlled trials or meta-analyses available to guide treatment. An important issue in the operative management of the overhead athlete is to address all of the pathology that is contributing to the athlete's elbow symptoms. Specifically, if valgus instability of the elbow is present, an ulnar collateral ligament reconstruction should be performed at the time of the ulnar nerve decompression. Additionally, significant tendinopathy or tearing of the flexor pronator tendon origin should be debrided and repaired. Failure to address the underlying pathology in the elbow can lead to recurrent elbow problems.[86]

SUMMARY

The throwing motion in baseball places significant and repetitive stress across the shoulder and elbow. These forces result in unique patterns of injuries seen in the overhead athlete. Specific nerve injuries identified in the overhead athlete include suprascapular neuropathy, quadrilateral space syndrome, and cubital tunnel syndrome. The principles of nonoperative management include cessation of throwing and symptomatic treatment. As the athletes' symptoms subside, they should be started in supervised rehabilitation that progresses to an interval throwing program. The goal of treatment is the resolution of nerve symptoms and the return to competitive throwing. In those overhead athletes who fail to improve with nonoperative treatment, surgery can result in a positive outcome in particular patients. Additional indications for surgery include more profound neuropathy and mass-lesion–induced nerve compression.

REFERENCES

1. Narakas A. Compression and traction neuropathies about the shoulder and arm. In: RHG, editor. Operative nerve repair and reconstruction. Philadelphia: JB Lippincott; 1991.
2. Meister K. Injuries to the shoulder in the throwing athlete: part one: biomechanics/pathophysiology/classification of injury. Am J Sports Med 2000;28:265–75.
3. Tullos H, King J. Throwing mechanism in sports. Orthop Clin North Am 1973;4: 709–20.
4. Fleisig G, Andrews J, Dillman C, et al. Kinetics of baseball pitching with implications about injury mechanism. Am J Sports Med 1995;23:233–9.
5. Pappas A, Zawacki R, Sullivan T. Biomechanics of baseball pitching. A preliminary report. Am J Sports Med 1985;13:216–22.
6. Jobe F, Moynes D, Tibone J, et al. An EMG analysis of the shoulder in pitching: a second report. Am J Sports Med 1984;12:218–20.
7. Jobe F, Tibone J, Perry J, et al. An EMG analysis of the shoulder in throwing and pitching: a preliminary report. Am J Sports Med 1983;11:3–5.
8. Kwan M, Wall E, Massie J, et al. Strain, stress and stretch of peripheral nerve. Rabbit experiment in vitro and in vivo. Acta Orthop Scand 1992;63:267–72.
9. Lundborg G, Rydevik B. Effects of stretching the tibial nerve of the rabbit. A preliminary study of the intraneural circulation and the barrier function of the perineurium. J Bone Joint Surg Br 1973;55:390–401.
10. Lundborg G. Structure and function of the intraneural microvessels as related to trauma, edema formation and nerve function. J Bone Joint Surg Am 1975;57: 938–48.
11. Ajmani M. The cutaneous branch of the human suprascapular nerve. J Anat 1994;185:439–42.
12. Bigliani L, Dalsey R, McCann P, et al. An anatomical study of the suprascapular nerve. Arthroscopy 1990;6:301–5.
13. Mestdagh H, Drizenko A, Ghestem P. Anatomical basis of suprascapular nerve syndrome. Anat Clin 1981;3:67–71.
14. Ozer Y, Grossman J, Gilbert A. Anatomical observations on the suprascapular nerve. Hand Clin 1995;11:539–44.
15. Cummins C, Anderson K, Bowen M, et al. Anatomy and histological characteristics of the spinoglenoid ligament. J Bone Joint Surg Am 1998;80:1622–5.
16. Plancher K, Peterson R, Johnston J, et al. The spinoglenoid ligament: anatomy, morphology, and histological findings. J Bone Joint Surg Am 2005;87:361–5.

17. Edeland H, Zachrisson B. Fracture of the scapular notch associated with lesion of the suprascapular nerve. Acta Orthop Scand 1975;46:758–63.
18. Berry H, Kong K, Hudson A, et al. Isolated suprascapular nerve palsy: a review of nine cases. Can J Neurol Sci 1995;22:301–4.
19. Travlos J, Goldberg I, Boome R. Brachial plexus lesions associated with dislocated shoulders. J Bone Joint Surg Br 1990;72:68–71.
20. Rengachary SS, Neff JP, Singer PA, et al. Suprascapular entrapment neuropathy: a clinical, anatomical and comparative study. Part 1: clinical study. Neurosurgery 1979;5:441–6.
21. Cummins C, Messer T, Schafer M. Infraspinatus muscle atrophy in professional baseball players. Am J Sports Med 2004;32(1):116–20.
22. Cummins C, Bowen M, Anderson K, et al. Suprascapular nerve entrapment at the spinoglenoid notch in a professional baseball pitcher. Am J Sports Med 1999;27: 810–2.
23. Ringel S, Treihaft M, Carr M, et al. Suprascapular neuropathy in pitchers. Am J Sports Med 1990;18:80–6.
24. Bryan W, Wild J. Isolated infraspinatus atrophy: a common cause of posterior shoulder pain and weakness in throwing athletes? Am J Sports Med 1989;17: 130–1.
25. Ferretti A, De Carli A, Fontana M. Injury of the suprascapular nerve at the spinoglenoid notch: the natural history of infraspinatus atrophy in volleyball players. Am J Sports Med 1998;26:759–63.
26. Ferretti A, Cerullo G, Russo G. Suprascapular neuropathy in volleyball players. J Bone Joint Surg Am 1987;69:260–3.
27. Sandow M, Ilic J. Suprascapular nerve rotator cuff compression syndrome in volleyball players. J Shoulder Elbow Surg 1998;7:516–21.
28. Chochole M, Senker W, Meznik C, et al. Glenoid-labral cyst entrapping the suprascapular nerve: dissolution after arthroscopic debridement of an extended SLAP lesion. Arthroscopy 1997;13:753–5.
29. Fehrman D, Orwin J, Jennings R. Suprascapular nerve entrapment by a ganglion cyst: a report of six cases with arthroscopic finding and review of the literature. Arthroscopy 1995;11:727–34.
30. Kullmer K, Sievers K, Reimers C, et al. Changes of sonographic, magnetic resonance tomographic, electromyographic and histopathologic findings within a 2-month period of examinations after experimental muscle denervation. Arch Orthop Trauma Surg 1998;117:228–34.
31. Palmer W, Brown J, Rosenthal D. Labral-ligamentous complex of the shoulder: evaluation with MR arthrography. Radiology 1994;190:645–51.
32. Gladstone J, Bishop J, Lo IK, et al. Fatty infiltration and atrophy of the rotator cuff do not improve after rotator cuff repair and correlate with poor functional outcome. Am J Sports Med 2007;35:719–28.
33. Post M, Mayer J. Suprascapular nerve entrapment. Diagnosis and treatment. Clin Orthop Relat Res 1987;223:126–36.
34. Hama H, Ueba Y, Morinaga T, et al. A new stategy for treatment of suprascapular entrapment neuropathy in athletes: shaving of the base of the scapular spine. J Shoulder Elbow Surg 1992;1:253–60.
35. Hagert C, Linder L. Entrapment neuropathy of the suprascapular nerve. Acta Orthop Scand 1984;55:107.
36. Lafosse L, Tomasi A, Corbett S, et al. Arthroscopic release of the suprascapular nerve entrapment at the suprascapular notch: technique and preliminary results. Arthroscopy 2007;23:34–42.

37. Barwood S, Burkhart S, Lo I. Arthroscopic suprascapular nerve release at the suprascapular notch in a cadaveric model: an anatomic approach. Arthroscopy 2007;23:221–5.
38. Moore T, Fritts H, Quick D, et al. Suprascapular nerve entrapment caused by supraglenoid cyst compression. J Shoulder Elbow Surg 1997;6:455–62.
39. Westerheide K, Dopirak R, Karzel R, et al. Suprascapular nerve palsy secondary to spinoglenoid cysts: results of arthroscopic treatment. Arthroscopy 2006;22: 721–7.
40. Iannotti J, Ramsey M. Arthroscopic decompression of a ganglion cyst causing suprascapular nerve compression. Arthroscopy 1996;12:739–45.
41. Pollack L, Davis L. Peripheral nerve injuries. Am J Surg 1932;17:462–71.
42. Gumina S, Postacchini F. Anterior dislocation of the shoulder in elderly patients. J Bone Joint Surg Br 1972;79:540–3.
43. Perlmutter G, Apruzzese W. Axillary nerve injury in contact sports; recommendations for treatment and rehabilitation. Sports Med 1998;26:351–61.
44. Toolanen G, Hildingsson T, Hedlund T, et al. Early complications after anterior dislocation of the shoulder in patients over 40 years; an ultrasonographic and electromyographic study. Acta Orthop Scand 1993;64:549–52.
45. Cahill B, Palmer R. Quadrilateral space syndrome. J Hand Surg Am 1983;8:65–9.
46. Sanders T, Tirman P. Paralabral cyst: an unusual case of quadrilateral space syndrome. Arthroscopy 1999;15:632–7.
47. Saha A. Surgery of the paralyzed and flail shoulder. Acta Orthop Scand 1967; 97(Suppl):5–90.
48. Wilson L, Sundaram M, Piraino D, et al. Isolated teres minor atrophy: manifestation of quadrilateral space syndrome or traction injury to the axillary nerve? Orthopedics 2006;29(5):447–50.
49. Mochizuki T, Isoda H, Masui T, et al. Occlusion of the posterior circumflex humeral artery; detection with MR angiography in healthy volunteers and in a patient with quadrilateral space syndrome. AJR Am J Roentgenol 1994;163:625–7.
50. Crameri R, Weston A, Rutkowski S, et al. Effects of electrical stimulation leg training during the acute phase of spinal cord injury: a pilot study. Eur J Appl Physiol 2000;83:409–15.
51. Dupont Salter A, Richmond F, Leob G. Prevention of muscle disuse atrophy by low-frequency electrical stimulation in rats. IEEE Trans Neural Syst Rehabil Eng 2003;11:218–26.
52. Lester B, Jeong G, Weiland A, et al. Quadrilateral space syndrome: diagnosis, pathology and treatment. Am J Orthop 1999;28:718–25.
53. Alnot J, Valenti P. Surgical reconstruction of the axillary nerve. In: Post M, MB, Hawkins RJ, editors. Surgery of the shoulder. St Louis (MO): Mosby; 1990. p. 330–3.
54. Petrucci F, Morelli A, Raimondi P. Axillary nerve injuries: 21 cases treated by nerve graft and neurolysis. J Hand Surg Am 1982;7:271–8.
55. Rochwerger A, Benaim L, Toledano E, et al. Surgical repair of the axillary nerve: results of a five-year follow up. Chir Main 2000;19:31–5.
56. Chen D, Cai P, Lao G, et al. Quadrilateral space syndrome. Chin Med J (Engl) 1995;108:109–12.
57. Kuang Y, Hou C. The diagnosis and tratment of quadrilateral space syndrome. Zhongguo Xiu Fu Chong Jian Wai Ke Za Zhi 2001;15:199–201, In Chinese.
58. Francel T, Dellon A, Campbell J. Quadrilateral space syndrome: diagnosis and operative decompression technique. Plast Reconstr Surg 1991;87:911–6.
59. Safran M. Nerve injuries about the shoulder in athletes, part 1: suprascapular nerve and axillary nerve. Am J Sports Med 2004;32:803–19.

60. Childress H. Recurrent ulnar-nerve dislocation at the elbow. Clin Orthop Relat Res 1975;108:168–73.
61. Apfelberg D, Larson S. Dynamic anatomy of the ulnar nerve at the elbow. Plast Reconstr Surg 1973;51:79–81.
62. Werner C, Ohlin P, Elmqvist D. Pressures recorded in ulnar neuropathy. Acta Orthop Scand 1985;56:404–6.
63. Miller R. The cubital tunnel syndrome: diagnosis and precise localization. Ann Neurol 1979;6:56–9.
64. Morrey B, Tanaka S, An K. Valgus stability of the elbow: a definition of primary and secondary constraints. Clin Orthop Relat Res 1991;265:187–95.
65. Schwab G, Bennett J, Woods G, et al. Biomechanics of elbow instability: the role of the medial collateral ligament. Clin Orthop Relat Res 1980;146:42–52.
66. Hotchkiss R, Weiland A. Valgus stability of the elbow. J Orthop Res 1987;5:372–7.
67. Morrey B, An K. Articular and ligamentous contributions to the stability of the elbow joint. Am J Sports Med 1983;11:315–9.
68. Morrey B, An K. Functional anatomy of the ligaments of the elbow. Clin Orthop Relat Res 1985;201:84–90.
69. Regan W, Korinek S, Morrey B, et al. Biomechanical study of ligaments around the elbow joint. Clin Orthop Relat Res 1991;271:170–9.
70. Andrews J, Timmerman L. Outcome of elbow surgery in professional baseball players. Am J Sports Med 1995;23:407–13.
71. Bennett G. Elbow and shoulder lesions of the professional baseball pitcher. Am J Surg 1959;98:484–92.
72. Pechan J, Julis I. The pressure measurement in the ulnar nerve: a contribution to the pathophysiology of the cubital tunnel syndrome. J Biomech 1975;8:75–9.
73. Upton A, McComas A. The double crush in nerve entrapment syndromes. Lancet 1973;2:359–62.
74. Sunderland S, editor. Nerve and nerve injuries. 2nd edition. New York: Churchill Livingstone; 1978.
75. Jobe F, Kvitne R. Elbow instability in the athlete. Instr Course Lect 1991;40:17–23.
76. Timmerman L, Andrews J. Undersurface tear of the ulnar collateral ligament in baseball players: a newly recognized lesion. Am J Sports Med 1994;22:33–6.
77. Posner M. Compressive ulnar neuropathies at the elbow: I. Etiology and diagnosis. J Am Acad Orthop Surg 1998;6:282–8.
78. Jabre J. Ulnar nerve lesions at the wrist: new techniques for recording from the sensory dorsal branch of the ulnar nerve. Neurology 1980;30:873–6.
79. Kincaid J. AAEE minimonograph #31: the electrodiagnosis of ulnar neuropathy at the elbow. Muscle Nerve 1988;11:1005–15.
80. Eisen A. Early diagnosis of ulnar palsy. Neurology 1974;24:256–62.
81. Miller C, Savoie FI. Valgus extension injuries of the elbow in the throwing athlete. J Am Acad Orthop Surg 1994;2:261–9.
82. Campbell W, Pridgeon R, Sahni K. Short segment incremental studies in evaluation of ulnar neuropathy at the elbow. Muscle Nerve 1992;15:1050–4.
83. Aoki M, Kanaya K, Aiki H, et al. Cubital tunnel syndrome in adolescent baseball players: a report of six cases with 3- to 5-year follow-up. Arthroscopy 2005;21(6):758.
84. Boatright J, D'Alessandro D, et al. Nerve entrapment syndromes at the elbow. In: Jobe FW, PM, Glousman RE, editors. Operative techniques in upper extremity sports injuries. St Louis (MO): Mosby-Year Book; 1996.
85. Del Pizzo W, Jobe F, Norwood L. Ulnar nerve entrapment syndrome in baseball players. Am J Sports Med 1977;5(5):182–5.

86. Glousman R. Ulnar nerve problems in the athlete's elbow. Clin Sports Med 1990;
9:365–77.
87. Rettig A, Ebben J. Anterior subcutaneous transfer of the ulnar nerve in the athlete.
Am J Sports Med 1993;21:836–40.
88. Rokito A, McMahon P, Jobe F. Cubital tunnel syndrome. Oper Tech Sports Med
1996;4:15–20.

Concussion in the National Football League: An Overview for Neurologists

Ira R. Casson, MD[a,b], Elliot J. Pellman, MD[a,c,d,e],
David C. Viano, Dr. med., PhD[a,f],*

KEYWORDS

• Football • Concussion • Head injury
• National Football League

Clinical neurologists often encounter a patient with concussion—mild traumatic brain injury (MTBI)—in the office weeks or months after the injury. In this setting, the physician's evaluation is frequently limited by a lack of information regarding the actual mechanisms of injury and the objectively determined clinical situation immediately following the injury. This makes it difficult to know the evolution of the clinical picture in the first few days to weeks after the traumatic event. The physician-scientist can use the athletic playing fields as a "laboratory" for the study of MTBI. The authors have been fortunate to have the opportunity to study concussions in such a setting—the National Football League (NFL).

The authors review the results of these studies here in the hope that this will help the clinical neurologist better understand the nature of MTBI, and thus improve the evaluation and treatment of all patients who have this condition. In the early 1990s, Al Toon and Merrill Hoge, two prominent NFL players, retired because of prolonged postconcussion syndrome. Commissioner Paul Tagliabue sanctioned the creation of a committee consisting of team physicians, team athletic trainers, and outside experts to objectively study and research MTBI.

This article originally appeared in *Neurologic Clinics*, Volume 26, Issue 1.

This work was supported in part by research sponsored by the NFL and NFL Charities.

[a] Mild Traumatic Brain Injury Committee, National Football League, 280 Park Avenue, New York, NY 10017, USA

[b] Department of Neurology, Long Island Jewish Medical Center, Albert Einstein College of Medicine, New Hyde Park, Bronx, NY, USA

[c] ProHEALTH Care Associates, LLP, 2800 Marcus Avenue, Lake Success, New York 11042, NY, USA

[d] Department of Medicine, Mount Sinai School of Medicine, New York, NY, USA

[e] Department of Orthopaedics, Mount Sinai School of Medicine, New York, NY, USA

[f] ProBiomechanics LLC, 265 Warrington Road, Bloomfield Hills, MI 48304-2952, USA

* Corresponding author. ProBiomechanics LLC, 265 Warrington Road, Bloomfield Hills, MI 48304-2952.

E-mail address: dviano@comcast.net (D.C. Viano).

Phys Med Rehabil Clin N Am 20 (2009) 195–214

doi:10.1016/j.pmr.2008.10.006

The committee's first several meetings were dedicated to developing a definition of MTBI that would be used by club medical staffs when diagnosing and reporting an injury. The definition was purposely broad, in hopes of allowing the committee to capture as much data as possible. The commissioner mandated that all MTBIs be reported, blinded, and deposited in a single repository for future analysis. Medical conferences were held with team physicians and athletic trainers.

After much discussion, the committee decided that research and data collection should focus on biomechanical and clinical analysis of the injury. Biomechanical analysis was critical because the ability of football helmets to prevent MTBI was poorly understood, and helmet manufacturer's biomechanical research was underfunded. Understanding of the biomechanical forces that result in MTBI would precipitate objective helmet improvements, higher design standards, and greater injury prevention. Collection and study of prospective data analysis would increase sensitivity to the injury and allow clinicians to make informed decisions on a potentially unique patient population, based upon objective data. The results of the research would be published in peer-reviewed medical literature.

BIOMECHANICS

The biomechanical information was generated from studies performed under the auspices of the NFL MTBI Committee, with the assistance of Biokinetics and Associates (Ottawa, Canada). The data were collected using video analysis of a number of NFL head impacts, some resulting in an MTBI and some not resulting in MTBI. After video analysis, the impacts were reconstructed in the laboratory using Hybrid III test dummies (General Motors, Detroit, Michigan).[1]

Regarding impacts that resulted in clinical MTBI, the authors' studies yielded the following findings. With concussion, the average impact speed was 9.3 ± 1.9 m/s (20.8 ± 4.2 mph).[1] No concussions or clinical MTBIs occurred in striking players. Our analysis showed that the striking player lines up his head, neck, and torso, and strikes the other player obliquely on the face mask or where the face mask attaches to the helmet, usually below the center of gravity of the head or on the side of the helmet above the center of gravity. The striking player has a higher effective mass than the struck player because the striking player uses his whole body in the impact, whereas the struck player's head only is involved in the impact. As a result, more momentum is transferred to the struck player, causing a rapid change in head velocity, delta V (ΔV). The peak head acceleration for concussed players averaged 98 ± 28 g, with duration of 15 msec.[1] The peak head acceleration for the uninjured struck players averaged 60 ± 24 g.[1] The difference in these peak head accelerations is statistically significant.

The authors' studies revealed that clinical concussion was primarily related to translational head acceleration.[1] Clinical concussion was strongly correlated with Severity Index (SI), Head Injury Criterion (HIC), peak translational acceleration, and head ΔV.[1] The incidence of clinical concussion was correlated to a lesser degree with peak rotational acceleration. As noted above, the average duration of the impact was 15 msec. ΔV increases with increased translational acceleration. Our findings indicate that impact speeds of more than 7 m/s (15.6 mph) and 90 g offer a line of delineation between the occurrence of clinical concussion and the absence of clinical concussion.[1]

The high impact speeds, ΔVs, head accelerations, and duration of 15 milliseconds are exceptionally high velocities, accelerations, and long durations compared with other types of head impacts.[1] The average peak force to the head in NFL impacts is in the range for cranial fractures with short duration impacts for the unprotected head. In view of these results, it appears clear that the helmet shell and padding were functioning well in distributing the load and lowering the risk for more serious brain injuries and cranial fractures from these impacts. These biomechanical data on NFL impacts have given the scientific community new insights on head tolerances for impacts of 15 msec duration. In view of the authors' findings, it appears that translational acceleration should be the primary measure for the assessment of helmet protection performance. Because our studies clearly showed that translational acceleration and rotational acceleration are related, efforts to decrease the peak translational acceleration, SI, or HIC will also result in proportional decreases in rotational acceleration.

As part of the authors' studies, we investigated the location and the direction of helmet impacts resulting in MTBI in the NFL.[2] Twenty-nine percent of the helmet impacts involved loading of the face mask (67% of these occurred between the angles of 0° and 45°). Seventy-one percent of the helmet impacts involved impacts to the helmet shell: 22% involved impacts with the ground, 20% involved impacts with another player's shoulder pad or arm, 7% involved impacts with the leg of another player, and 50% involved impacts with another player's helmet.[2] Overall, 61% of all NFL MTBI impacts involved collision with the other player's helmet. Seventy-six percent of face mask impacts occurred below the center of gravity of the head. More than 80% of all the impacts to the helmet shell occurred above the head center of gravity. Impacts to the face mask occurring between 0° and 45° below the head center of gravity exhibited the highest average impact velocity of all NFL impacts, and the lowest ΔVs of all NFL MTBI impacts.[2]

Falls in which the back of the helmet struck the ground resulted in the lowest average impact velocities and the highest ΔVs.[2] This occurs because when the back of the helmet hits the ground, the closing velocity only is coming from the one player, but the ΔV is highest because it is increased by the rebound off of the ground. The lowest translational accelerations with MTBI occur with face mask impacts; the highest translational accelerations occur with falls to the back of the head. Falls to the ground in which the back of the helmet strikes the ground exhibit the lowest rotational accelerations and velocities of all NFL impacts.

For the striking player, impact velocities were just as high as the impact velocities for the struck players, but the ΔV and peak translational accelerations were lower than for the struck players who sustained concussion.[2] The reason for this is that the effective mass of the striking player is much greater than that of the struck player, because the effective mass of the striking player includes a greater mass from the torso. The striking player hits the other player using the top of the helmet because he lowers his head and aligns his head, neck, and torso to impact the head of the struck player. This procedure results directly in more effective mass and energy transfer to the struck player. The rotational velocities and accelerations of the striking player, in contrast, are very similar to those of the concussed struck player. The authors' data also indicated that with face mask impacts, there was a horizontal direction of loading. Impacts to the face mask from an oblique angle twist the head (head rotation with eyes right or left) while accelerating it, resulting in an increased lateral component of acceleration.

Further analysis of the biomechanics of the striking player indicates that the key to the concussive blow is the head-down position, which increases the mass of the striking player by 67% as a result of the coupling of his torso into the collision.[3] This results in the transfer of more momentum to the struck player. The biomechanical analysis of the striking player suggested ways to possibly diminish the risk of concussion in helmet to helmet collisions. Stricter enforcement of rules against head-down tackling techniques can lower the risk of concussion.

Players by rule are supposed to tackle with their heads up. Tackling in the head-up position results in diminished torso inertia in the striking player, which imparts diminished impact force to the struck player, which should lower the risk of concussion.[3] Diminishing the stiffness of the top crown region of the helmet should result in lower impact force from the striking player, leading to diminished head acceleration for the struck player and increased duration of impact when the top of the helmet is used in making the tackle. This should also lower the risk of concussion. Finally, diminishing the mass of the helmet should result in lower inertia of the striking player. If the helmet weight were to be decreased by 20%, this would result in a 6% reduction in the mass of the striking player's head and a 6% decrease in the collision impact resulting from head-down impact.

The authors also performed biomechanical analyses of the struck player in MTBI collisions.[4] In the impact phase of these collisions, the peak head acceleration of the struck player is 94 ± 28 g and ΔV (velocity change) is 7.2 ± 1.8 m/s. During the impact phase, the movement of the struck player's head is only 20.2 ± 6.8 mm and $6.9° \pm 2.5°$ near the end of the impact (time 10 msec). After the impact phase, there occurs a phase of rapid head displacement in the struck player. During this phase, there is a fourfold increase in head displacement.[4] The head displacement increases to 87.6 ± 21.2 mm and $29.9° \pm 9.5°$, and results in neck tension and bending. This phase of rapid head displacement occurs at approximately 20 msec following initial impact.[4] Impacts to the front of the helmet result in rotation around the superior-inferior axis of the struck player's head because the impact is forward of the neck centerline. Rotation about the superior-inferior axis averages $17.6° \pm 12.7°$, with a twist moment of 17.7 ± 3.3 Nm and neck tension of $1,704 \pm 432$ N at 20 msec.

As noted earlier, the authors' studies have shown that HIC correlates best with NFL concussion risk. Mathematical analysis reveals that HIC is proportional to ΔV to the fourth power divided by head displacement to the 1.5th power ($\Delta V^4/d^{1.5}$).[4] Therefore, relatively small decreases in head ΔV will have a large effect on HIC and concussion risk because the change in ΔV affects HIC by a factor to the fourth power. This suggests that players who have stronger necks will have decreased concussion risk. Stronger necks result in diminished head accelerations in the struck player, decreased ΔV in the struck player, and decreased displacement of the head and neck in the struck player. This has a significant effect on lowering HIC and concussion because of the mathematical equation noted above. As a result of this mathematical relationship, a 10% reduction in head ΔV will result in a 34% reduction in HIC if the head displacement (d) is constant.[4] A 10% increase in head displacement (such as would occur with increased padding and thickness of the helmet) would result in a 15% decrease in HIC, but because the ΔV is often increased by the change in head displacement, the actual decrease in HIC is often less than would be expected.

During the late response (approximately 20 msec after impact), head displacement and rotation loads the neck, resulting in increased neck tension.[4] The largest neck moments are caused by increased rotational moments, and these occur at 40 msec after impact. An increase in neck stiffness will result in decreased peak head acceleration and head ΔV, leading to a large decrease in HIC and concussion risk. Differing neck strengths may help explain the increased susceptibility to concussion seen in younger athletes, because of their relatively weaker neck muscles. This may also play a role in the increased susceptibility to concussion in some female athletes. Differing neck strengths and stiffness may also be an individual difference between NFL players, which can help to explain why some players sustain a clinical concussion and others do not, even though they experience similar impact speeds and accelerations. This suggests that strength training programs aimed at increasing the strength of the neck muscles that resist head rotation and lateral bending might help lower HIC via the mechanism of lowering head ΔV.

Impacts to the face mask result in larger head rotations in the struck player than do impacts directly to the helmet shell.[4] Impacts to the face mask result in a greater head rotation than those to the shell because the face mask is further from the head center of gravity and SI axis of the neck than the shell itself.

The authors further analyzed the biomechanical data using a finite element computer model that simulates the fine anatomic detail and tissue level characteristics of the human head and brain to study head impacts.[5] This model is well-suited for the investigation of strain and strain-rates (tissue deformation) in the brain following head impacts. Our finite element studies of NFL impacts reveal some interesting results. High mid-to-late time-frame strain and strain rate in the midbrain and fornix regions correlated strongly with the occurrence of clinical MTBI.[5] Our computer analysis revealed that the areas of high strain and strain-rates move to the midbrain later in the brain response than the first 10 msec during the impact phase. The average mid-to-late time frame strain was higher in athletes who sustained clinical MTBI than in those who did not sustain clinical MTBI. These findings indicate that the occurrence of clinical MTBI (concussion) is related to brain deformation that occurs after the primary head impact and momentum transfer.[5] This mid-to-late phase of the brain response involves rapid displacement and rotation of the head after the ΔV and rotational velocity changes have occurred.

The authors also found a number of significant correlations between the finite element brain responses and the signs, symptoms, and outcome of clinical MTBI.[5] High strains and strain rates in the mid-to-late time period in the fornix and the corpus callosum correlated with players not returning to play on the day of the injury. High strains and strain rates in the mid-to-late time period in the fornix and the midbrain also correlated with the occurrence of memory and cognition problems.[5] High strain rates occurring in the mid-to-late time period in the midbrain correlated with the occurrence of loss of consciousness.[5] Dizziness correlated with high strain rates in the early time period in the temporal lobes and the orbital frontal cortex. These findings provide strong evidence of a link between the biomechanical effects of NFL impacts to the head and the clinical picture of MTBI.

The biomechanics of the finite element brain responses revealed further insights into the mechanism of MTBI in NFL impacts.[5] The results indicated that there is a delayed response of the brain resulting from impact acceleration of the cranium. Immediately after the impact there is a low strain response in brain regions near the impact site (coup) areas. Because NFL impacts are primarily oblique or lateral, the early regions of these strains are often in the temporal lobe. A short time later, in what is termed the "mid-time phase response," the areas of increased strain move to the opposite side of the brain from the area of initial impact loading (contrecoup areas). In NFL impacts, this is usually the opposite temporal lobe. These finite element model findings offer insight into a possible mechanism to explain coup-contrecoup injuries.

During the late time phase (approximately 20 msec after impact) the areas of high strains and strain rates move to the midbrain and other midline regions. This migration of areas of high strain and strain rates is not caused by wave propagation, which occurs over much shorter time durations than those seen in this model. The migration of the areas of increased strain and strain rate results from the motion of the head secondary to the ΔV and the resultant rapid free-motion displacement and rotation of the cranium. This also offers some insights into further means of preventing clinical MTBI. It suggests that attention should be paid to reducing the mid-to-late strains and strain rates in the midbrain as a new area of prevention. Perhaps this could be done by focusing on the role of the neck musculature. Taken in conjunction with the authors' findings in the biomechanical analysis of the struck player, this supports the notion that strength training to increase neck strength and stiffness may be a means of lowering the risk of MTBI.

Over the past 10 years, helmet performance has been improved by the manufacturers installing thicker padding and providing fuller coverage over larger regions of the helmet shell. Pendulum testing of different helmets demonstrates that the newer helmet designs and padding reduced the risk of concussion in 7.4 m/s (16.6 mph) and 9.3 m/s (20.8 mph) impacts oblique on the face mask or on the helmet shell.[6] Testing also showed that at the highest impacts of 11.2 m/s (25.1 mph), the helmet padding in the newer helmets bottomed out and the head responses increased dramatically, resulting in no improvement in concussion risk. Studies on the newer football helmets have demonstrated that they reduce concussion risk by 10% to 20% in collisions representative of the NFL player experience.[7] By using thicker, more energy-absorbent padding and more padding lower on the side and back of the helmets and around the ears, the helmet manufacturers have improved the safety of NFL players. Their changes have resulted in increased energy absorption by the helmet, decreased head accelerations, and therefore diminished risk of concussion.

EPIDEMIOLOGY

The authors performed a 6-year clinical study of MTBI in the NFL. Data were collected prospectively. We collected complete injury data, initial clinical evaluation data, and follow-up clinical evaluation data for 787 MTBIs that occurred in preseason, regular, or playoff games for 6 seasons between 1996 and 2001. One hundred additional MTBIs from practice sessions were included in the database as well. Data were collected from forms filled out by team physicians and athletic trainers at the time of the initial clinical examination and at the time of follow-up examinations. Clinical symptoms and signs and treatments were recorded.

The definition introduced by the MTBI Committee in 1996 and used for the remainder of the study is as follows.[8] A reportable concussion was defined as a traumatically induced alteration in brain function, which is manifested by:

- Alteration of awareness or consciousness, including but not limited to being dinged, dazed, stunned, woozy, foggy, amnesic, or unconscious.[8]
- Signs and symptoms commonly associated with postconcussion syndrome, including persistent headaches, vertigo, light-headedness, loss of balance, unsteadiness, syncope, near syncope, cognitive dysfunction, memory disturbance, hearing loss, tinnitus, blurred vision, diplopia, visual loss, personality change, drowsiness, lethargy, fatigue, and inability to perform usual daily activities.[8]

The definition of concussion used by the MTBI Committee is a natural extension of a much earlier one from the Committee of the Congress of Neurological Surgeons in 1966 that defined concussion as "a clinical syndrome characterized by immediate transient impairment of neural function such as alteration of consciousness, disturbance of vision, equilibrium, etc, due to mechanical forces."[9]

In the 1913 games (two teams per game) over the 6 years there were 787 MTBIs. The average annual incidence of MTBIs was 131.2 ± 26.8 MTBIs per year. The average rate of occurrence was 0.41 MTBIs per game.[8]

Positions played had a significant impact upon the incidence of MTBIs. The offensive team players had more MTBIs than defensive team players. More concussions occurred among defensive secondary (18.2%), kicking unit players (16.6%), and wide receivers (11.9%) than other position players.[8] The authors determined the injury rates per 100 game positions to determine the relative risks of MTBI according to position. The risk was highest for quarterbacks (1.62 concussions per 100 game positions).[8] It was somewhat lower for wide receivers (1.23), tight ends (0.94), and defensive secondary players (0.93).[8] Punters, return unit players, kickers, and holders had relatively low risks. All backs had three times the relative risk of MTBI compared with all linemen.[8]

The highest frequency of injury occurred in passing plays (35.8%), followed by rushing plays (31.3%), kickoffs (15.9%), and punts (9.5%).[8] When injuries rates per 1000 plays were considered, the relative risk of MTBI on kickoff plays (9.29 per 1000 plays) was four times the risk in rushing plays and passing plays, and 2.5 times that in punting plays;[8] 60.5% of MTBIs were associated with tackling, and 29.5% were associated with blocking. In the majority of the cases (67.7%), MTBI was related to striking of the helmet by the helmet of another player.[8]

On initial clinical evaluation following MTBI, the three most common symptoms that occurred were headaches (55.0%), dizziness (41.8%), and blurred vision (16.3%).[8] At least one symptom of cognitive or memory dysfunction was experienced by 45.9% of players. 16.1% of players returned to the game immediately, 35.6% returned to play later in the same game, 44% did not return to the same game but were not hospitalized, and 2.4% were hospitalized.[8]

Players who did not return to play on the day of the injury statistically had an increased number of symptoms compared with the players who did return to play on the day of injury.[8] The occurrence of any memory or cognitive problem was statistically associated with the player not returning to play on the day of the injury. Loss of consciousness occurred in 9.3% of the cases.[8] The occurrence of loss of consciousness was related to the player missing a longer period of time before returning to play. Players who sustained loss of consciousness average 5.0 ± 7.5 lost days following injury, which was 2.6 times longer than those who did not have loss of consciousness (1.9 ± 5.3 days).[8]

This 6-year study was unique in that it was prospective. It cast a wide net, using a broad definition of MTBI to be very inclusive. A standardized reporting form for all teams was used. All of the players were evaluated by team physicians and trainers and had forms filled out by team physicians and athletic trainers, therefore increasing confidence in the validity and reliability of the medical information. All of the reporting forms from team doctors and athletic trainers were completed at the time of the evaluation of the player, and therefore were not subject to the vagaries of recall at a later time. None of the subjects was lost to follow-up.

Results of the authors' clinical studies help to validate the results of our biomechanical analyses.[8] The players who had the highest risk of MTBI in our study are the same players who make up most of the cases in the video analysis (open-field, high-velocity impacts). There are clear correlations between the biomechanical features and the epidemiologic findings of our study. Quarterbacks have the highest risk of MTBI because they are immobile or slowly moving, and are struck at high velocities by other players while the quarterback is often unaware of the impending impact. As a result, the high velocity of the striking player is transferred to the head of the quarterback, resulting in large ΔV and large accelerations of the head of the quarterback. Defensive backs and wide receivers have a higher relative risk of MTBI as well because they are moving at higher speeds. They are more often struck in high-velocity, high-acceleration impacts. They are often struck in midair, resulting in a fall backward and hitting the back of the helmet on the ground. These high head accelerations often exceed tolerance levels. As noted, linemen have a lower risk of MTBI. This is because they move at slower velocities over shorter distances, resulting in lower head ΔVs and accelerations.

When one compares the clinical symptoms of MTBI in the NFL and MTBI in non-athletes and other athletes, one concludes that the symptoms and signs are generally similar.[8] As noted, 55% of NFL players complained of headache on initial evaluation.

Literature review revealed that 30% to 90% of non-athletes complain of headache and 40% to 85% of other athletes complain of headaches.[8]

Dizziness occurred in 45% of NFL players after MTBI. Other studies have shown that 53% of non-athletes complained of dizziness on initial evaluation.[8] Blurred vision occurred in 16% of NFL players and was found in 14% of non-athletes in other studies. Photophobia occurred in 4.1% of NFL athletes and was found in 7.2% of non-athletes.[8] Cognitive and memory problems occurred in 45.9% of NFL players. Impairment of immediate recall was much more frequent than disorientation. This has important clinical implications for the sideline physician. It is not enough to ask the player only the year, month, and date; the physician must specifically test for immediate recall when evaluating MTBI patients on the sideline. The 39.5% incidence of memory problems in NFL players on initial evaluation is consistent with the results in non-athletes examined 4 weeks after injury: 19% had memory problems, 21% had concentration problems.[8] This is also consistent with the extensive literature on neuropsychological testing in high school and college players.[8]

Somatic complaints such as fatigue, anxiety, personality change, irritability, and sleep disturbance were found in 20.1% of NFL players following MTBI.[8] Similar complaints were found in 50% to 84% of non-athletes, and fatigue specifically was found in 29% of non-athletes 4 weeks after injury.[8] Only one player experienced a seizure following MTBI. This was a generalized tonic-clonic seizure that occurred in the locker room about 30 minutes following the injury. That player made a full recovery. The clinical course of MTBI in the NFL is somewhat different than in the general population. For the great majority of NFL players there is no prolonged disability or prolonged absence from play. Only 2.9% of NFL players missed more than 9 days before returning to play.[8] Most of the MTBIs were self-limiting, and the players made a full spontaneous and rapid recovery. It is also important to note that only 9.3% of the authors' MTBI cohort sustained loss of consciousness. It is thus clear that loss of consciousness is not a common occurrence in NFL MTBIs. If the physicians and athletic trainers only diagnose MTBI when loss of consciousness is present, over 90% of MTBIs will be missed.

Repeat Concussions

The authors performed a more detailed analysis of players who had repeat MTBIs.[10] Of the 887 total MTBIs occurring in 6 years during games or practices, we found that 650 players were involved. One hundred and sixty players (24.6%) had repeat concussions during the 6-year period, 51 players (7.9%) had three or more concussions, and 1 player had seven concussions.[10] The median duration between the first and second MTBI was 374.5 days. Of the 38 repeat MTBIs that occurred within a 90-day window, the median time interval was 31.5 days. Thirty-six of these 38 injuries occurred during regular games in the same season. Only six repeat MTBIs occurred within 2 weeks of the initial injury.[10] The risk of repeat concussion is statistically increased in quarterbacks only. The risk is decreased in offensive linemen.

The authors' analysis revealed that the signs and symptoms were essentially the same for players experiencing only one MTBI and those whose first MTBI later turned out to be the first of repeat MTBIs.[10] The repeat MTBI was different from the first only by the presence of increased somatic complaints, but was otherwise similar to the initial MTBI. There was no difference in the frequency of loss of consciousness for more than 1 minute in single or repeat concussions.[10] There was no difference in the total number of signs or symptoms between single or repeat concussions. There was no difference in the total number of signs or symptoms in single or repeat concussions related to the time interval between the initial and repeat events. There was no difference in the time interval to return to play between single, initial, or repeat concussions. There was no significant difference in the incidence of postconcussion syndrome (missing more than 7 days) between single injury, initial injury and repeat injury.

The authors also evaluated players who had three or more concussions over the 6-year period, and compared them with players who had two or one concussions during the 6-year period.[10] The average duration between concussions was 1 year. There was no difference seen compared with those who had two or one concussions in any clinical characteristic. Our studies thus reveal that the incidence of repeat concussions in the NFL is relatively low: 160 of the 3228 players in the NFL during this 6-year period sustained multiple MTBIs (5%). There were no cases of second impact syndrome seen in our study, and in fact the second impact syndrome has never been seen in the NFL.[10]

The authors' clinical examinations did not reveal an increased frequency of cognitive or memory impairments in players who had multiple concussions compared with players who had single concussions. We also found that cognitive or memory impairments occurred at the same frequency in the group who had three more concussions compared with the group who had two or fewer concussions.[10]

Players Out 7 or More Days

The authors performed an analysis of the 72 cases of a player missing more than 7 days following an MTBI.[11] These account for 8.1% of all NFL MTBIs. Quarterbacks had the highest odds ratio of such prolonged postconcussion syndrome, but this was not statistically significant. Players who were out for more than 7 days had more signs and symptoms on initial evaluation than those who ultimately were out less than 7 days.[11] Certain symptoms are statistically correlated with a player ultimately being out for more than 7 days. These symptoms include disorientation to time, loss of consciousness for greater than 1 minute, the presence of retrograde amnesia, fatigue, overall cognition problems, problems with immediate recall, and general memory problems.[11] Players who were out for more than 7 days also had more total number of symptoms on initial evaluation compared with players who were out for less than 7 days. The players who were out for more than 7 days averaged 4.64 symptoms or signs, versus those who were out for less than 7 days, who averaged 2.58 symptoms or signs on initial evaluation.[11] Of the players who ultimately were out for more than 7 days, 72.2% had been removed from play and not returned to play on the day of the injury. An additional 12.5% had been hospitalized following the injury. Only 6.9% of these players had returned to play immediately.[11]

The clinical course of players who ultimately were out for more than 7 days was evaluated by the authors. The initial examination usually occurred on the sideline or in the locker room, and the first follow-up usually occurred the next day (median 19 hours later). Most of the symptoms started to decrease between the initial and first follow-up, except for memory problems, fatigue, irritability, and sleep disturbance.[11] By the fourth follow-up (median 4.7 days after injury) all memory and cognition problems had resolved. At that time, 17.7% of the group who ultimately would be out for more than 7 days still had headaches, 16.7% had dizziness, and 25% had photophobia. By the seventh follow-up examination all of the symptoms except for headaches had resolved.[11]

Video analysis of some of the cases who ultimately were out for 7 days revealed that most of these were caused by open-field, high-speed impacts. The impacts of two of the players who were ultimately out for more than 7 days had been reconstructed in the laboratory as part of our biomechanical studies. These two cases had very high impact speeds, well above the median.[11]

The authors' analysis revealed that postconcussion symptoms resolve much more quickly in NFL players than in non-athletes.[11] A large percentage of NFL players recover fully from MTBI within minutes to 1 hour. A smaller percentage has symptoms for up to 2 days before recovery. In the authors' opinion, these players fall into the recovery phase of concussion, not postconcussion syndrome. Our analysis indicates that post-concussion syndrome occurs in only 8.1% of NFL MTBIs.[11] We define this as the group having persistent symptoms or signs for 3 to 5 days or longer, who are thus out for more than 7 days. The majority of these players (80.5%) become fully asymptomatic in 7 to 11 days, and therefore are out for less than 14 days. A very small number of players (19.5% of the more than 7day-out group) ultimately missed more than two games.[11]

There are thus four groups of NFL MTBIs that can be characterized by clinical course of recovery:[11] (1) the immediate recovery group (56.0%) become asymptomatic in less than 1 hour, and return to play on the day of the injury; (2) the early recovery group (35.9%) have symptoms and signs for 1 hour to 2 days, and then become asymptomatic and return to play in less than 7 days; (3) the short-duration postconcussion syndrome group (6.5%) have symptoms for 3 to 10 days, and are held out of play for more than 7 and less than 14 days—they miss one game; and (4) the prolonged postconcussion syndrome group (1.6%) have symptoms for more than 10 days, and miss two or more games.

The authors' studies found that there were certain early predictors on initial evaluation that a player might fall into the group that ultimately would be out for more than 7 days.[11] Loss of consciousness for more than 1 minute was associated with increased risk of being out for 7 days. Memory problems at the onset, disorientation to time or general cognitive difficulties on initial evaluation all were associated with increased risk of being out for more than 7 days.[11] The total number of signs and symptoms on initial evaluation was also a good predictor of ultimate 7 days plus out. The group that ultimately would be out for 7 or more days had an average of 4.64 symptoms or signs at the time of initial evaluation. The group that ultimately would be out for less than 7 days had an average of 2.58 symptoms and signs at the time of initial evaluation. We also found that players who were hospitalized after the injury had an increased chance of ultimately being out for more than 7 days.[11]

Only 6.9% of players who were eventually out for more than 7 days had been allowed to return to play on the day of the injury.[11] This indicates that team physicians and athletic trainers in the NFL are effective in screening out the most severely injured players on the sidelines shortly after injury. The authors also found that photophobia at initial evaluation was associated with increased risk of being out for more than 7 days. Results also indicate that the symptom of fatigue at the first follow-up evaluation is associated with an increased risk of being out for more than 7 days. Other findings on follow-up evaluations that were associated with increased risk of being out for more than 7 days were memory or cognitive impairments.[11] Our results indicate that persistent headaches are the most common reason for extended delays in return to play in NFL players.

Return to Play on the Day of Injury

The authors' results indicated that 49.5% of players return to play on the day of injury. No players were considered for return to play until and unless they were asymptomatic and had completely normal clinical neurological examinations, including mental status. The final decision regarding medical clearance to return to play was made by the team physician using clinical expertise and judgment. The median time interval between injury and return to play was 5 minutes in the group that immediately returned, and 17 minutes in the group that was removed from the game for a period of time, rested, and then returned later to the game.[12] Forty-one percent of the players return-ing to the same game or practice were out from play for more than 15 minutes.

The authors found no relationship between repeat concussions and the timing of the player's return to play.[12] Of all the players returning to play in the same game, only 12% had a second concussion the same season involving more than 7 days out. This number is similar to the 10% of cases of 7 plus days out among those who did not return to play that day. Forty-five total players had a repeat concussion in the same season; 20 of these had been removed from play on the day of the injury or hospitalized, and 25 had returned to play on the same day.

Players who returned to play immediately had the lowest mean total number of signs and symptoms (1.52) followed by those who rested and returned (2.07 signs and symp-toms).[12] There was a significantly lower incidence of cognitive or memory problems in those who returned to play on the same day compared with players who did not return to play on the day of the injury. None of the players who returned to play on the day of the injury had experienced loss of consciousness for more than 1 minute.[12]

There were nine cases (in 8 players) in which the player experienced loss of con-sciousness for less than 1 minute and subsequently returned to play on the day of the injury.[12] All but 2 of these had injuries near the end of the game. Six of these 8 players had injuries in later seasons, but these numbers are too small for a statistical analysis. Of the 439 injured players who returned to play on the day of the injury, only 10 subse-quently were out for more than 7 days.[12] This group had more signs and symptoms on average than the 429 other players who had returned to play on the day of the injury.

In the group of players who returned to play on the day of the injury, there were no cases of subdural hematoma, epidural hematoma, or other intracranial hematoma or cerebral edema.[12] There were no cases of second impact syndrome. Compared to the players who did not return to play on the day of the injury, there was no increased risk of the players ultimately being out for more than 7 days (prolonged postconcussion syndrome) or of having a repeat concussion.[12] There were a small number of players in this group who ultimately were out for more than 7 days, which emphasizes the im-portance of follow-up medical evaluation in the days after MTBI, even in those players who had returned to play on the day of the injury.

Based on the results of the authors' 6-year study and the experience of NFL team physicians and certified athletic trainers, the League has recently reaffirmed current NFL medical practice regarding the evaluation and treatment of players who sustain MTBI (**Box 1**). As noted previously, loss of consciousness is infrequent in NFL MTBIs. Over the course of our study, only nine players who sustained brief loss of conscious-ness returned to play on the day of the injury.[12] Only one of those nine players returned to play on the day of the injury in each of the 2000 and 2001 seasons. None of those nine players returned to play on the day of the injury during the 1999 season. Although there is no evidence that any of these players experienced any adverse consequences as a result of returning to play on the day of the injury, NFL team physicians have adop-ted a conservative approach to these cases. The League has recently reaffirmed that those players who are determined by team physicians to be unconscious as the result of head impact should not return to play on the day of the injury (see **Box 1**). In order to further the NFL players' understanding of concussion, the League has also recently developed and disseminated to all its players an information sheet on the subject (**Box 2**).

Neuropsychological Testing

Between 1996 and 2001 neuropsychological testing was done with written tests. The NFL program consisted of testing for attention, visual scanning, information

---

Box 1
NFL statement on return to play after concussion (August 10, 2007)

- Team physicians and athletic trainers should continue to exercise their clinical judgment and expertise in the treatment of each player who sustains a concussion, and to avail themselves of additional expert consultation when clinically indicated. We encourage team physicians and athletic trainers to continue to take a conservative approach to treating concussion.

- Team physicians and athletic trainers should continue to take the time to obtain a thorough history, including inquiring specifically about the common symptoms of concussion, and to conduct a thorough neurological examination, including mental status testing at rest and post-exertion, before making return-to-play decisions in a game or practice.

- The essential criteria for consideration of return to play remain unchanged. The player should be completely asymptomatic and have a normal neurologic examination, including mental status testing at rest and post-exertion, before being considered for return to play.

- Team physicians and athletic trainers should continue to take into account certain symptoms and signs that have been associated with a delayed recovery when making return-to-play decisions. These include confusion, problems with immediate recall, disorientation to time, place, and person, anterograde and retrograde amnesia, fatigue, blurred vision, and presence of three or more signs and symptoms of concussion.

- If the team medical staff determines a player was unconscious, the player should not be returned to the same game or practice.

- Team physicians and athletic trainers should continue to consider the player's history of concussion, including number and time between incidents, type and severity of blow, and time to recover.

- Team physicians and athletic trainers should continue to educate players about concussion and to emphasize the need for players to be forthright about physical and neurological complaints associated with concussion. Player input assists the medical staff and athletic trainers to render appropriate care.

---

processing, visual and verbal memory, speech fluency, and visual motor coordination. These are the cognitive functions most likely to be affected by MTBI.[13] Baseline testing was performed for many players, but not all. After MTBI, initial follow-up neuropsychological testing was done within 24 to 48 hours. If the results were abnormal or there were other postconcussion symptoms, follow-up neuropsychological testing was repeated 5 to 7 days after injury. Analysis of baseline results of 655 NFL players revealed similar findings to baseline results in 386 college athletes.

Neuropsychological testing of NFL players after MTBI revealed that there were no significant differences from baseline to follow-up testing on any of the individual tests.[13] The post-MTBI group scored better on some tests, most likely because of practice effects. The subgroup of athletes who had memory dysfunction on initial clinical evaluation following MTBI performed more poorly on memory tests than those who did not have on field memory symptoms or signs during their initial evaluation.[13] The speed test scores were not different between these groups.

The authors also compared the subgroup of athletes who had three or more concussions over 6 years with those who had two or fewer concussions, and there was no difference in neuropsychological testing between these two groups.[13] We also analyzed the neuropsychological test results of players who were out for more than 7 days, and found that there was no difference compared with those players who were out for less than 7 days, and no difference compared with the baseline norms of the NFL.[13] This analysis of neuropsychological testing indicates that when the team doctor finds memory problems during the initial sideline evaluation, these

Box 2
NFL letter to the players about concussion (August 10, 2007)

What is a concussion? It's more than a "ding."

- Concussions are caused by a hard hit to the head. The hit is typically from another player's helmet, shoulder pad, or knee, or from a fall to the ground. The effects usually last a short time, but it's important that they are treated properly and promptly by you, your team doctors, and your athletic trainers.

- You shouldn't decide if it is just a "ding." Instead, you should report any symptom from the list below to your medical staff. This will help determine whether or not you have had a concussion.

- "Ding" is not a medical term. It doesn't describe specific symptoms and won't help your medical staff. Try to describe your symptoms from the list below.

How do I know if I have had a concussion?

- These are some of the symptoms you may experience immediately or within a few days of having a concussion. Every concussion is different; players may react differently, and not all players will experience the same symptoms.

- The most common symptoms are:

Imbalance: you may feel a change in your sense of balance, feel dizzy or unsteady on your feet.

Headache: this is the most common symptom with concussion. It may be mild to severe in intensity and you may feel like there is pressure in your head. This may be accompanied by nausea and vomiting.

Confusion: you may be confused about where you are, about a play, the score or game situation. You may not remember the play you are running.

Memory loss: you may lose memory about things that happened before or after you were hit. You may not remember what happened during the play or the quarter before your collision, or you can't remember what happened on the field or on the sidelines after your hit. You may ask the same questions over and over again.

Loss of consciousness: you may black out or get knocked out, even for a second or two.

Vision change: You may become sensitive to light, have blurred vision, double vision or feel like lights seem brighter. Some athletes also report "seeing stars" or other objects following a hard hit.

Hearing change: you may feel a change in your hearing so sounds suddenly seem very loud, or you may hear a high-pitched tone in your ears.

Mood change: you may have a sudden change in your mood, or a teammate may notice a change in your mood following a collision. For example, you might suddenly start to laugh or cry for no reason. You may not know this is happening but teammates, coaches, or the medical staff may see it. After a game, you may feel more irritable, anxious, or cranky than usual.

Fatigue: you may feel more exhausted than usual after a game when you had a hard hit to the head. Some athletes report that they need to sleep many more hours after a concussion.

Malaise: You may just "not feel right" but can't point to a specific problem.

- Not every hard hit to the head leads to a concussion, and whether or not you have a concussion can only be determined by your team doctors and athletic trainers. If the team medical staff does not know that you are injured, they can't help you!

- You may not always recognize your symptoms. But your teammates, coaches or family members may see a difference in you that you don't. If someone sees a change in you, take it seriously and report it to your team medical staff.

What should you report to your team medical staff?

(continued on next page)

> **Box 2**
> (*continued*)
>
> - Don't try to make a diagnosis yourself. A concussion needs to be diagnosed by your team medical staff. If you have had a hard hit to the head and have symptoms, you should immediately report your symptoms to your team doctors and athletic trainers, who will conduct a thorough evaluation on the sideline.
> - On occasions, symptoms from concussion will be more obvious or noticeable hours after the impact. Symptoms should be reported to your medical staff regardless when you become aware of them.
> - If you see any symptoms in a teammate, tell your team doctors or athletic trainers, because your teammate may not always realize he has had a concussion.
>
> *Return to play following a concussion*
>
> - After a concussion, all return-to-play decisions should be made by your team medical staff. These decisions should never be made by players or coaches. You should be free of symptoms before you return to play.
>
> *Am I at risk for further injury if I have had a concussion?*
>
> - Current research with professional athletes has shown that you should not be at greater risk of further injury once you receive proper medical care for a concussion and are free of symptoms.
>
> *If I have had more than one concussion, am I at increased risk for another injury?*
>
> - Current research with professional athletes has not shown that having more than one or two concussions leads to permanent problems if each injury is managed properly. It is important to understand that there is no magic number for how many concussions is too many.
> - Research is currently underway to determine if there are any long-term effects of concussion in NFL athletes.
>
> *What is the treatment for a concussion?*
>
> - The treatment for concussion usually consists of rest. Medication may sometimes be prescribed by your team doctors for symptoms such as headaches and dizziness. If your team doctor prescribes medication, be sure to follow his directions and those provided with the prescription.
> - It is important that you avoid drinking alcohol. Also, if you intend to use over-the-counter medication, vitamins, or supplements, tell your team doctor. He may want you to stop taking them.
> - You should avoid caffeine and make sure that you do not become dehydrated.

players will usually have memory impairments on neuropsychological testing performed 1 to 2 days later.

When the team physician does not find clinical cognitive or memory symptoms or signs on the initial sideline evaluation, these players did not have abnormal neuropsychological test results 1 to 2 days later. One can conclude from these data that the clinical examination by the team medical staff on the sideline in the NFL does not miss subtle cognitive or memory dysfunctions. The authors' analysis also indicates that NFL athletes recover within 1 to 2 days following MTBI, which is different than the neuropsychological test results reported in college or high school athletes, who tend to take up to 7 days to recover.[13] The results of neuropsychological testing corroborate our clinical findings that players who sustained three or more concussions or were out for more than 7 days following an MTBI had normal cognitive and memory function, and that there was no evidence of permanent or cumulative effects of MTBI in this group of contemporary NFL players.

In a second evaluation of neuropsychological testing in the NFL, the authors compared the results of computerized neuropsychological testing to those in a group of high school players. NFL players performed better than high school players on initial and follow-up evaluations following MTBI.[14] This analysis supports our conclusion from neuropsychological testing using paper and pencil that NFL players recover relatively quickly compared with younger athletes.

CONCUSSION MANAGEMENT GUIDELINES

A number of practitioners have developed and promoted guidelines for the evaluation and management of concussion in sport.[15-18] Based on the authors' experience in the NFL and our studies of concussion in the NFL, we do not believe that any of these guidelines are applicable or relevant to the NFL experience. The rationale for these guidelines is flawed. The authors of the guidelines indicate that the reasons why such guidelines are necessary include the prevention of second impact syndrome, the prevention of intracranial hemorrhage secondary to trauma, and the prevention of chronic brain damage related to head injuries in sports.[15]

In fact, none of these rationales is applicable to the NFL experience. There has never been a case of second impact syndrome in the NFL. There have been no cases of intracranial hemorrhage, subdural hemorrhage, epidural hemorrhage, or cerebral edema occurring in the NFL for over 20 years, and none were seen in our studies. There is presently no valid evidence that a chronic encephalopathy exists for contemporary professional football players.

The proposed guidelines start by grading the severity of concussions. Up until the past few years, concussion grading was done by assessing the presence or absence of symptoms such as loss of consciousness and post-traumatic amnesia, and tracking the number of concussions that the player had sustained.[15-17] The use of such a limited number of criteria limits these grading systems significantly. The authors' NFL studies have confirmed that loss of consciousness and post-traumatic confusion or cognitive or memory impairments are predictors of longer recovery after MTBI;[11] however, our studies also show that there are a number of other prognostic factors of equal importance that have never been included in the concussion guideline grading systems. Such factors include photophobia, fatigue, and the total number of signs and symptoms present on initial evaluation.[11]

The authors' studies also demonstrated that the position played by the injured athlete and the type of play during which the injury occurred also have prognostic value, and these are not included in the concussion grading systems. Our results also demonstrate that signs and symptoms on follow-up examinations a day after injury also had significant prognostic usefulness.[11] Such signs include fatigue, sleep disturbance, irritability, and cognitive or memory impairments. None of the concussion grading systems use any results from examinations other than those on the day of the injury. Thus, the grading systems are limited in scope and fail to incorporate numerous factors that can be seen as predictors of delayed recovery in the NFL.

An attempt to grade concussion severity immediately after the injury is prone to error. In the authors' studies, there were a number of players who had signs and symptoms suggesting a poor prognosis who in fact recovered quickly and returned to play on the day of the injury, or were cleared to return to play within a few days of the injury. Conversely, there were a few players who had minimal signs or symptoms immediately following the injury suggesting a good prognosis, but who ultimately had delayed recovery and did not return to play for more than 7 days. The authors' statistical analysis showed clearly that none of the prognostic factors noted or any combination of the prognostic factors was 100% accurate in predicting delayed recovery.

The authors' data show that the presence of any of the following five signs or symptoms correctly identified 72% of players who had delayed recovery:[11] (1) loss of consciousness for 1 minute or more, (2) fatigue, (3) photophobia, (4) disorientation to time, or (5) retrograde amnesia. There were also 216 players who had one or more of the signs or symptoms who did not have a delayed recovery, however.[11] Using the above signs and symptoms for grading concussion and relating it to prognosis identifies a large number of players, but only 19% of them would actually go on to have a delayed recovery. The results of our studies, with the delineation of four different groups of recovery type following NFL concussion, indicate that the most reliable way to grade concussion severity is retrospectively, based on how long it actually takes the player to make a full recovery.[11]

Some recent concussion grading systems have adopted the authors' approach and now state that concussion severity can only be graded retrospectively.[18] This is scientifically valid, but obviously cannot be used to determine prognosis for any individual player, and therefore has no value to the clinician in the form of a guideline helping to make appropriate management decisions at the time of the injury or shortly following the injury.

Some current guidelines indicate that all players who sustain loss of consciousness should be removed from play for at least 7 days.[15,18] The authors' studies show that, although loss of consciousness is one factor related to prognosis, it certainly is not the only factor, and that some players who experience brief loss of consciousness can safely return to play on the day of the injury. Focusing solely on loss of consciousness is a problem because there are a number of other signs and symptoms equally as important in determining prognosis that guidelines tend to overlook.

Concussion management guidelines have until recently been based upon concussion grading systems. Various guidelines have linked management decisions to the grade of concussion.[15,16] As the authors have noted, the grading system that is most consistent with the evidence is one that has no prognostic usefulness, and in fact indicates that concussions cannot be graded until after the player has fully recovered. Therefore management decisions based on concussion grade in the old system using loss of consciousness or amnesia are flawed.

Rigid, arbitrary guideline-determined decision-making stands in contrast to the NFL experience, in which every player who sustains MTBI must be cleared by the team physician and athletic trainer. Team medical staffs only allow the player to return to play when they believe that it is safe for the player to do so. In the NFL experience, there are 6 years of data demonstrating that these medical decisions by the team medical personnel are valid and reliable, and that adult professional football players returned to play on the day of the injury under such circumstances have no risk of second impact syndrome, cerebral edema, or intracranial bleeding, and have no increased risk of repeat MTBI or prolonged postconcussion syndrome or any other adverse consequences, compared with adult professional football players who are not cleared to return to play of the day of the injury.[12]

The concussion management guidelines were developed to assist the treating physicians in making clinical management decisions, but their rationale is flawed. The system of grading concussions was not scientifically valid until recently, and the new system of grading concussions that does have scientific validity is of no prognostic usefulness. The concussion management recommendations under the various guidelines are not consistent with NFL practice or the results of the authors' prospective 6-year study on MTBI in the NFL. It is the authors' recommendation that NFL team physicians and trainers continue to make return-to-play decisions based upon their professional judgment, their clinical expertise, and individual evaluation of each case of MTBI, without resorting to or being limited by general guidelines that are not relevant to this specific patient population.

CHRONIC TRAUMATIC ENCEPHALOPATHY

That there is a chronic traumatic encephalopathy (CTE) of boxers is not in doubt. The same, however, cannot be said about CTE of football players. There is an extensive medical literature documenting the clinical picture (ie, combinations of dysarthria, cerebellar dysfunction, extrapyramidal dysfunction, pyramidal dysfunction, cognitive-behavioral impairments), radiologic findings (ie, enlarged third and lateral ventricles, cerebral atrophy, cavum septum pellucidum) and distinctive neuropathologic features (abnormalities of the septum pellucidum, depigmentation of the substantia nigra with neuronal loss, cerebellar scarring, and numerous neurofibrillary tangles [NFTs] with a sparsity of amyloid plaques on routine histology but the presence of such plaques with more modern antibody immunofluorescent techniques) associated with CTE of boxers.[19–25] This stands in stark contrast to the scant evidence of a CTE in American football players found in isolated case reports and survey type studies of retired players.

Omalu and colleagues[26,27] have published two papers in the literature purported to document cases of CTE in former professional football players. The first case is that of a player who had a long NFL career and who reportedly had a "neuropsychiatric history that resembled dysthymic disorder," deficits in memory and judgment, and "Parkinsonian symptoms."[26] The brain neuropathology consisted of decreased pigmentation of the substantia nigra, "many diffuse amyloid plaques," "sparse NFTs," and "sparse" neuritic threads.[26] The study stated that the neuropathology met the criteria for CTE in boxers, especially as described by Corsellis and colleagues.[19] There are numerous problems with this paper that the authors have detailed in two letters to the editor.[28,29]

Briefly, these problems include the fact that the neuropathology in this case was not at all consistent with the CTE of boxers as described by Corsellis;[19] the absence of any objective medical, neurologic, or psychiatric reports or studies from any physician who ever saw the patient while he was alive (the history as presented in the paper came from postmortem interviews with the patient's family); and the failure of Omalu and colleagues to consider the possible role of the patient's multiple medical illnesses and possible steroid use during his playing career on his clinical or neuropathological findings.[28,29]

The second case reported by Omalu and colleagues[27] is that of a former NFL player who developed a psychiatric disorder characterized by paranoia, agitation, unpredictable fluctuations in mood and personality, "extreme highs and lows," business failures, multiple suicide attempts, multiple psychiatric hospitalizations, and ultimately death by suicide. The neuropathology reportedly consisted of a cavum septum pellucidum, mild depigmentation of the substantia nigra, mild dropout of cerebellar neurons, and absence of amyloid plaques and moderate-to-marked density of NFTs and neuropil threads in many brain regions.[27] Among the problems with this case report are that the history was obtained only from a second family, and that there is no objective verification or reports from the multiple psychiatrists or other physicians who must have evaluated the patient during his many psychiatric hospitalizations.

Omalu and colleagues[27] are intent upon demonstrating that this player's psychiatric problems only developed after his retirement. This is inconsistent with the fact reported in the paper that the player had attempted suicide at least once before his retirement and was diagnosed with major depression during his playing career. The attempt by Omalu and colleagues[27] to link head injuries in professional football to this player's neuropathological findings ignores the concussion that the player sustained in an automobile accident during his career and de-emphasizes the fact that he played almost as many years of football in college and the military as he did in the NFL. It is also important to note that the neuropathology in their second case is much different from the neuropathology in the first case.[26,27]

Omalu and colleagues[27] also failed to take into account the possible effects of the player's severe thyroid disease and history of steroid usage during his playing career on his clinical or neuropathological picture. Thus, the linkage of the clinical and neuropathological findings solely to his career in the NFL is clearly in doubt. Subsequent to these case reports, Omalu has reported two further "cases" to the media rather than in a scientific journal. As scientists and physicians, the authors cannot objectively evaluate reports that do not appear in the appropriate scientific formats.

The results of two recent mail survey studies of retired NFL players have suggested that players who have a history of three or more concussions during their NFL career have an increased incidence of depression, and that retired NFL players are at increased risk of developing mild cognitive impairment (MCI) or early-onset Alzheimer's disease compared with the general population.[30,31] These studies relied solely on the reports of the players themselves, with no objective verification from physician reports or examinations, and relied upon the players themselves to give an accurate concussion history for events occurring many decades before the survey was completed.[30,31] In view of these obvious methodological problems, the results must be seen as preliminary and inconclusive, although raising important questions. More research and study is needed to determine the long-term effects, if any, of a career in professional football on the brain.

SUMMARY

The authors' studies have yielded a great deal of data regarding the biomechanics of head injury and the clinical picture of MTBI in the NFL. The research has demonstrated the link between the effects of biomechanical forces on the brain and the clinical symptomatology of the concussed players. New insights into the mechanisms of injury are leading to new ways of protecting football players from the effects of MTBI. Our clinical data validate the effectiveness of the current NFL physician approach to the evaluation and treatment of the player who sustains MTBI. There are still many more questions to answer and much more knowledge to be gained from continuing research in this area.

REFERENCES

1. Pellman EJ, Viano DC, Tucker AM, et al. Concussion in professional football: reconstruction of game impacts and injuries. Neurosurgery 2003;53:799–814.
2. Pellman EJ, Viano DC, Tucker AM, et al. Concussion in professional football: location and direction of helmet—part 2. Neurosurgery 2003;53:1328–41.
3. Viano DC, Pellman EJ. Concussion in professional football: biomechanics of the striking player—part 8. Neurosurgery 2005;56:266–80.
4. Viano DC, Casson IR, Pellman EJ. Concussion in professional football: biomechanics of the struck player—part 14. Neurosurgery 2007;61:313–28.
5. Viano DC, Casson IR, Pellman EJ, et al. Concussion in professional football: brain responses by finite element analysis—part 9. Neurosurgery 2005;57:891–916.

6. Pellman EJ, Viano DC, Withnall C, et al. Concussion in professional football: helmet testing to assess impact performance–part 11. Neurosurgery 2006; 58(1):78–96.

7. Viano DC, Pellman EJ, Withnall C, et al. Concussion in professional football: newer helmet performance in reconstructed NFL impacts—part 13. Neurosurgery 2006; 59:591–606.

8. Pellman EJ, Powell JW, Viano DC, et al. Concussion in professional football: epidemiological features of game injuries and review of the literature—part 3. Neurosurgery 2004;54:81–97.

9. Congress of Neurological Surgeons. Proceedings of the Congress of Neurological Surgeons: Report of the Ad Hoc Committee to Study Head Injury Nomenclature. Clin Neurosurg 1996;16:386–94.

10. Pellman EJ, Viano DC, Casson IR, et al. Concussion in professional football: repeat injuries—part 4. Neurosurgery 2004;55:860–76.

11. Pellman EJ, Viano DC, Casson IR, et al. Concussion in professional football: injuries involving 7+ days out—part 5. Neurosurgery 2004;55:1100–19.

12. Pellman EJ, Viano DC, Casson IR, et al. Concussion in professional football: players returning to the same game—part 7. Neurosurgery 2005;56:79–92.

13. Pellman EJ, Lovell MR, Viano DC, et al. Concussion in professional football: neuropsychological testing—part 6. Neurosurgery 2004;55:1290–305.

14. Pellman EJ, Lovell MR, Viano DC, et al. Concussion in professional football: recovery of NFL and high school athletes assessed by computerized neuropsychological testing—part 12. Neurosurgery 2006;58:263–74.

15. American Academy of Neurology: Practice parameter: the management of concussion in sports (summary statements). Neurology 1997;48:581–5.

16. Cantu RC. Classification and clinical management of concussion. In: Bailes JE, Day AL, editors. Neurological sports medicine: a guide for physicians and athletic trainers. Park Ridge (IL): AANS; 2001. p. 25–33.

17. Colorado Medical Society: Report of the Sports Medicine Committee: guidelines for the management of concussion in sports. Denver (CO): Colorado Medical Society; 1991.

18. McCrory P, Johnston K, Meeuwisse W, et al. Summary and agreement statement of the 2nd International Conference on Concussion in Sport, Prague 2004. Br J Sports Med 2005;39(4):196–204, review.

19. Corsellis JA, Bruton CJ, Freeman-Browne D. The aftermath of boxing. Psychol Med 1973;3:270–303.

20. Casson IR, Siegel O, Sham R, et al. Brain damage in modern boxers. JAMA 1984; 251:2663–7.

21. Martland HS. Punch drunk. JAMA 1928;91:1103–7.

22. Morrison R. Medical and public health aspects of boxing. JAMA 1986;255: 2475–80.

23. Payne E. Brains of boxers. Neurochirurgia (Stuttg) 1968;11:173–88.

24. Roberts AH. Brain damage in boxers. London: Pitman Medical and Scientific Publishing; 1969.

25. Ross RJ, Cole M, Thompson JS, et al. Boxers: computed tomography, EEG, and neurological evaluation. JAMA 1983;249:211–3.

26. Omalu BI, DeKosky ST, Minster RL, et al. Chronic traumatic encephalopathy in a National Football League player:I. Neurosurgery 2005;57(1):128–34 [discussion: 128–34].

27. Omalu BI, Dekosky ST, Minster RL, et al. Chronic traumatic encephalopathy in a National Football League player: II. Neurosurgery 2006;58(5):E1003.

28. Casson IR, Pellman EJ, Viano DC. Chronic traumatic encephalopathy in a National Football League player [letter to the editor]. Neurosurgery 2006;59(5):E1152.
29. Casson IR, Pellman EJ, Viano DC. Chronic traumatic encephalopathy in a National Football League player [letter to the editor]. Neurosurgery 2006;58(5):E1003.
30. Guskiewicz KM, Marshall SW, Bailes J, et al. Association between recurrent concussion and late-life cognitive impairment in retired professional football players. Neurosurgery 2005;57:719–26.
31. Guskiewicz KM, Marshall SW, Bailes J, et al. Recurrent concussion and risk of depression in retired professional football players. Med Sci Sports Exerc 2007; 39(6):903–9.

Neurologic Injuries in Hockey

Richard A. Wennberg, MD, MSc, FRCPC[a],*, Howard B. Cohen, DDS, MA, PhD[b],
Stephanie R. Walker, MA, MLS[c]

KEYWORDS

• Hockey • Head injury • Concussion • Spinal cord injury

What they worry about most is injuries,…[in] this combination of ballet and murder…

Al Purdy, Hockey Players, 1965

References to hockey injuries can be found not only in poetry but also in the medical literature, where authors have described the game as a combination of "finesse and controlled aggression".[1,2] Hockey players attain skating speeds of more than 30 miles per hour and may shoot the puck at more than 100 miles per hour, all in the setting of a contact sport played on an ice surface enclosed by unyielding boards and glass.[1] There is an understandable risk for injuries, and many of these affect the nervous system.

Epidemiologic studies of hockey have reported overall injury rates using heterogeneous methods that prevent direct comparisons.[1–7] A recent large study of United States college hockey revealed an injury rate of approximately 16 injuries per 1000 athlete exposures.[7] Injuries occur much more commonly during games than practices[1,2,4,6–8] and most injuries (80%–90%) are the result of direct trauma, including collisions with other players, the ice surface, the boards and glass, goal posts, sticks, and the puck.[1,7] Injury rates increase with age and level of play;[1,4,6,9,10] based on age, the number of hours of playing time per injury is reported as 100 hours per injury for 11 to 14 year olds, 16 hours per injury for 15 to 18 year olds, 11 hours per injury for 19- to 21-year-old college players, and 7 hours per injury for professional players.[4] Children and youths playing in leagues permitting body checking have higher injury rates than players in noncontact leagues.[5,6,11,12] A study of Canadian University hockey showed no significant difference in injury rates between male and female players;[13] however,

---

This article originally appeared in *Neurologic Clinics*, Volume 26, Issue 1.

[a] Division of Neurology, Toronto Western Hospital, University of Toronto, 399 Bathurst Street, 5W444, Toronto, ON, Canada M5T 2S8

[b] Dufferin Rogers Dental, 2032 Dufferin Street, Toronto, ON, Canada M6E 3R5

[c] Brooklyn College of the City University of New York, 2900 Bedford Avenue, Library, Room 147, Brooklyn, NY 11210-2889, USA

* Corresponding author.

E-mail address: r.wennberg@utoronto.ca (R.A. Wennberg).

Phys Med Rehabil Clin N Am 20 (2009) 215–226
doi:10.1016/j.pmr.2008.10.005
1047-9651/08/$ – see front matter © 2009 Elsevier Inc. All rights reserved.

more recent studies of United States college hockey showed female athletes to have game injury rates less than 60% that of male athletes.[7,14] Most female hockey injuries result from collisions, even though intentional body checking is not permitted in women's hockey.[7,13,14] Neurologic injuries seem to account for 5% to 25% of all injuries in these various epidemiologic studies, with concussions making up the majority of neurologic injuries.

This article presents an overview of neurologic injuries occurring in hockey. More common or serious injuries are given extra attention. The articles by Boden and Jarvis; Tator; Park and Levy; and Lovell specifically devoted to sports-related spinal injuries and sports-related head injuries elsewhere in this issue are also relevant for researchers and clinical personnel caring for injured hockey players.

Information used in this article was obtained from searches of the following databases: Medline, SportDiscus, Scopus, CINAHL, Health Reference Center Academic, and CSA Biological and Medical Sciences. The majority of pertinent, nonduplicate citations were found in Medline (MeSH "Hockey" AND [MeSH "Brain Concussion+" OR {(MeSH "Trauma+" OR MeSH "Wounds and Injuries+") AND MeSH "Central Nervous System+"}]) and CSA Biological and Medical Sciences (keywords: Hockey AND [wound* OR injur* OR trauma*] AND [neuro* OR nervous system OR brain]). References within these citations were used to identify additional relevant articles.

A presentation of the injuries formally described in the medical literature does not provide a complete picture of neurologic injuries in hockey. For example, there are no articles describing lumbosacral disc disease/radiculopathy or the more rare thoracic radiculopathy in hockey, despite the fact that a perusal of public injury data from professional hockey teams shows diagnoses of back strain, back spasms, herniated disc in back, and surgery for herniated disc in back as among the most common injuries accounting for lost time from play (personal observations). This may reflect not only a difficulty in attributing this particular injury to any specific incident, but also an understanding that this injury is common and certainly likely to occur in active athletes playing a contact sport, such that there is no great interest or novelty in reporting on it in the medical literature. Uncommon injuries that could occur as a result of similar, non–sports-related trauma also are unlikely to be reported formally and, therefore, escape inclusion in this review.

Neurologic injuries that have been described in the scientific literature are discussed in a peripheral-to-central direction—considering muscle, nerve, plexus, root, cord, and brain—beginning with injuries affecting the peripheral nervous system and followed by injuries affecting the central nervous system. Additional points regarding diagnosis, investigation, and treatment are included if novel or unusual, and a section on injury prevention concludes this article.

INJURIES OF THE PERIPHERAL NERVOUS SYSTEM
Muscle

The broad category of "muscle strain" is discussed both for completeness and because "muscle strain" injuries of one sort or another make up a large percentage of overall hockey injuries.[1–5,7,8] Muscle strains may occur about the shoulder region but more common are strains about the region of the lower abdomen, upper leg, hip, and pelvis, especially the "groin strain," likely the result of overuse of the hip adductors, which can be a cause of significant lost time from play.[1,7,15] It seems that the incidence of groin strains, abdominal strains, and "sports hernias" (with symptoms possibly related to iliohypogastric nerve compression) has increased in professional players in recent years; a history of previous similar injury and a less intense off-season sport-specific training regimen are identified as risk factors for injury occurrence.[15,16]

Peripheral Nerve

In the lower extremity, peroneal nerve lesions are described as resulting from direct blunt trauma or, in one case, laceration of the nerve with a skate blade.[17–19] A single case of a reversible plantar neuropathy was reported in a recreational hockey player, caused by compression from a skate boot fitted with an inflatable lining.[20]

In the upper extremity, axillary neuropathies are described as a result of direct trauma and compression and with shoulder dislocations.[17,21–23]

Plexus and Nerve Root

The so-called "stinger" or "burner" occurs acutely after trauma to the shoulder region and is associated with pain, numbness, or tingling radiating down one upper limb, sometimes associated with transient weakness, typically recovering over a period of minutes.[17,21,24] This injury is most common in American football but is also reported in hockey.[17,21,24] It is considered to represent upper cervical nerve root injury or transient dysfunction affecting the upper trunk of the brachial plexus.[17,21,24]

INJURIES OF THE CENTRAL NERVOUS SYSTEM
Spinal Cord

Traumatic spinal cord injury is probably the most devastating injury in hockey.[6] Although rare, the risk for catastrophic spinal cord injury is never absent from hockey and the possibility of incurring a sports injury resulting in permanent quadriplegia is a sobering consideration.

The vast majority of spinal cord injuries in hockey occur in the cervical spine region, especially between the C5 and C7 levels.[6,25,26] Collisions with the boards account for most spinal injuries, usually occuring when a player is body checked or pushed from behind into the boards head first.[6,25–29] The risk for catastrophic outcome is greatest if a player's neck is flexed in posture at the time of impact with the boards, a posture greatly increasing the risk for a vertebral burst fracture and associated cervical cord compression.[6,30,31] The sequence of images in the top row of **Fig. 1** shows an example of this type of collision: in this case, the player suffered only a concussion with no associated cervical spine injury, likely protected by the slight neck extension apparent before impact.

Data from a Canadian registry suggests an increase in the incidence of hockey-related spinal injuries between 1981 and 1996 compared with the preceding 15 years, although this apparent increase may have been related to better diagnosis and reporting.[25] Encouragingly, subsequently reported data from the same registry suggest a decline in the number of spinal injuries in more recent years, especially those causing paralysis resulting from checking from behind.[32]

Another, less serious, spinal cord injury is the so-called "cervical cord neurapraxia" or "transient quadriplegia" phenomenon, wherein reversible four-extremity weakness and/or sensory loss occurs as a result of transient cord compression.[33–35] In adults, it is most common in individuals who have sagitally narrowed cervical canals;[33] however, cervical stenosis usually is not found in injured children, where the mobility of the pediatric spine is postulated as the most relevant anatomic risk factor.[36] Like the stinger, this injury is most common in American football but also can occur in hockey.[33,36] Recurrence is common in adult athletes who return to contact sports, and the risk for recurrence is correlated with the degree of cervical stenosis.[33–35]

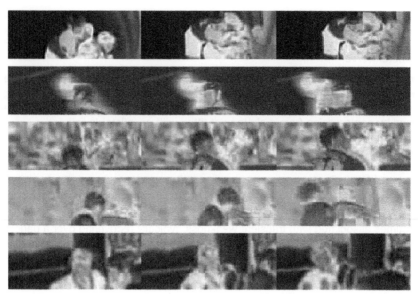

Fig. 1. Different mechanisms of injury causing concussion in hockey. (*Top row*) Deceleration impact as player moving at high speed collides head first into end boards and glass. Mild extension posture of neck before (*left*) and at impact (*middle*) affords protection against cervical spine injury. This type of collision with the neck flexed can result in catastrophic cervical spinal cord injury. (*Second row*) Rotational impact about vertical axis as player's head is struck by opponent's shoulder in open ice collision. (*Middle row*) Combination of deceleration and rotational impact about vertical and horizontal axes as player moving at high speed is body checked in an open ice collision. The rotational component of impact results from the opponent's shoulder hitting the player's head. (*Fourth row*) Rotational neck flexion/extension impact (whiplash injury) occurring without direct head contact. Before impact, neck posture is neutral (*left*). Impact occurs as player is body checked in the chest by opponent's shoulder (*middle*), resulting in rapid neck flexion (*middle*) and subsequent extension (*right*). (*Bottom row*) Rotational impact about horizontal axis occurs as player is struck under the jaw by an uppercut punch (*middle*).

Brain

Severe brain injuries, such as epidural or subdural hematomas and fatalities associated with skull fractures, are known to have occurred throughout the history of hockey, and occasional cases are reported in the scientific literature.[6,37–39] Such injuries, however, have become exceedingly rare as a result of the introduction of mandatory helmet use in recent decades.[40,41]

There are two case reports describing extraordinary brain injury mortalities triggered by hockey trauma; in the first, a blow to the neck was followed by delayed embolization from a traumatic pseudoaneurysm of the common carotid artery, resulting in fatal cerebral infarction;[42] in the second, a man struck by a puck in the mastoid region just below his helmet suffered a fatal rupture of a vertebral artery berry aneurysm.[43]

In contrast to the few reports of severe sports-related brain injury, mild traumatic brain injury, or concussion, is without doubt the most written about neurologic sports injury of the past decade.[44–73] Most of the published information regarding diagnosis, management, investigations, neuropsychologic testing, return-to-play guidelines, concussive convulsions, second impact syndrome, and recent research into the poorly understood pathophysiology of concussion is not specific to hockey and is not summarized in this article. The high incidence of concussions in modern hockey, however, is now appropriately recognized as an important issue and certain hockey-specific aspects are discussed.

In parallel with increased recognition of sports-related concussions during the past decade, it is suggested that the incidence of concussions in hockey is increasing.[2,74] There are few data, however, validating this claim. A prospective study of Swedish Elite League hockey showed no change in concussion frequency over four seasons from 1988–1989 through 1991–1992.[40] Concussion incidence in a single Swedish Elite League team followed over a period of 17 years, however, suggests an increasing rate of concussion in recent years.[75] A study of reported concussions in professional National Hockey League (NHL) players between 1986–1987 and 2001–2002 found a tripling in the concussion rate around 1997, followed by a subsequent plateau.[76] This abrupt increase in reported concussions in the NHL occurred during a time of increased awareness of sports-related concussions and during the initiation of the NHL Concussion Program, a project developed to monitor the occurrence of concussions and help guide return-to-play decisions.[76,77] Therefore, much of this apparent increase in the NHL concussion rate is likely related to improved recognition and reporting.[62,76] Nonetheless, the high incidence of concussions across all levels of hockey remains cause for concern.

More than 10% of 9- to 17-year-old players sustain a concussion in a given season.[6,41] Different studies report concussion rates of up to 0.8 per 1000 player hours in 5- to14-year-olds, 2.7 per 1000 player hours in high school players, 4.2 per 1000 player hours in university players, and 6.6 per 1000 player hours in elite players.[6,37] The annual risk for concussion in professional players in the Swedish Elite League is approximately 5% per player.[40] Perhaps unexpectedly, recent studies of United States college hockey show female athletes to have a higher game concussion rate (2.72/1000 athlete exposures) than male athletes (1.47/1000 athlete exposures). This female preponderance of concussion could be related to a greater disparity in the abilities of individual female players or to a larger number of unexpected collisions, given that volitional body checking is not permitted.[7,14] Weighted by position, forwards are more likely to suffer concussions than defense players, and goalies are far less likely to suffer concussions than either forward or defense.[7,58] It also must be acknowledged, with respect to all of these published injury rates, that the true incidence of hockey concussions is almost certainly is higher because of under-reporting.[76,78,79]

Biomechanical studies show that concussion may result from either translational (linear) motion of the brain imparted by a direct head impact or from rotational mechanisms, where an impact rotates the brain in a circular motion about some axis.[80,81] Concussion-inducing rotational forces may be imparted to the brain without direct head impact (ie, with whiplash injury).[80–82] Hockey-related concussions may result from any of these mechanisms.[83,84]

A collision of some sort is invariably the cause of a concussion in hockey. Different studies report that 45% to 60% of concussions result from player-player collisions and that 26% to 34% result from collisions of players with the boards or glass. The remainder of concussions are the result of collisions with the ice surface or goal posts or direct impacts from sticks or the puck.[6,7,10] It is reported that fighting (in leagues that permit fighting) is not a common cause of concussion in hockey;[6,58] however, more recent evidence suggests otherwise,[84] and it seems that concussions related to fighting are particularly likely to be under-reported in the NHL (personal observation).

Representative examples of the different mechanisms of injury causing concussions in hockey are presented in **Fig. 1**, with detailed explanations given in the legend.

PREVENTION

Prevention of head and neck injuries is a paramount concern in hockey. The personal and social costs of chronic spinal cord and brain injury are extensive.[41,85] The absence of effective medical interventions to reverse the effects of spinal cord and mild traumatic brain injury, combined with the potential severity of the former and the great incidence of the latter, make prevention efforts for these two injuries crucial. Injury prevention methods are considered under different headings of equipment, rules, training, education, and environment.[85]

Equipment

The introduction of mandatory helmet use essentially eliminated catastrophic brain injury at all levels of hockey, and the later introduction of mandatory facial protection in youth hockey has virtually eliminated ocular, facial, and dental injuries.[41,86,87] Early concerns that the weight of the helmet and face mask combination might increase the risk for cervical spine injuries[86,88] are not supported by biomechanical studies,[89,90] although a hypothesis that the increased protection afforded to players by helmets and face masks has led to an increase in illegal and injurious behavior is not disproved.[86,88]

There is no available hockey equipment that protects against cervical spine injury. Helmet development and testing is a complex issue not discussed in this article.[89–94] There is a belief, however, that the continued modifications made to helmet designs in recent years have failed to have much, if any, effect on the incidence of concussions in hockey (personal observation). There is not a single study in the scientific literature documenting the efficacy of helmets in prevention of concussion.[85]

The effect of full facial or half facial (visor) protection on concussion incidence is reported by several investigators.[95–100] Neither form of facial protection has decreased concussion incidence; however, decreased severity of concussions in players wearing full-face shields, as reflected by time lost from play, is suggested in some studies.[95,96,99]

The potential for mouth guards to protect against concussions in hockey is also controversial. There is some evidence suggesting that mouthguard usage decreases concussion severity in hockey.[95] Most studies examining the effects of mouthguards, however, fail to demonstrate conclusively decreased incidence or severity of sports-related concussion.[101,102]

There is concern that the design of shoulder pads and elbow pads has changed over the years to incorporate harder materials that may increase the risk for concussion in players struck by these pieces of hard protective equipment. The NHL created an injury analysis panel in 2000, which recommended that manufacturers should cover exposed hard plastic surfaces with softer padding.[76]

Rules

Vigorous enforcement of existing rules and the introduction of stiffer penalties to prevent deliberate blows to the head have been advocated and instituted across multiple levels of hockey in recent years.[58,76,103]

There is some evidence that the introduction of new rules and stiffer penalties to eliminate checking from behind may be starting to have a beneficial effect on reduction of the number of catastrophic cervical cord injuries.[32,41]

Because of clear evidence of an increased incidence of concussion in youth minor hockey leagues that permit body checking,[5,6,11,12] recommendations have arisen from within the medical community for the further restriction of body checking in youth hockey.[104]

Training

It is suggested that sport-specific training programs might be able to limit the risk for concussion or spinal cord injury through neck strengthening or the improvement of avoidance skills.[85,105] The potential benefit of such training, however, has not been addressed formally.[85]

Education

There is some recent evidence that educational programs of various sorts may be beneficial in reducing the incidence of spinal cord injury and concussion by reducing players' tendencies to injurious behavior and by increasing their knowledge of personal safety.[106,107]

Environment

Given that most head and neck injuries are caused by collisions, changes in the playing environment that would decrease the frequency of collisions, or lessen the force of impact, could provide direct prevention against spinal cord injury and concussion. Fewer collisions of all sorts, including head impacts, occur in elite hockey played on the larger international ice surfaces, compared with the smaller NHL rinks.[108,109] Therefore, enlarging the playing surface could presumably decrease the incidence of concussions. The same effect of reduced collisions would presumably also accrue from reducing the number of players on the ice, for example, switching to four-on-four play, although this would alter the nature of the game significantly.[108]

ACKNOWLEDGMENT

Text from the Al Purdy poem, *Hockey Players*, (*courtesy of* Harbour Publishing, Madeira Park, BC, Canada; with permission).

REFERENCES

1. Daly PJ, Sim FH, Simonet WT. Ice hockey injuries. A review. Sports Med 1990; 10(2):122–31.
2. Biasca N, Simmen HP, Bartolozzi AR, et al. Review of typical ice hockey injuries. Survey of the North American NHL and hockey Canada versus European leagues. Unfallchirurg 1995;98(5):283–8.
3. Hornof Z, Napravnik C. Analysis of various accident rate factors in ice hockey. Med Sci Sports 1973;5(4):283–6.
4. Sutherland GW. Fire on ice. Am J Sports Med 1976;4(6):264–9.
5. Roberts WO, Brust JD, Leonard B. Youth ice hockey tournament injuries: rates and patterns compared to season play. Med Sci Sports Exerc 1999;31(1):46–51.
6. Toth C, McNeil S, Feasby T. Central nervous system injuries in sport and recreation: a systematic review. Sports Med 2005;35(8):685–715.
7. Agel J, Dompier TP, Dick R, et al. Descriptive epidemiology of collegiate men's ice hockey injuries: National Collegiate Athletic Association injury surveillance system, 1988–1989 through 2003–2004. J Athl Train 2007;42(2):241–8.

8. Lorentzon R, Wedren H, Pietila T. Incidence, nature, and causes of ice hockey injuries. A three-year prospective study of a Swedish elite ice hockey team. Am J Sports Med 1988;16(4):392–6.
9. Wattie N, Cobley S, Macpherson A, et al. Injuries in Canadian youth ice hockey: the influence of relative age. Pediatrics 2007;120(1):142–8.
10. Gerberich SG, Finke R, Madden M, et al. An epidemiological study of high school ice hockey injuries. Childs Nerv Syst 1987;3(2):59–64.
11. Hagel BE, Marko J, Dryden D, et al. Effect of bodychecking on injury rates among minor ice hockey players. CMAJ 2006;175(2):155–60.
12. Macpherson A, Rothman L, Howard A. Body-checking rules and childhood injuries in ice hockey. Pediatrics 2006;117(2):e143–7.
13. Schick DM, Meeuwisse WH. Injury rates and profiles in female ice hockey players. Am J Sports Med 2003;31(1):47–52.
14. Agel J, Dick R, Nelson B, et al. Descriptive epidemiology of collegiate women's ice hockey injuries: National Collegiate Athletic Association injury surveillance system, 2000–2001 through 2003–2004. J Athl Train 2007;42(2):249–54.
15. Emery CA, Meeuwisse WH, Powell JW. Groin and abdominal strain injuries in the National hockey league. Clin J Sport Med 1999;9(3):151–6.
16. Emery CA, Meeuwisse WH. Risk factors for groin injuries in hockey. Med Sci Sports Exerc 2001;33(9):1423–33.
17. Toth C, McNeil S, Feasby T. Peripheral nervous system injuries in sport and recreation: a systematic review. Sports Med 2005;35(8):717–38.
18. MacDonald PB, Strange G, Hodgkinson R, et al. Injuries to the peroneal nerve in professional hockey. Clin J Sport Med 2002;12(1):39–40.
19. Shevell MI, Stewart JD. Laceration of the common peroneal nerve by a skate blade. CMAJ 1988;139(4):311–2.
20. Watson BV, Algahtani H, Broome RJ, et al. An unusual presentation of tarsal tunnel syndrome caused by an inflatable ice hockey skate. Can J Neurol Sci 2002; 29(4):386–9.
21. Feinberg JH, Nadler SF, Krivickas LS. Peripheral nerve injuries in the athlete. Sports Med 1997;24(6):385–408.
22. Perlmutter GS, Leffert RD, Zarins B. Direct injury to the axillary nerve in athletes playing contact sports. Am J Sports Med 1997;25(1):65–8.
23. Perlmutter GS, Apruzzese W. Axillary nerve injuries in contact sports: recommendations for treatment and rehabilitation. Sports Med 1998;26(5):351–61.
24. Feinberg JH. Burners and stingers. Phys Med Rehabil Clin N Am 2000;11(4):771–84.
25. Tator CH, Carson JD, Cushman R. Hockey injuries of the spine in Canada, 1966–1996. CMAJ 2000;162(6):787–8.
26. Molsa JJ, Tegner Y, Alaranta H, et al. Spinal cord injuries in ice hockey in Finland and Sweden from 1980 to 1996. Int J Sports Med 1999;20(1):64–7.
27. Tator CH, Edmonds VE, Lapczak L, et al. Spinal injuries in ice hockey players, 1966–1987. Can J Surg 1991;34(1):63–9.
28. Tator CH, Carson JD, Edmonds VE. New spinal injuries in hockey. Clin J Sport Med 1997;7(1):17–21.
29. Tator CH, Carson JD, Edmonds VE. Spinal injuries in ice hockey. Clin Sports Med 1998;17(1):183–94.
30. Tator CH, Ekong CE, Rowed DW, et al. Spinal injuries due to hockey. Can J Neurol Sci 1984;11(1):34–41.
31. Torg JS. Epidemiology, pathomechanics, and prevention of athletic injuries to the cervical spine. Med Sci Sports Exerc 1985;17(3):295–303.

32. Tator CH, Provvidenza CF, Lapczak L, et al. Spinal injuries in Canadian ice hockey: documentation of injuries sustained from 1943–1999. Can J Neurol Sci 2004;31(4):460–6.

33. Torg JS, Corcoran TA, Thibault LE, et al. Cervical cord neurapraxia: classification, pathomechanics, morbidity, and management guidelines. J Neurosurg 1997;87(6):843–50.

34. Cantu RC. Stingers, transient quadriplegia, and cervical spinal stenosis: return to play criteria. Med Sci Sports Exerc 1997;29(7 Suppl):S233–5.

35. Cantu RV, Cantu RC. Current thinking: return to play and transient quadriplegia. Curr Sports Med Rep 2005;4(1):27–32.

36. Boockvar JA, Durham SR, Sun PP. Cervical spinal stenosis and sports-related cervical cord neurapraxia in children. Spine 2001;26(24):2709–12.

37. Honey CR. Brain injury in ice hockey. Clin J Sport Med 1998;8(1):43–6.

38. Benoit BG, Russell NA, Richard MT, et al. Epidural hematoma: report of seven cases with delayed evolution of symptoms. Can J Neurol Sci 1982;9(3):321–4.

39. Fekete JF. Severe brain injury and death following minor hockey accidents: the effectiveness of the "safety helmets" of amateur hockey players. Can Med Assoc J 1968;99(25):1234–9.

40. Tegner Y, Lorentzon R. Concussion among Swedish elite ice hockey players. Br J Sports Med 1996;30(3):251–5.

41. Biasca N, Wirth S, Tegner Y. The avoidability of head and neck injuries in ice hockey: an historical review. Br J Sports Med 2002;36(6):410–27.

42. Pretre R, Kursteiner K, Reverdin A, et al. Blunt carotid artery injury: devastating consequences of undetected pseudoaneurysm. J Trauma 1995;39(5):1012–4.

43. Sahjpaul RL, Abdulhak MM, Drake CG, et al. Fatal traumatic vertebral artery aneurysm rupture. Case report. J Neurosurg 1998;89(5):822–4.

44. Aubry M, Cantu R, Dvorak J, et al. Summary and agreement statement of the First International Conference on Concussion in Sport, Vienna 2001. Recommendations for the improvement of safety and health of athletes who may suffer concussive injuries. Br J Sports Med 2002;36(1):6–10.

45. McCrory P, Johnston K, Meeuwisse W, et al. Summary and agreement statement of the 2nd International conference on concussion in sport, Prague 2004. Br J Sports Med 2005;39(4):196–204.

46. Biasca N, Maxwell WL. Minor traumatic brain injury in sports: a review in order to prevent neurological sequelae. Prog Brain Res 2007;161:263–91.

47. Bloom GA, Horton AS, McCrory P, et al. Sport psychology and concussion: new impacts to explore. Br J Sports Med 2004;38(5):519–21.

48. Johnston KM, Bloom GA, Ramsay J, et al. Current concepts in concussion rehabilitation. Curr Sports Med Rep 2004;3(6):316–23.

49. Cantu RC. Reflections on head injuries in sport and the concussion controversy. Clin J Sport Med 1997;7(2):83–4.

50. Cantu RC, Aubry M, Dvorak J, et al. Overview of concussion consensus statements since 2000. Neurosurg Focus 2006;21(4):E3.

51. Cantu RC. Athletic concussion: current understanding as of 2007. Neurosurgery 2007;60(6):963–4.

52. Cantu RC. Recurrent athletic head injury: risks and when to retire. Clin Sports Med 2003;22(3):593–603.

53. Dupuis F, Johnston KM, Lavoie M, et al. Concussions in athletes produce brain dysfunction as revealed by event-related potentials. Neuroreport 2000;11(18):4087–92.

54. Lavoie ME, Dupuis F, Johnston KM, et al. Visual p300 effects beyond symptoms in concussed college athletes. J Clin Exp Neuropsychol 2004;26(1):55–73.
55. Echemendia RJ, Putukian M, Mackin RS, et al. Neuropsychological test performance prior to and following sports-related mild traumatic brain injury. Clin J Sport Med 2001;11(1):23–31.
56. Echemendia RJ, Cantu RC. Return to play following sports-related mild traumatic brain injury: the role for neuropsychology. Appl Neuropsychol 2003; 10(1):48–55.
57. Gaetz M, Goodman D, Weinberg H. Electrophysiological evidence for the cumulative effects of concussion. Brain Inj 2000;14(12):1077–88.
58. Goodman D, Gaetz M, Meichenbaum D. Concussions in hockey: there is cause for concern. Med Sci Sports Exerc 2001;33(12):2004–9.
59. Goodman D, Gaetz M. Return-to-play guidelines after concussion: the message is getting through. Clin J Sport Med 2002;12(5):265.
60. Johnston KM, McCrory P, Mohtadi NG, et al. Evidence-based review of sport-related concussion: clinical science. Clin J Sport Med 2001;11(3):150–9.
61. Johnston KM, Ptito A, Chankowsky J, et al. New frontiers in diagnostic imaging in concussive head injury. Clin J Sport Med 2001;11(3):166–75.
62. Johnston KM. Hockey concussion reporting improved. Can J Neurol Sci 2003; 30(3):183.
63. Johnston KM, McCrory P. Predicting slow recovery from sport-related concussion: the new simple-complex distinction. Clin J Sport Med 2007;17(4):330–1.
64. Kissick J, Johnston KM. Return to play after concussion: principles and practice. Clin J Sport Med 2005;15(6):426–31.
65. Koh JO, Cassidy JD, Watkinson EJ. Incidence of concussion in contact sports: a systematic review of the evidence. Brain Inj 2003;17(10):901–17.
66. Leclerc S, Lassonde M, Delaney JS, et al. Recommendations for grading of concussion in athletes. Sports Med 2001;31(8):629–36.
67. Collins MW, Lovell MR, Iverson GL, et al. Cumulative effects of concussion in high school athletes. Neurosurgery 2002;51(5):1175–9.
68. Iverson GL, Brooks BL, Lovell MR, et al. No cumulative effects for one or two previous concussions. Br J Sports Med 2006;40(1):72–5.
69. Lovell MR, Iverson GL, Collins MW, et al. Measurement of symptoms following sports-related concussion: reliability and normative data for the post-concussion scale. Appl Neuropsychol 2006;13(3):166–74.
70. Lovell MR, Collins MW, Iverson GL, et al. Grade 1 or "ding" concussions in high school athletes. Am J Sports Med 2004;32(1):47–54.
71. Maroon JC, Lovell MR, Norwig J, et al. Cerebral concussion in athletes: evaluation and neuropsychological testing. Neurosurgery 2000;47(3):659–69.
72. McCrory P, Johnston KM, Mohtadi NG, et al. Evidence-based review of sport-related concussion: basic science. Clin J Sport Med 2001;11(3):160–5.
73. Perron AD, Brady WJ, Huff JS. Concussive convulsions: emergency department assessment and management of a frequently misunderstood entity. Acad Emerg Med 2001;8(3):296–8.
74. Groger A. Ten years of ice hockey-related-injuries in the German ice hockey federation - a ten year prospective study/523 international games. Sportverletz Sportschaden 2001;15(4):82–6.
75. Tegner Y. Concussion experience: Swedish elite ice hockey league. Br J Sports Med 2001;35(5):376–7.
76. Wennberg RA, Tator CH. National Hockey League reported concussions, 1986–87 to 2001–02. Can J Neurol Sci 2003;30(3):206–9.

77. Meeuwisse W, Burke C. NHL concussion program. Br J Sports Med 2001;35(5): 375.

78. Bailes JE, Cantu RC. Head injury in athletes. Neurosurgery 2001;48(1):26–45.

79. Williamson IJ, Goodman D. Converging evidence for the under-reporting of concussions in youth ice hockey. Br J Sports Med 2006;40(2):128–32.

80. Goldsmith W. The state of head injury biomechanics: past, present, and future: part 1. Crit Rev Biomed Eng 2001;29(5–6):441–600.

81. Shaw NA. The neurophysiology of concussion. Prog Neurobiol 2002;67(4): 281–344.

82. Zumsteg D, Wennberg R, Gutling E, et al. Whiplash and concussion: similar acute changes in middle-latency SEPs. Can J Neurol Sci 2006;33(4):379–86.

83. Scott DJ, Puni V, Rouah F. Mechanisms of injury for concussions in university football, ice hockey, and soccer: a pilot study. Clin J Sport Med 2006;16(2): 162–5.

84. Hynes LM, Dickey JP. Is there a relationship between whiplash-associated disorders and concussion in hockey? A preliminary study. Brain Inj 2006;20(2): 179–88.

85. McIntosh AS, McCrory P. Preventing head and neck injury. Br J Sports Med 2005;39(6):314–8.

86. Murray TM, Livingston LA. Hockey helmets, face masks, and injurious behavior. Pediatrics 1995;95(3):419–21.

87. Biasca N, Simmen HP, Trentz O. [Head injuries in ice hockey exemplified by the National hockey league "Hockey Canada" and European teams]. Unfallchirurg 1993;96(5):259–64 [In German].

88. Reynan PD, Clancy WG. Cervical spine injury, hockey helmets, and face masks. Am J Sports Med 1994;22(2):167–70.

89. Bishop PJ, Norman RW, Wells R, et al. Changes in the centre of mass and moment of inertia of a headform induced by a hockey helmet and face shield. Can J Appl Sport Sci 1983;8(1):19–25.

90. Smith AW, Bishop PJ, Wells RP. Alterations in head dynamics with the addition of a hockey helmet and face shield under inertial loading. Can J Appl Sport Sci 1985;10(2):68–74.

91. Bellow DG, Mendryk S, Schneider V. An investigation into the evaluation of hockey helmets. Med Sci Sports 1970;2(1):43–9.

92. Bishop PJ. Head protection in sport with particular application to ice hockey. Ergonomics 1976;19(4):451–64.

93. Norman RW, Bishop PJ, Pierrynowski MR. Puck impact response of ice hockey face masks. Can J Appl Sport Sci 1980;5(4):208–14.

94. Kis M, Saunders F, ten Hove MW, et al. Rotational acceleration measurements—evaluating helmet protection. Can J Neurol Sci 2004;31(4):499–503.

95. Benson BW, Rose MS, Meeuwisse WH. The impact of face shield use on concussions in ice hockey: a multivariate analysis. Br J Sports Med 2002;36(1):27–32.

96. Benson BW, Mohtadi NG, Rose MS, et al. Head and neck injuries among ice hockey players wearing full face shields vs half face shields. JAMA 1999; 282(24):2328–32.

97. LaPrade RF, Burnett QM, Zarzour R, et al. The effect of the mandatory use of face masks on facial lacerations and head and neck injuries in ice hockey. A prospective study. Am J Sports Med 1995;23(6):773–5.

98. Stevens ST, Lassonde M, De Beaumont L, et al. The effect of visors on head and facial injury in National hockey league players. J Sci Med Sport 2006;9(3): 238–42.

99. Meeuwisse WH. Full facial protection reduces injuries in elite young hockey players. Clin J Sport Med 2002;12(6):406.

100. Stuart MJ, Smith AM, Malo-Ortiguera SA, et al. A comparison of facial protection and the incidence of head, neck, and facial injuries in Junior A hockey players. A function of individual playing time. Am J Sports Med 2002;30(1):39–44.

101. Mihalik JP, McCaffrey MA, Rivera EM, et al. Effectiveness of mouthguards in reducing neurocognitive deficits following sports-related cerebral concussion. Dent Traumatol 2007;23(1):14–20.

102. Knapik JJ, Marshall SW, Lee RB, et al. Mouthguards in sport activities: history, physical properties and injury prevention effectiveness. Sports Med 2007; 37(2):117–44.

103. Pashby T, Carson JD, Ordogh D, et al. Eliminate head-checking in ice hockey. Clin J Sport Med 2001;11(4):211–3.

104. Marchie A, Cusimano MD. Bodychecking and concussions in ice hockey: should our youth pay the price? CMAJ 2003;169(2):124–8.

105. Cross KM, Serenelli C. Training and equipment to prevent athletic head and neck injuries. Clin Sports Med 2003;22(3):639–67.

106. Cook DJ, Cusimano MD, Tator CH, et al. Evaluation of the ThinkFirst Canada, smart hockey, brain and spinal cord injury prevention video. Inj Prev 2003; 9(4):361–6.

107. Goodman D, Bradley NL, Paras B, et al. Video gaming promotes concussion knowledge acquisition in youth hockey players. J Adolesc 2006;29(3):351–60.

108. Wennberg R. Collision frequency in elite hockey on North American versus international size rinks. Can J Neurol Sci 2004;31(3):373–7.

109. Wennberg R. Effect of ice surface size on collision rates and head impacts at the World Junior Hockey Championships, 2002 to 2004. Clin J Sport Med 2005; 15(2):67–72.

Section 5

Neurologic Injuries in Individual Sports

Neurologic Injuries in Boxing and Other Combat Sports

Tsharni R. Zazryn, BAppSci (Human Movement)[a],*,

Paul R. McCrory, MBBS, PhD, FRACP, FACSP, FASMF, FACSM, FRSM, GradDipEpidStats[b],

Peter A. Cameron, MBBS, MD, FACEM[c]

KEYWORDS

- Boxing • Concussion • Head injury
- Chronic traumatic encephalopathy

Boxing and other combat sports (including kickboxing, contact karate, tae kwon do, judo, and the like) are different from other sporting pursuits because the head is a legitimate place of contact. Other sporting activities have incidental contact to the head that may result in neurological injury; however, the rules and close settings associated with combat sports allow contact to the head region, and thus a potential for neurological injuries of both an acute and chronic nature exists. Although each combat sport is different in terms of which regions of the body can be used for contact and how scoring is conducted, they are similar in terms of the exposure time experienced by competitors, and in many cases competitors will compete in more than one combat sport style in their lifetimes. Additionally, it has been shown that acute injury rates during competition are similar between professional boxing and other combat sports, indicating that these groups are appropriate to consider together for injury purposes.[1]

Injuries of all types occur to combat sport participants, with between one fifth to one half of all fights in boxing, karate, and tae kwon do resulting in an injury.[2-7] In boxing, the majority of these injuries are to the head and neck region, with studies in other combat sports consistently reporting the head and neck region as the first or, more often, the second most common site of injury (following the lower limbs).[4,5,8-11]

This article originally appeared in *Neurologic Clinics*, Volume 26, Issue 1.

[a] Department of Health Science, Monash University, McMahons Road, Frankston, Melbourne, Victoria, Australia, 3199

[b] Centre for Health, Exercise and Sports Medicine and the Brain Research Institute, University of Melbourne, 202 Berkeley Street, Carlton, Melbourne, Victoria, Australia, 3010

[c] Department of Epidemiology and Preventive Medicine, Monash University, The Alfred Hospital, Commercial Road, Melbourne, Victoria, Australia 3004

* Corresponding author.

E-mail address: tsharni.zazryn@med.monash.edu.au (T.R. Zazryn).

Phys Med Rehabil Clin N Am 20 (2009) 227–239

doi:10.1016/j.pmr.2008.10.004

1047-9651/08/$ – see front matter © 2009 Elsevier Inc. All rights reserved.

MECHANISMS OF NEUROLOGICAL INJURIES IN COMBAT SPORTS

The mechanism of neurological injury varies depending upon the combat sport discipline. In boxing, head injuries generally occur because of contact between the fist and head, head and head, or head and some part of the boxing ring. In other combat sport disciplines, head contact can occur in all of those manners, and also as a result of striking other surfaces (the palms, fingers, elbows, legs, feet, and so forth). In boxing it is thought that the more serious neurological injuries result from punches that cause rotational movements of the head, whereas in the other combat sports it is believed that these injuries result from incorrect throwing techniques (judo), or erroneous kicks, especially those involving rotation.[12–16] A number of factors that affect the outcome of neurological injury in combat sports have been assessed in a laboratory setting. These include the region of the head that receives the contact, the magnitude, force, and direction of the contact, the use of gloves and their associated weights, and the use of any other barriers for protection (eg, headgear) whose use depends on the combat sport rules.[17–24] The impact of these factors during competition, however, is yet to be determined because of difficulties measuring the effect occurring with two moving people.

ACUTE NEUROLOGICAL INJURIES

Acute neurological injuries (ANI) occurring to combat sport participants have been studied extensively, especially in the sport of boxing. Numerous case studies of particular ANI types have been published (for example, a number of case reports relating to vertebral or carotid artery dissections exist in the combat sport literature);[25–27] however, the ANI leading to fatalities and those of concussion have been the focus of the majority of the literature, and are discussed here.

Fatalities Resulting from Combat Sport Participation

Deaths as a result of participation in combat sports have received plenty of media attention; however, validated epidemiological data are less commonly reported. Although there is no doubt that some deaths do occur, the frequency and circumstances of these deaths are not available from any formal international, validated dataset. Instead, many of the reported fatality data have been obtained from a combination of media sources, industry reports, and coronial inquests, and rarely are these deaths reported as anything other than individual case reports that offer little information on how those deaths may represent all combat sport participations.

Deaths to boxing participants have been reported in a more comprehensive manner than deaths as a result of any other combat sport type. In fact, very limited data exist for deaths occurring in other combat sports.[14] Although a small number of deaths in other combat sports have been the subject of a few case reports, rates of death in those sports certainly cannot be determined based upon the available literature.[12,13] The majority of deaths from boxing participation result from a subdural hematoma, and are often associated with an immediate loss of consciousness during a fight.[28,29] Subdural hematomas have also been reported in judo and tae kwon do.[13,30–32]

The most comprehensive review of boxing fatalities was published in 1998 based upon newspaper sources.[33,34] That review included deaths that had occurred "worldwide" that had been reported in newspapers since World War I. To the end of 1996, the review stated that 659 boxing-fatalities had been recorded, for an average of fewer than 9 deaths per year over the 78-year period.[33,34]

Despite the addition of better reporting over the more recent decades of that study, a reduced death rate in boxing was seen, most likely resulting from a real decrease in the number of deaths rather than a decrease in the number of active boxers over the time period.[35] It is also probable that the data from the newspaper records may have been inaccurate, and that the earlier reports may have misrepresented deaths as being caused by boxing. The published work of Ryan[33,34] is supplemented by an on-line database of boxing deaths that have occurred worldwide since the 19th century.[36] Similar decreases in the number of deaths in recent times have been shown in that dataset, although without population numbers in either of these datasets, information related to the risk of death caused by boxing participation cannot be ascertained. In Australia, a recent review of 20 years of professional boxing competition data determined a death rate for that cohort of 0.2 per 100 bouts.[1]

When attempting to compare the number of fatalities occurring as a result of combat sport participation as opposed to other sports, a paucity of data exists. One study calculating fatality rates during sporting activities in England and Wales included boxing within the 8 years of data collection.[37] In that study, climbing sports (<793), air sports (>640), and motor (146) or water sports (67.5) dominated the estimated fatality rate per 100 million participation days. Boxing and wrestling were reported in one category, with three fatal incidents over the 8 years studied, rating it the tenth most common cause of sport or recreation death, with a fatality rate of 5.2 per 100 million participation days.[37] This rate was one third of that of the only other contact sport in the top ten of this list—rugby.

Concussions in Combat Sports

Concussions in the combat sports are the subject of major methodological differences in reporting and definition. Depending on the combat sport being described, concussions may be reported in a number of different ways. For example, in boxing a concussion could be reported as a direct medical diagnosis from the ringside physician, or could be inferred as a result of either a knockout (KO), technical knockout (TKO), or the referee stopping the contest as a result of a head injury (RSC-H). As a result of these discrepancies in defining a concussion, reported incidences of boxing-related concussions vary greatly. For professional boxers, the literature reports that between 15.9% and 69.7% of all injuries are ANI.[38–40] In amateur boxing, studies have reported the incidence of ANI to be between 6.5% and 51.6% of all injuries.[41–45]

In terms of other combat sports, medically reported concussions occur infrequently. In adult karate competition concussions have been reported to account for between 0.9% and 5.4% of all injuries.[4,5,46,47] In studies of younger karate competitors or studies in which age was not specified or various ages were studied, concussions have been reported to account for between 1.2% and 8.8% of all injuries.[3,11,48] In adult tae kwon do competitions, between 4.3% and 7.5% of injuries are concussions.[6,9] For younger tae kwon do participants, concussion accounts for 8.6% to 24.4% of all injuries.[49,50] In kickboxing, a high incidence of concussion has been reported, both for amateur and professional competition (65.2% and 17.5%, respectively).[10,51] In other studies that have documented concussion rates in various martial arts, between 1.1% and 2.5% of injuries are concussions.[52–54]

Concussion rates per 100 participants and per 1000 athletic exposures (whereby one bout is equal to two athletic exposures) are shown in **Tables 1** and **2**, respectively. The majority of the studies used to determine these concussion rates have involved prospective data collection; however, they have reported prospective data only for concussions that occurred during competition. No prospective collection has thus far determined rates of concussion occurring during training or sparring times, and the studies that report such retrospective data are hindered by issues related to recall. This is an area of research need within the combat sports.

Table 1
Concussion rates per 100 participants in combat sports

Reference	Participants, Setting Injury Occurred	Injury Rate Per 100 Participants
Tae kwon do		
Beis et al[98]	Adults, competition	0.2
Oler et al[12]	Children, competition	0.3
Oler et al[12]	Adults, competition	0.4
Pieter et al[99]	Children, competition	0.5
Beis et al[98]	Children, competition	0.6
Pieter et al[99]	Adults, competition	0.8
Pieter and Zemper[49]	Children, competition	0.9
Pieter and Zemper[100]	Adults, competition	1.2
Koh et al[16]	Adults, competition	1.4
Pieter et al[101]	Adults, competition	5.2
Koh and Cassidy[102]	Children, competition	9.8
Karate		
Stricevic et al[4]	Adults, competition	0.4
Destombe et al[48]	Not specified, not specified	0.5
Zetaruk et al[46]	Adults, competition	0.9
Critchley et al[11]	Various, competition	0.9
McLatchie et al[47]	Not specified, not specified	2.8
Martial arts		
Birrer[52]	Various, not specified	0.3
Buschbacher and Shay[54]	Not specified, not specified	1.7
Birrer and Birrer[53]	Not specified, competition	3.5
Boxing		
Welch et al[44]	Adults (amateur), competition	14.0
Porter and O'Brien[45]	Various (amateur), various	20.4
McCown, 1958[38]	Adults (professional), competition	21.0
Jordan and Campbell[39]	Adults (professional), competition	41.5
Zazryn et al 2006[2]	Adults (both), various	44.7

RISK FACTORS FOR ACUTE NEUROLOGICAL INJURIES IN THE COMBAT SPORTS

Risk factors for the development of any injuries in the combat sports are not well-established.[55] This is also true for ANI. Although a number of potential risk factors have been hypothesized, well-designed epidemiological studies have not been completed.[14,56] The majority of factors of interest are anecdotal rather than evidence-based. Some factors common to all combat sport styles have been noted for further attention that may relate to ANI occurrence. These include age, gender, experience, and various measures of exposure.[56,57] **Table 3** summarizes the available evidence for risk factors for ANI in combat sports.

CHRONIC NEUROLOGICAL INJURIES

Along with deaths, chronic neurological injuries (CNI) associated with combat sport participation have dominated the published international literature. In particular,

Table 2
Concussion rates per 1000 athletic exposures in combat sports

Reference	Participants, Setting Injury Occurred	Injury Rate per 1000 Athletic Exposures
Tae kwon do		
Beis et al[98]	Adults, competition	0.7
Pieter et al[99]	Children, competition	3.1
Beis et al[98]	Children, competition	3.2
Pieter et al[99]	Adults, competition	4.5
Zemper and Pieter[6]	Adults, competition	4.6
Pieter and Zemper[100]	Adults, competition	5.5
Pieter and Zemper[50]	Children, competition	5.0
Kazemi and Pieter[9]	Adults, competition	6.9
Koh et al[16]	Adults, competition	7.9
Pieter et al[101]	Adults, competition	13.4
Koh and Cassidy,[102,a]	Children, competition	50.2
Karate		
Stricevic et al[4]	Adults, competition	1.6
Critchley et al[11]	Various, competition	3.4
Arriaza and Leyes[5]	Adults, competition	6.0
McLatchie[3]	Not specified, competition	11.9
Kick boxing		
Zazryn et al[10]	Adults (professional), competition	19.2
Buse and Wood[51]	Adults (military), competition	101.4
Boxing		
Porter and O'Brien[45]	Various (amateur), competition	11.4
Estwanik et al[41]	Adults (amateur), competition	77.7
Bledsoe et al[103]	Adults (professional), competition	186.1
Zazryn et al[40]	Adults (professional), competition	250.6

[a] Had a specific focus on concussions and head blows.

boxing has again received the most attention, and such injuries in this sport led to the coining of a term synonymous with CNI in boxing—the "punch-drunk syndrome." When first coined in 1928 by a physician in the *Journal of the American Medical Association*, the condition was known in boxing circles and was largely "diagnosed" by those who knew the boxer before any symptoms became apparent.[58] In this first publication of the condition, only 5 of the 23 retired boxers who were reported as being punch drunk or having symptoms of the condition were personally examined by the doctor, and various confounding factors for the reasons such symptoms were being exhibited existed.[58] Since that publication, the signs and symptoms associated with punch-drunk syndrome have been progressively recognized, and it is now understood that the condition is not specific to boxing. As such, this condition, formerly called dementia pugilistica, is now known as chronic traumatic encephalopathy (CTE).[59–61]

Table 3 Summary of available evidence of risk factors for acute neurological injuries in the combat sports	
Risk Factors for Acute Neurological Injury	Evidence
Age[46,48,49,98,99,102,104]	±
Gender[5,9,48–50,52,100]	±
Skill/experience/fighting style[46,48,52,89–91,105–109]	±
Exposure	
Number of bouts[52,72,74,75,78,79,81,82,86,89–91,104,110,111]	±
Duration of career[52,72,75,78,81–83]	−
Training/sparring[44,46,48,52,79,81,82,108]	±
Number of knockouts[81,83,84]	−

Abbreviations: ±, studies report conflicting results; −, studies that have been completed indicate there is no evidence of increased risk.
Adapted from Zazryn T. The epidemiology of injury in Australian boxing [PhD dissertation]. Melbourne (Australia): Monash University 2007; with permission.

The clinical, radiological, neurophysiological, and pathological features of CTE in boxing populations have recently been extensively reviewed.[62] The clinical evidence does not support the idea that CTE has a set of predictable or sequential stages. Rather, a constellation of symptoms are present in the early stage of the condition as a result of lesions that affect the cerebellar, pyramidal, and extra-pyramidal systems.[35] Approximately one third of CTE cases are progressive, with cognitive impairment becoming the major neurological feature as this occurs, and various neuropsychiatric and behavioral symptoms presenting at different times.[55,63–70] The pathological features of CTE include abnormalities of the septum pellucidum associated with fenestration and forniceal atrophy, cerebellar and other scarring of the brain, substantia nigral degeneration, and the occurrence of neurofibrillary tangles in the cerebral cortex and temporal horn areas.[71]

It is well-established that there are few prospective epidemiological studies that allow an accurate estimation of the prevalence or incidence of CNI in any combat sport. Although boxing has been extensively researched, the majority of that research has focused on anecdotal case reports of retired boxers seen late in life, who fought in times and conditions that have little relevance to modern participants, and with limited reference to potential confounders.[35,62] The most often quoted (and best estimate based on methodological quality) is a prevalence of 16.5% in professional boxers who were registered to fight between 1929 and 1955 in the United Kingdom.[65] For amateur boxers, only small-sample, cross-sectional studies of neuropsychological performance and a variety of other tests have been performed to show indications of CNI. In one such study, 87% of the 15 retired amateurs showed abnormal results on at least two of the four tests that were completed.[72] Despite there not being an accurate measure of CNI prevalence in amateur boxers, it has been shown that compared with professionals, amateurs have milder neuropsychological and neuroimaging evidence of CNI.[73–79] In other combat sports, only one published case report of CNI exists.[80]

RISK FACTORS FOR CHRONIC NEUROLOGICAL INJURIES IN THE COMBAT SPORTS

Table 4 demonstrates the results of the studies undertaken to determine the effect of certain factors on CNI development in the combat sports. These results relate to the

Table 4
Summary of available evidence for risk factors that have been studied for chronic neurological injury in boxing

Risk Factors for Chronic Neurological Injury	Evidence
Age[81,91,104]	±
Weight class (division)[90]	−
Exposure	
Number of bouts[65,72,74,75,78,79,81,82,86,89–91,104,110,111]	±
Duration of career[65,72,75,78,81–83]	+
Training/sparring[44,79,81,82]	−
Number of knock-outs[81,83,84]	+
Boxing skill/experience/fighting style[89–91,105–107]	−
Genetics[85,86]	+

Abbreviations: ±, studies report conflicting results; −, studies that have been completed indicate there is no evidence of increased risk; +, studies that have been completed indicate an increased susceptibility/risk.
From Zazryn T. The epidemiology of injury in Australian boxing [PhD dissertation]. Melbourne (Australia): Monash University 2007; with permission.

sport of boxing, because no studies in other combat sports have been designed to document CNI risk factors. In boxing, studies have shown that having a boxing career greater than 10 years, a greater number of bouts (more than 150), and the presence of the apolipoprotein E4 phenotype all increase the likelihood of chronic neurological symptoms being present.[65,72,75,78,81–86]

The following two sections discuss the risk factors that have been the main foci in the literature in relation to CNI in boxing: exposure and genetics.

Exposure as a Risk Factor for Chronic Neurological Injury in Boxing

There are many different aspects of exposure that may increase the risk of CNI in boxing. Both the competition and training aspects of participation in the sport must be considered, including the number of bouts/sessions, the length of the career, the results of any bouts, and any KOs or TKOs sustained in either setting. Although studies have shown a greater relationship to CNI in boxers who have had more fights (greater than 20 professional bouts) than to the number of KOs or TKOs they may have sustained, this is still an important aspect to consider because not all KOs or TKOs may have been recalled in these largely retrospective studies.[33,65,87–91]

Certainly injuries to the head during training and sparring are one of the least understood risks of CNI. The one study that has examined head injuries occurring during sparring[81] suggests that cognitive impairment can develop through this mechanism, even in the absence of formal competitive bouts. If an association between CNI and boxing is to be fully understood, greater attention must be given to the head injuries occurring during training and sparring. This is especially important given that the vast amount of boxing participation is in a training setting.[2]

Genetics as a Risk Factor for Chronic Neurological Injury in Boxers

Genetic factors and their relationships to sporting performance and injury development have become an important research area in recent years. In terms of genetic risk factors for CNI, the focus has been on an apolipoprotein that functions to transport lipids that aid the repair and construction of cell membranes, neuritis, and synapses.[92,93] In particular, the apolipoprotein E ϵ4 gene (ApoE4), increases the susceptibility for late-onset familial and sporadic Alzheimer's disease, and has been shown to be significantly associated with death and poor outcomes following acute traumatic brain injury.[93–96] The mechanisms by which this particular polymorphism results in CNI is believed to involve the deposition of amyloid-γ protein in patients with ApoE4 resulting in an impaired ability to recover from a head injury.[85,93] Within boxers, the presence of an ApoE4 phenotype has been clearly associated with an increased risk of CNI in retrospective studies; however, no prospective cohort studies have been conducted to confirm these results.[85,86,92,97] As such, genetic screening of participants is not yet warranted as a routine preparticipation tool, but may become more likely into the future as more detail about the apolipoprotein is discovered.

PREVENTION OF NEUROLOGICAL INJURIES IN THE COMBAT SPORTS

The limited evidence of causes and mechanisms for neurological injuries in the combat sports hinders the ability to make widespread changes that may reduce their likelihood; however, a number of potential strategies have been suggested by various authors, although limited prospective evidence of their effectiveness currently exists.

Table 5 lists some of the commonly suggested injury prevention methods for combat sports, and an evaluation of their current state of evidence.

Table 5
Level of evidence for suggested injury prevention strategies to reduce neurological injuries in the combat sports

Suggested Prevention Measure	Studies Conducted	Level of Evidence
Education and training		
Education of athletes, coaches, referees about injuries	Pieter and Zemper,[49] Oler et al[12]	±
Better training and advice on appropriate technique	Pieter et al,[99] Pieter and Zemper,[50] Koh and Cassidy[102]	±
Coaching and officiating		
Minimum standards of referee and coach certifications	Birrer,[52] Oler et al,[12] Critchley et al[11]	±
Minimum referee experience requirements	McLatchie et al[112]	±
Equipment		
Allowing of foot padding and other protective equipment	Beis et al,[98] McLatchie and Morris[7]	±
Use of headgear	McLatchie and Morris,[7] Schmidt-Olsen et al[113]	±
Use of mouth guards	Tuominen[109]	±
Glove weight standardization	Unterharnscheidt,[17] Schmidt-Olsen et al[113]	±
Alterations to flooring of ring/sport surfaces	Unterharnscheidt[17]	−
Sport policies and regulations		
Reduction in head blows through rule & scoring changes	Birrer,[52] Oler et al,[12] Tuominen.[109] Pieter and Zemper,[50] Burke et al,[114] Macan et al[115]	±

Abbreviations: ±, studies report conflicting results; −, no studies have been conducted.

SUMMARY

Neurological injuries of both an acute and chronic nature have been reported in the literature for various combat sport styles; however, the incidence and prevalence of these injury types vary greatly within the literature, and where they have been measured accurately, limited evidence exists for the causes and mechanisms of these injuries. This hinders any programs aimed at reducing neurological injury occurrence in these sports. Systematic ongoing surveillance systems that detail causes of injuries are needed across all combat sport disciplines. Additionally, further biomechanical analyses detailing forces produced during competition and training activities, and the effectiveness of all types of protective equipment in dissipating that force are needed before evidence-based injury prevention strategies can be developed and implemented to reduce neurological injuries in the combat sports.

REFERENCES

1. Zazryn T. The epidemiology of injury in Australian boxing. [PhD dissertation]. Melbourne (Australia): Monash University; 2007.
2. Zazryn T, Cameron P, McCrory P. A prospective cohort study of injury in amateur and professional boxing. Br J Sports Med 2006;40(8):670–4.
3. McLatchie G. Analysis of karate injuries sustained in 295 contests. Injury 1976; 8(2):132–4.
4. Stricevic M, Patel M, Okazaki T, et al. Karate: historical perspective and injuries sustained in national and international tournament competitions. Am J Sports Med 1983;11(6):320–4.
5. Arriaza R, Leyes M. Injury profile in competitive karate: prospective analysis of three consecutive World Karate Championships. Knee Surg Sports Traumatol Arthrosc 2005;13:603–7.
6. Zemper E, Pieter W. Injury rates during the 1988 US Olympic team trials for taekwondo. Br J Sports Med 1989;23(3):161–4.
7. McLatchie G, Morris E. Prevention of karate injuries—a progress report. Br J Sports Med 1977;11:78–82.
8. Gartland S, Malik M, Lovell M. Injury and injury rates in Muay Thai kick boxing. Br J Sports Med 2001;35:308–13.
9. Kazemi M, Pieter W. Injuries at a Canadian National Taekwondo Championships: a prospective study. BMC Musculoskelet Disord 2004;5:22–9.
10. Zazryn T, Finch C, McCrory P. A 16-year study of injuries to professional kickboxers in the state of Victoria, Australia. Br J Sports Med 2003;37(5):448–51.
11. Critchley G, Mannion S, Meredith C. Injury rates in Shotokan karate. Br J Sports Med 1999;33:174–7.
12. Oler M, Tomson W, Pepe H, et al. Morbidity and mortality in the martial arts: a warning. J Trauma 1991;31(2):251–3.
13. Jackson F, Earle K, Beamer Y, et al. Blunt head injuries incurred by marine recruits in hand-to-hand combat (judo training). Mil Med 1967;132(10):803–8.
14. Birrer R. Martial arts. In: Jordan B, editor. Sports neurology. 2nd edition. Philadelphia: Lippincott-Raven Publishers; 1998. p. 423–8.
15. Wilkerson L. Martial arts injuries. J Am Osteopath Assoc 1997;97(4):221–6.
16. Koh J, de Freitas T, Watkinson E. Injuries at the 14th World Taekwondo Championships in 1999. International Journal of Applied Sports Sciences 2001;13(1): 33–48.

17. Unterharnscheidt F. A neurologist's reflections on boxing. 1: Impact mechanics in boxing and injuries other than central nervous system damage. Rev Neurol 1995;23(121):661–74.
18. Schwartz M, Hudson A, Fernie G, et al. Biomechanical study of full-contact karate contrasted with boxing. J Neurosurg 1986;64:248–52.
19. Walilko T, Viano D, Bir C. Biomechanics of the head for Olympic boxer punches to the face. Br J Sports Med 2005;39:710–9.
20. Atha J, Yeadon M, Sandover J, et al. The damaging punch. BMJ 1985;291: 1756–7.
21. Smith P, Hamill J. The effect of punching glove type and skill level on momentum transfer. Journal of Human Movement Studies 1986;12:153–61.
22. Smith M, Dyson R, Hale T, et al. Development of a boxing dynamometer and its punch force discrimination efficacy. J Sports Sci 2000;18(6):445–50.
23. Walker J. Karate strikes. Am J Phys 1975;43(10):845–9.
24. Serina E, Lieu D. Thoracic injury potential of basic competition Taekwondo kicks. J Biomech 1991;24(10):951–60.
25. Pary L, Rodnitzky R. Traumatic internal carotid artery dissection associated with taekwondo. Neurology 2003;60(8):1392–3.
26. Lannuzel A, Moulin T, Amsallem S, et al. Vertebra-artery dissection following a judo session: a case report. Neuropediatrics 1994;25:106–8.
27. Malek A, Halbach V, Phatouros C, et al. Endovascular treatment of a ruptured intra-cranial dissecting vertebral aneurysm in a kickboxer. J Trauma 2000;48(1):143–5.
28. Unterharnscheidt F. A neurologist's reflection on boxing. 3:Vascular injuries. Revision Neurology 1995;23(122):847–55.
29. Cantu R. Head injuries in sport. Br J Sports Med 1996;30(4):289–96.
30. DeVera-Reyes J. Three cases of chronic subdural hematoma caused by the practice of judo. Actas Luso Esp Neurol Psiquiatr 1970;29:53–6.
31. Nakamura N. Judo and karate—do. In: Schneider R, Kennedy J, Plant M, editors. Sports injuries; mechanisms, prevention and treatment. Baltimore (MD): Williams & Wilkins; 1985. p. 417–30.
32. Koiwai E. Fatalities associated with judo. Phys Sportsmed 1981;9:61–6.
33. Ryan A. Intracranial injuries resulting from boxing: a review (1918–1985). Clin Sports Med 1987;6(1):31–9.
34. Ryan A. Intracranial injuries resulting from boxing. Clin Sports Med 1998;17(1): 155–68.
35. Clausen M, Anderson V, McCrory P. The risk of chronic traumatic brain injury in professional boxing—change in exposure variables in professional boxing over the past century. Br J Sports Med 2005;39:661–5.
36. Svinth J. Death under the spotlight: the Manuel Velazquez boxing fatality collection. Available at: http://ejmas.com/jcs/jcsart_svinth_a_0700.htm. Accessed July 1, 2007.
37. Nicholl J, Coleman P, Williams B. Injuries in sport and exerise: main report. A national study of the epidemiology of exercise-related injury and illness. London (UK): Sports Council; 1993.
38. McCown I. Boxing injuries. Am J Surg 1958;98:509–16.
39. Jordan B, Campbell E. Acute injuries among professional boxers in New York: a two-year survey. Phys Sportsmed 1988;16(1):87–91.
40. Zazryn T, Finch C, McCrory P. A 16-year study of injuries to professional boxers in the state of Victoria, Australia. Br J Sports Med 2003;37:321–4.
41. Estwanik J, Boitano M, Ari N. Amateur boxing injuries at the 1981 and 1982 USA/ ABF national championships. Phys Sportsmed 1984;12:123–8.

42. Larsson L, Melin K, Nordstrom-Ohrberg G, et al. Acute head injuries in boxers: clinical and electroencephalographic studies. Acta Psychiatr Neurol Scand 1954;95(Suppl):1–42.

43. Jordan B, Voy R, Stone J. Amateur boxing injuries at the US Olympic Training Center. Phys Sportsmed 1990;18(2):81–90.

44. Welch M, Sitler M, Kroeten H. Boxing injuries from an instructional program. Phys Sportsmed 1986;14(9):81–9.

45. Porter M, O'Brien M. Incidence and severity of injuries resulting from amateur boxing in Ireland. Clin J Sport Med 1996;6(2):97–101.

46. Zetaruk M, Violan M, Zurakowski D, et al. Injuries in martial arts: a comparison of five styles. Br J Sports Med 2005;39:29–33.

47. McLatchie G, Davies J, Caulley J. Injuries in karate—a case for medical control. J Trauma 1980;2:956–8.

48. Destombe C, Lejeune L, Guillodo Y, et al. Incidence and nature of karate injuries. Joint Bone Spine 2006;73:182–8.

49. Pieter W, Zemper E. Injury rates in children participating in taekwondo competition. J Trauma 1997;43(1):89–95.

50. Pieter W, Zemper E. Head and neck injuries in young taekwondo athletes. J Sports Med Phys Fitness 1999;39:147–53.

51. Buse G, Wood R. Safety profile of amateur kickboxing among military and civilian competitors. Mil Med 2006;171(5):443–7.

52. Birrer R. Trauma epidemiology in the martial arts. The results of an 18-year international survey. Am J Sports Med 1996;24(Supp 6):S72–9.

53. Birrer R, Birrer C. Unreported injuries in the martial arts. Br J Sports Med 1983; 17(2):131–4.

54. Buschbacher R, Shay T. Martial arts. Phys Med Rehabil Clin N Am 1999;10(1):35–47.

55. Jordan B. Boxing. In: Jordan B, Tsaris P, Warren R, editors. Sports neurology. 2nd edition. Philadelphia: Lippincott-Raven; 1998. p. 351–67.

56. Jordan B. Boxing. In: Caine D, Caine C, Lindner K, editors. Epidemiology of sports injuries. Champaign (IL): Human Kinetics Publishers, Inc.; 1996. p. 113–23.

57. Pieter W. Martial arts injuries. Med Sport Sci 2005;48:59–73.

58. Martland H. Punch drunk. JAMA 1928;91:1103–7.

59. Millspaugh J. Dementia pugilistica. US Naval Medical Bulletin 1937;35:297–303.

60. Parker H. Traumatic encephalopathy of professional pugilists. J Neurol Psychopathol 1934;15:20–8.

61. Critchley E. Nervous disorders in boxers. Med Annu 1937;318–20.

62. McCrory P, Zazryn T, Cameron C. The evidence for chronic traumatic encephalopathy in boxing. Sports Med 2007;37(6):467–76.

63. Guterman A, Smith R. Neurological sequelae of boxing. Sports Med 1987;4: 194–210.

64. Jordan B. Chronic traumatic brain injury associated with boxing. Semin Neurol 2000;20(2):179–85.

65. Roberts A. Brain damage in boxers. A study of prevalence of traumatic encephalopathy among ex-professional boxers. London: Pitman Medical Scientific Publishing Co.; 1969.

66. Jordan B, editor. Medical aspects of boxing. Boca Raton (FL): CRC Press; 1993.

67. LaCava G. Boxer's encephalopathy. J Sports Med 1963;3:87–92.

68. Cantu R, editor. Boxing and medicine. Champaign (IL): Human Kinetics; 1995. p. 19–32.

69. Johnson J. Organic psychosyndromes due to boxing. Br J Psychiatry 1969;115: 45–53.

70. Jordan B. Neurologic aspects of boxing. Arch Neurol 1987;44:453–9.
71. Corsellis J, Bruton C, Freeman-Browne D. The aftermath of boxing. Psychol Med 1973;3:270–303.
72. Casson I, Siegel O, Sham R, et al. Brain damage in modern boxers. JAMA 1984; 251(20):2663–7.
73. Haglund Y, Edman G, Murelius O, et al. Does Swedish amateur boxing lead to chronic brain damage? 1. A retrospective medical, neurological and personality trait study. Acta Neurol Scand 1990;82:245–52.
74. Haglund Y, Bergstrand G. Does Swedish amateur boxing lead to chronic brain damage? 2. A retrospective study with CT and MRI. Acta Neurol Scand 1990; 82(5):297–302.
75. Haglund Y, Persson H. Does Swedish amateur boxing lead to chronic brain damage? 3. A retrospective clinical neurophysiological study. Acta Neurol Scand 1990;82(6):353–60.
76. Haglund Y, Eriksson E. Does amateur boxing lead to chronic brain damage? A review of some recent investigations. Am J Sports Med 1993;21(1):97–109.
77. Kemp P, Houston A, Macleod M. Cerebral perfusion and psychometric testing in amateur boxers and controls. Eur J Nucl Med 1994;21(Suppl):S33.
78. Kemp P, Houston A, Macleod M, et al. Cerebral perfusion and psychometric testing in military amateur boxers and controls. J Neurol Neurosurg Psychiatr 1995;59:368–74.
79. Stewart W, Gordon B, Selnes O, et al. Prospective study of central nervous system function in amateur boxers in the United States. Am J Epidemiol 1994; 139(5):573–88.
80. Aotsuka A, Kojima S, Furumoto H, et al. Punch drunk syndrome due to repeated karate kicks and punches. Rinsho Shinkeigaku 1990;30(11):1243–6.
81. Jordan B, Matser E, Zimmerman R, et al. Sparring and cognitive function in professional boxers. Phys Sportsmed 1996;24(5):87–98.
82. Porter M, Fricker P. Controlled prospective neuropsychological assessment of active experienced amateur boxers. Clin J Sport Med 1996;6(2):90–6.
83. Brooks N, Kupshik G, Wilson L, et al. A neuropsychological study of active amateur boxers. J Neurol Neurosurg Psychiatr 1987;50:997–1000.
84. Sironi V, Ravagnati L. Brain damage in boxers. Lancet 1983;1:244.
85. Jordan B, Kanik A, Horwich M, et al. Apolipoprotein E ε4 and fatal cerebral amyloid angiopathy associated with dementia pugilistica. Ann Neurol 1995;38(4):698–9.
86. Jordan B, Relkin N, Ravdin L, et al. Apolipoprotein E ε4 associated with chronic traumatic brain injury in boxing. JAMA 1997;278(2):136–40.
87. Casson I, Sham R, Campbell E, et al. Neurological and CT evaluation of knocked-out boxers. J Neurol Neurosurg Psychiatr 1982;45:170–4.
88. Ross R, Ochsner M, Boyd C. Acute intracranial boxing-related injuries in U.S. Marine Corps recruits: report of two cases. Mil Med 1999;164(1):68–70.
89. Drew R, Templer D, Schuyler B, et al. Neuropsychological deficits in active licensed professional boxers. J Clin Psychol 1986;42:520–5.
90. Sironi V, Scotti G, Ravagnati L, et al. CT-scan and EEG findings in professional pugilists: Early detection of cerebral atrophy in young boxers. J Neurosurg Sci 1982;26:165–8.
91. Jordan B, Jahre C, Hauser W, et al. CT of 338 active professional boxers. Neuroradiology 1992;185:509–12.
92. Jordan B. Genetic susceptibility to brain injury in sports: a role for genetic testing in athletes. Phys Sportsmed 1998;26(2):25–6.

93. Teasdale G, Nicoll J, Murray G, et al. Association of apolipoprotein E polymorphism with outcome after head injury. Lancet 1997;350:1069–71.
94. Nicoll J, Roberts G, Graham D. Apolipoprotein E ε4 allele is associated with deposition of amyloid β-protein following a head injury. Nat Med 1995;1(2):135–7.
95. Friedman G, Froom P, Sazbon L, et al. Apolipoprotein E-e4 genotype predicts a poor outcome in survivors of traumatic brain injury. Neurology 1999;52(2):244–8.
96. Liberman J, Stewart W, Wesnes K, et al. Apolipoprotein E e4 and short term recovery from predominantly mild brain injury. Neurology 2002;58(7):1038–44.
97. Nicholl J, Coleman P, Williams B. The epidemiology of sports and exercise related injury in the United Kingdom. Br J Sports Med 1995;29(4):232–8.
98. Beis K, Tsaklis P, Pieter W, et al. Taekwondo competition injuries in Greek young and adult athletes. Eur J Sports Traumatol Rel Res 2001;23:130–6.
99. Pieter W, Bercades L, Heijmans J. Competition injuries in Olympic taekwondo. Kinesiology 1998;30:22–30.
100. Pieter W, Zemper E. Incidence of reported cerebral concussion in adult taekwondo athletes. J R Soc Health 1998;118(5):272–9.
101. Pieter W, van Ryssegem G, Lufting R, et al. Injury situation and injury mechanism at the 1993 European Taekwondo Cup. Journal of Human Movement Studies 1995;28:1–24.
102. Koh J, Cassidy JD. Incidence study of head blows and concussions in competitive taekwondo. Clin J Sport Med 2004;14:72–9.
103. Bledsoe G, Li G, Levy F. Injury risk in professional boxing. South Med J 2005;98(10):994–9.
104. McLatchie G, Brooks N, Galbraith S, et al. Clinical neurological examination, neuropsychology, electroencephalography and computed tomographic head scanning in active amateur boxers. J Neurol Neurosurg Psychiatr 1987;50:96–9.
105. Jordan B, Jahre C, Hauser W, et al. Serial computed tomography in professional boxers. J Neuromag 1992;2:181–5.
106. Cabanis E, Perez G, Tamraz J, et al. Cephalic magnetic resonance imaging of boxers: preliminary results. Acta Radiol 1986;369(Suppl):365–6.
107. Noble C. Hand injuries in boxing. Am J Sports Med 1987;15(4):342–6.
108. Zetaruk M, Violan M, Zurakowski D, et al. Karate injuries in children and adolescents. Accid Anal Prev 2000;32:421–5.
109. Tuominen R. Injuries in national karate competitions in Finland. Scand J Med Sci Sports 1995;5:44–8.
110. Ross R, Cole M, Thompson J, et al. Boxers—computed tomography, EEG and neurological evaluation. JAMA 1983;249(2):211–3.
111. Butler R, Forsythe W, Beverly D, et al. A prospective controlled investigation of the cognitive effects of amateur boxing. J Neurol Neurosurg Psychiatr 1993;56:1055–61.
112. McLatchie G, Commandre F, Zakarian H, et al. Injuries in the martial arts. In: Renstrom P, editor. Clinical practice of sports injury prevention and care. Oxford (England): Blackwell Scientific Publications; 1994. p. 609–23.
113. Schmidt-Olsen S, Kallund Jensen S, Mortensen V. Amateur boxing in Denmark. The effect of some preventive measures. Am J Sports Med 1990;18(1):98–100.
114. Burke D, Barfoot K, Bryant S, et al. Effect of implementation of safety measures in tae kwon do competition. Br J Sports Med 2003;37:401–4.
115. Macan J, Bundalo-Vrbanac D, Romic G. Effects of the new karate rules on the incidence and distribution of injuries. Br J Sports Med 2006;40:326–30.

Neurologic Injuries in Cycling and Bike Riding

James Kennedy, MD, PhD

KEYWORDS

• Cycling • Biking • Bicycle • Nerve entrapment
• Head injury • Pudendal nerve

Bicycling is one of the most popular means of transportation, recreation, fitness, and sport among millions of people of all ages. The bicycle has undergone extensive refinements since its initial beginnings as the velocipede in 1817 by Karl von Drais, remaining a readily available form of aerobic nonimpact exercise with established beneficial cardiovascular effects. Bicycling also continues to be a popular means of city transport, especially within Asian and European countries. Commercial interests, such as the postal service and law enforcement, continue to use cycling for transportation. Additionally, in the past, bicycles were an effective vehicle for mobilizing soldiers and supplies to combat zones during World Wars I and II.

Cycling was part of the inaugural first modern Olympic Games in 1896. Since this time, the International Olympic Committee has recognized the popularity of various forms of cycling and included mountain biking in the 1996 games in Atlanta with plans to incorporate bicycle motocross (BMX) in the 2008 games in Beijing. Bicycle sales have steadily increased in each decade, with mountain bikes currently accounting for 62% of new bicycle sales in the United States.[1] The increasing attractiveness is not limited to the adult population, however. In 1994, the Centers for Disease Control and Prevention estimated that 73% of children aged 5 to 14 years ride bicycles.[2]

Cycling is not generally considered a high-risk activity. Given the increased number of people riding bicycles and the development of "extreme forms" of the activity, such as mountain biking, however, there has been a continued increase in injury incidence. Generally, bike-related injuries can be classified into acute physical trauma or chronic overuse patterns. The annual incidence of bicycle deaths has been reported as 900, with 23,000 hospital admissions, 580,000 emergency department visits, and greater than 1.2 million physician consults per year.[3] Bicycle crashes rank second only to riding animals as a sports- or recreation-associated cause of serious injury. Although injuries to mountain bikers of all ages account for only 3.7% of bike injuries overall, up to

This article originally appeared in *Neurologic Clinics*, Volume 26, Issue 1.

Division of Plastic Surgery, Department of Surgery, University of Calgary; Foothills Hospital, Resident's Mailroom, 1403 29th Street NW, Calgary, Alberta, Canada T2N 2T9
E-mail address: jmckenne@ucalgary.ca

Phys Med Rehabil Clin N Am 20 (2009) 241–248
doi:10.1016/j.pmr.2008.10.015
1047-9651/08/$ – see front matter © 2009 Elsevier Inc. All rights reserved.

51% of recreational and 85% of competitive mountain bikers sustain injuries each year.[4,5] The peak incidence of bike-related injuries and fatalities is within the group aged 9 to 15 years, whereas 20- to 39-year-old riders comprise the group incurring the most mountain bike injuries.[5,6] Mortality and morbidity rates attributable to bicycle accidents remain highest in older individuals, male cyclists, and cyclists involved in collisions with motor vehicles.[7]

Most bicycle-related injuries involve superficial trauma, such as abrasions, contusions, and lacerations. Significant trauma to the upper and lower extremities and to the head, face, abdomen, and thorax are also commonly seen.[3,6,8] Neurologic involvement, unfortunately, may represent a large proportion of the more severe injury patterns. Head injuries, in particular, often involve collision with a motor vehicle and are responsible for more than 60% of all bicycle-related deaths and most long-term disabilities.[9,10]

CENTRAL NERVOUS SYSTEM INJURIES
Head Injuries

Off-road cyclists seem to have a lower incidence of head, facial, and dental injuries compared with on-road cyclists. This is presumably attributable to physical segregation from vehicular traffic and the tendency to more frequent helmet use.[4,5,8] A recent report analyzed severe cycling injuries over a 10-year period and found that 18% involved a head injury with 10% spinal involvement.[11] Principal risk factors for head injury include not wearing a helmet, crashes involving motor vehicles, an unsafe riding environment, and male gender.[5,6] The effect of rider errors, such as losing control, performing stunts, inexperience, or bike mechanical failure, remains unclear. Elevated riding speeds do seem to be linked to more severe head injury, however.

Severe head injuries, such as intracranial hemorrhage and contusions, generally have a low incidence among cyclists but do remain the top culprit contributing to mortality.[5,12–14] Intracranial hemorrhage and contusions, if present, typically involve the cerebral cortex, followed by the cerebellum and brain stem.[15] Conversely, the most common head injury is a closed head injury without an overt structural lesion, presenting as a brief loss of consciousness. Given the relative infrequent nature of structural closed head injuries, it is not unexpected that only 1.5% of all cases require operative intervention.[15]

Helmets are known to reduce the risk for head injuries by 69% to 85% and are strongly advocated by various preventative health and government agencies.[16–18] It has been estimated that although nearly 50% of children have helmets, only 15% to 25% wear them consistently or correctly.[2,19] Proposed barriers to helmet use include poor fit, cost, discomfort, and negative pressure from peers, particularly among school-aged children. Helmet legislation has been shown to be effective for increasing helmet use and for decreasing the frequency of head injuries.[20,21] Strong community-based programs designed to provide free or subsidized helmets are also effective for promoting helmet use among children.[22] Most cycling organizations now mandate bicycle helmet use, and many state jurisdictions in the United States have added mandatory use legislation, but with restrictions only applied to children.[23]

Further preventative measures have aimed to educate riders to anticipate the errors of motorists and to become familiar with the risks of different road surfaces and weather conditions. Younger children are encouraged to avoid riding in the vicinity of traffic. Environmental solutions have centered around separating cyclists from road traffic by the use of designated cycle lanes on streets. Furthermore, the design of bike pathways has included the use of smoother surfaces, avoidance of obstacles, and discouraging "wrong-way" riding. The impact of these design strategies so far has been unclear. Recently, Aultman-Hall and Kaltenecker[24] have indicated that riding on sidewalks and dedicated bicycle paths may actually be more detrimental than riding on roads, presumably because of less adherence to "road safety rules."

Spinal Cord Injuries

Like head injuries, spinal cord injuries are, fortunately, less common compared with acute musculoskeletal or chronic overuse injuries. Kim and colleagues[15] found a 12% incidence rate of spinal injuries occurring in a population of patients experiencing cycling injuries. The cervical cord was the most frequently involved spinal region. Typically, severe cervical injury results from being propelled over the handlebars after loss of control or collision with an obstacle.[25] Injuries can range from simple vertebral fracture patterns to more severe injuries, such as central cord injury and overt cord disruption. Cord injury leading to para- or quadriplegia is not infrequent.[15] Unlike head injuries, the severity of cord involvement in cycling injuries frequently necessitates immediate operative intervention.

PERIPHERAL NERVOUS SYSTEM INJURIES
Upper Extremity

Ulnar nerve
Anatomy The ulnar nerve arises from the medial cord of the brachial plexus and is composed of fibers from the anterior rami of C8 and T1. In the upper arm, the ulnar nerve is posteromedial to the brachial artery, posterior to the intermuscular septum, and anterior to the medial head of the triceps. The ulnar nerve passes posterior to the medial epicondyle of the humerus and medial to the olecranon before entering the cubital tunnel at the elbow. Once through the cubital tunnel, the ulnar nerve travels deep into the forearm immediately innervating flexor carpi ulnaris and flexor digitorum profundus to the ring and small fingers. It then descends the forearm along the ulnar side of the ulnar artery to pass through Guyon's canal. Guyon's canal is formed by the pisiform bone ulnarly, the volar carpal ligament radially and superficially, and the transverse carpal ligament as its deep surface. Once exiting Guyon's canal, the ulnar nerve divides into superficial and deep branches. The superficial branch provides sensation to the small finger and the ulnar half of the ring finger, whereas the deep branch supplies motor fibers to the hypothenar muscles, the third and fourth lumbricals, the dorsal and volar interossei, the deep head of flexor pollicis brevis, and the adductor pollicis.

Etiology Common sites of ulnar nerve compression attributable to trauma, anomalous muscles, or overt masses include the thoracic outlet, the medial intermuscular septum in the arm, the cubital tunnel, and Guyon's canal. Compression in Guyon's canal is typically seen after repetititive trauma, such as with prolonged grip pressures on bicycle handlebars or as a result of the unique position of the wrists during cycling, often leading to "cyclist's palsy".[26,27]

Clinical presentation Cyclist's palsy is classically described as numbness and paresthesias in the small finger and ulnar half of the ring finger, with motor findings like weakness on abduction or adduction of fingers or adduction of the thumb. Patterson and colleagues[28] reported that 92% of long-distance cyclists experience motor or sensory symptoms, whereas 24% had both modalities involved. Furthermore, the incidence was independent of handlebar design. Despite the predominance of sensory symptoms in cyclist's palsy, Capitani and Beer[26] have reported cases of isolated motor palsy affecting the ulnar-innervated intrinsic muscles. Akuthota and colleagues[29] found significantly increased distal motor latencies in the deep branch of the ulnar nerve after a long-distance cycling event, suggesting the possibility of acute trauma.

Treatment Although decompression of Guyon's canal directly or in combination with carpal tunnel release is a viable surgical option, it is rarely indicated. Typically, most cases resolve spontaneously after transient avoidance of cycling, albeit symptoms may not subside for several months. Additionally, the use of gloves, padded handlebars, and frequent changes in hand position have been advocated as measures to prevent or alleviate symptoms of cyclist's palsy.[30,31] The effectiveness of these preventative strategies remains to be substantiated, however.

Median nerve

Anatomy The median nerve is formed from branches of the medial and lateral cords of the brachial plexus. It travels distally between the brachialis muscle and the medial intermuscular septum before passing through the antecubital fossa and under the bicipital aponeurosis. The nerve then travels into the forearm between the deep and superficial heads of pronator teres while providing innervation to the palmaris longus, flexor carpi radialis, and flexor digitorum superficialis. After exiting pronator teres, it gives off the anterior interosseous nerve, which supplies the flexor pollicis longus, flexor digitorum profundus to the index and long fingers, and pronator quadratus. The main branch of the median nerve descends vertically behind the flexor digitorum superficialis, and before passing through the carpal tunnel, gives off the palmar cutaneous branch to supply sensation to the thenar eminence. Once through the carpal tunnel, the median nerve divides into five branches: a recurrent motor branch to supply the thenar muscles and four digital branches to supply sensation to the thumb, index finger, long finger, and radial half of the ring finger. The second and third branches also give off motor branches to the first and second lumbricals.

Etiology Typical sites of median nerve compression include at the medial intermuscular septum, where the nerve travels through pronator teres leading to pronator syndrome as well as to two clinical entities distally: anterior interosseous nerve entrapment and carpal tunnel syndrome at the wrist. Similar to ulnar nerve involvement, cycling has been implicated primarily in entrapment at the wrist, causing carpal tunnel syndrome. Although not as well documented as cyclist palsy, the presentation of median nerve compression at the wrist is analogous to the prototypical carpal tunnel syndrome.

Clinical presentation Although rarely reported, the typical symptoms of carpal tunnel syndrome, such as numbness in the lateral digits after cycling, have been observed.[32,33] Akuthota and colleagues[29] did not demonstrate any significant electrophysiologic abnormality in median motor and sensory functions, however.

Treatment Similar to ulnar nerve compression, median nerve symptoms seem to improve after a change in handlebar and riding position. Once again, if these measures fail to provide symptomatic relief, brief cessation from cycling or surgical decompression may be needed in some cases.

Lower Extremity

Pudendal nerve

Anatomy The pudendal nerve arises from the sacral plexus (S2–S4) and comprises a mixed nerve transmitting somatosensory impulses from the genitalia and motor impulses to the perineal muscles, such as the ischiocavernosus and bulbocavernosus. The major trunk of the nerve passes caudally between the sacrospinal and sacrotuberous ligaments ("the clamp region") near the ischial spine before penetrating the obturator muscle aponeurosis, often called Alcock's canal. Subsequently, the nerve emerges below the pubic bone to innervate the perineum and genitalia.

Etiology Three potential sites for pudendal nerve compression exist. Proximally, as the nerve crosses between the sacrospinal and sacrotuberous ligaments, it can be stretched repeatedly during pedaling. Additionally, increased friction within Alcock's canal can arise as the result of increased perineal pressure during prolonged sitting on a hard bicycle saddle. Finally, once the nerve escapes the protection of the bony pelvis, it is prone to compression from direct pressure on the perineum and symphysis, such as from the nose of the riding saddle.[34]

Clinical presentation Because the pudendal nerve can be compressed at various locations along its course, its entrapment often leads to varying clinical presentations. The most common symptoms involve genital numbness and erectile dysfunction. Numbness may only involve the penis if the nerve is compressed distally or could present with mixed symptoms of penile, scrotal, or perianal anesthesia if compression is proximal within Alcock's canal.[34,35] Other symptoms may include difficulty in achieving orgasm and a reduced sensation of defecation.[36] Through pressure mapping, Schrader and colleagues[37] found that the pressures applied to the perineum of cyclists by the saddle are double the threshold value known to cause ischemic injury.

Sommer and colleagues[38] reported genital numbness in 61% and erectile dysfunction in 24% of male cyclists whose weekly training program exceeded 400 km, with similar prevalence rates also found among amateur recreational cyclists.[37,39,40] The Massachusetts Male Aging Study (MMAS) investigated the incidence of erectile dysfunction among cyclists from a variety of riding backgrounds[41] and seemed to demonstrate a protective effect of moderate amounts of cycling on the occurrence of erectile dysfunction. A recent survey of 688 cyclists also did not find a significant correlation between erectile dysfunction and several cycling parameters.[42] Despite these discrepant reports, an increased risk for erectile dysfunction and genital numbness has been linked to age older than 50 years, elevated body weight, more than 10 years of cycling history, and a high intensity of training.[41]

Although most research into pudendal nerve involvement and cycling has been limited to the male population, women are equally affected. This is not surprising, because the anatomic course of the pudendal artery and nerve within Alcock's canal is roughly homologous in men and women. Lasalle and colleagues[43] reported that approximately one third of female members of a cycling club had experienced signs or symptoms of perineal trauma, such as numbness.

Treatment Most cases require no treatment and resolve spontaneously after cessation of cycling for a brief period. Once again, preventative measures are the most effective strategy. Prevention aims to change the riding style and schedule but also modifies the design of the saddle and its positioning. The goal is to minimize the strain on the neurovascular structures in the perineum during vigorous cycling. The large variety of bicycle saddles on the market today are designed to shift the weight bearing from the perineum and to distribute the pressure over a wider area of the buttocks and the ischial tuberosities. Overall, the optimal saddle seems to be wide and heavily padded with a flexible or absent nose. Heavier riders seem to benefit the most from such wider saddles.[37]

Positioning of the saddle also remains highly pertinent. A downward tilt of the nose of the saddle and a limited height difference between the seat and the top of the handlebar are crucial to avoid vigorous pressure directly on the perineum. Changes in riding styles, such as taking frequent breaks during long outings and regularly alternating between riding in sitting and standing positions, are also imperative.

Surgical options are rarely indicated. Pudendal nerve decompression, primarily of Alcock's canal, was successful in reducing pain and incontinence recently in a female population.[44] Three main surgical approaches for pudendal nerve decompression, including transgluteal, transischiorectal, and transperineal, have been proposed.

Other lower extremity peripheral nerves

Although most lower extremity peripheral nerves could potentially be hampered by means of direct trauma secondary to orthopedic involvement, there have only been a few documented cases of lesions other than that of the pudendal nerve associated with cycling. Kho and colleagues[45] describe a lone case of meralgia paresthetica involving the lateral femoral cutaneous nerve after long-distance cycling. The patient described a painful sensation on the lateral aspect of the thigh, with an objective sensory deficit noted on clinical examination.

SUMMARY

Cycling is often considered a leisurely activity with minimal potential for severe or chronic injury. Acute head and spinal trauma can be devastating and can predominantly contribute to all-cause mortality in injuries attributed to cycling. Chronic overuse injuries primarily affecting the ulnar, median, and pudendal nerves are also a cause of significant morbidity for the cyclist.

REFERENCES

1. Pfeiffer RP, Kronisch RL. Off-road cycling injuries. An overview. Sports Med 1995; 19:311–25.
2. Sacks JJ, Kresnow M, Houston B, et al. Bicycle helmet use among American children, 1994. Inj Prev 1996;2:258–62.
3. Bijur PE, Trumble A, Harel Y, et al. Sports and recreation injuries in US children and adolescents. Arch Pediatr Adolesc Med 1995;149:1009–16.
4. Chow TK, Bracker MD, Patrick K. Acute injuries from mountain biking. West J Med 1993;159:145–8.
5. Rivara FP, Thompson DC, Thompson RS. Epidemiology of bicycle injuries and risk factors for serious injury. Inj Prev 1997;3:110–4.
6. Thompson MJ, Rivara FP. Bicycle-related injuries. Am Fam Physician 2001;63: 2007–14.
7. Bostrom L, Nilsson B. A review of serious injuries and deaths from bicycle accidents in Sweden from 1987 to 1994. J Trauma 2001;50:900–7.
8. Kronisch RL, Chow TK, Simon LM, et al. Acute injuries in off-road bicycle racing. Am J Sports Med 1996;24:88–93.
9. Li G, Baker SP, Fowler C, et al. Factors related to the presence of head injury in bicycle-related pediatric trauma patients. J Trauma 1995;38:871–5.
10. Nakayama DK, Gardner MJ, Rogers KD. Disability from bicycle-related injuries in children. J Trauma 1990;30:1390–4.
11. Konkin DE, Garraway N, Hameed SM, et al. Population-based analysis of severe injuries from nonmotorized wheeled vehicles. Am J Surg 2006;191:615–8.
12. Jeys LM, Cribb G, Toms AD, et al. Mountain biking injuries in rural England. Br J Sports Med 2001;35:197–9.
13. Mellion MB. Common cycling injuries. Management and prevention. Sports Med 1991;11:52–70.

14. Noakes TD. Fatal cycling injuries. Sports Med 1995;20:348–62.
15. Kim PT, Jangra D, Ritchie AH, et al. Mountain biking injuries requiring trauma center admission: a 10-year regional trauma system experience. J Trauma 2006;60:312–8.
16. Thompson DC, Rivara FP, Thompson RS. Effectiveness of bicycle safety helmets in preventing head injuries. A case-control study. JAMA 1996;276:1968–73.
17. Thompson RS, Rivara FP, Thompson DC. A case-control study of the effectiveness of bicycle safety helmets. N Engl J Med 1989;320:1361–7.
18. Elford RW. Prevention of motor vehicle accident injuries. In: Canadian Task Force on the Periodic Health Examination Canadian guide to clinical preventative health care. Ottawa (Canada): Health Canada; 1994. p. 514–24.
19. Liller KD, Morissette B, Noland V, et al. Middle school students and bicycle helmet use: knowledge, attitudes, beliefs, and behaviors. J Sch Health 1998;68:325–8.
20. Karkhaneh M, Kalenga JC, Hagel BE, et al. Effectiveness of bicycle helmet legislation to increase helmet use: a systematic review. Inj Prev 2006;12:76–82.
21. Macpherson A, Spinks A. Bicycle helmet legislation for the uptake of helmet use and prevention of head injuries. Cochrane Database Syst Rev 2007;4: CD005401.
22. Royal ST, Kendrick D, Coleman T. Non-legislative interventions for the promotion of cycle helmet wearing by children. Cochrane Database Syst Rev 2007;4: CD003985.
23. Graitcer PL, Kellermann AL, Christoffel T. A review of educational and legislative strategies to promote bicycle helmets. Inj Prev 1995;1:122–9.
24. Aultman-Hall L, Kaltenecker MG. Toronto bicycle commuter safety rates. Accid Anal Prev 1999;31:675–86.
25. Apsingi S, Dussa CU, Soni BM. Acute cervical spine injuries in mountain biking: a report of 3 cases. Am J Sports Med 2006;34:487–9.
26. Capitani D, Beer S. Handlebar palsy—a compression syndrome of the deep terminal (motor) branch of the ulnar nerve in biking. J Neurol 2002;249:1441–5.
27. Converse TA. Cyclist's palsy. N Engl J Med 1979;301:1397–8.
28. Patterson JM, Jaggars MM, Boyer MI. Ulnar and median nerve palsy in long-distance cyclists. A prospective study. Am J Sports Med 2003;31:585–9.
29. Akuthota V, Plastaras C, Lindberg K, et al. The effect of long-distance bicycling on ulnar and median nerves: an electrophysiologic evaluation of cyclist palsy. Am J Sports Med 2005;33:1224–30.
30. Munnings F. Cyclist's palsy making changes brings relief. Phys Sportsmed 1991; 19:113–9.
31. Richmond DR. Handlebar problems in bicycling. Clin Sports Med 1994;13: 165–73.
32. Braithwaite IJ. Bilateral median nerve palsy in a cyclist. Br J Sports Med 1992;26: 27–8.
33. Chan RC, Chiu JW, Chou CL, et al. [Median nerve lesions at wrist in cyclists]. Zhonghua Yi Xue Za Zhi (Taipei) 1991;48:121–4 [in Chinese].
34. Leibovitch I, Mor Y. The vicious cycling: bicycling related urogenital disorders. Eur Urol 2005;47:277–86.
35. Silbert PL, Dunne JW, Edis RH, et al. Bicycling induced pudendal nerve pressure neuropathy. Clin Exp Neurol 1991;28:191–6.
36. Doursounian M, Salimpour P, Adelstein M, et al. Sexual and urinary tract dysfunction in bicyclists. J Urol 1998;159(S):30.
37. Schrader SM, Breitenstein MJ, Clark JC, et al. Nocturnal penile tumescence and rigidity testing in bicycling patrol officers. J Androl 2002;23:927–34.

38. Sommer F, Konig D, Graft C, et al. Impotence and genital numbness in cyclists. Int J Sports Med 2001;22:410–3.

39. Schwarzer UWW, Bin-Saleh A, Lotzerich H, et al. Genital numbness and impotence rates in long distance cyclists. J Urol 1999;161(S):178.

40. Andersen KV, Bovim G. Impotence and nerve entrapment in long distance amateur cyclists. Acta Neurol Scand 1997;95:233–40.

41. Marceau L, Kleinman K, Goldstein I, et al. Does bicycling contribute to the risk of erectile dysfunction? Results from the Massachusetts Male Aging Study—MMAS. Int J Impot Res 2001;13:298–302.

42. Taylor JA 3rd, Kao TC, Albertsen PC, et al. Bicycle riding and its relationship to the development of erectile dysfunction. J Urol 2004;172:1028–31.

43. Lasalle M, Salimpour PI, Adelstein M, et al. Sexual and urinary tract dysfunction in female bicyclists. J Urol 1999;161(S):269.

44. Beco J, Climov D, Bex M. Pudendal nerve decompression in perineology: a case series. BMC Surg 2004;4:15.

45. Kho KH, Blijham PJ, Zwarts MJ. Meralgia paresthetica after strenuous exercise. Muscle Nerve 2005;31:761–3.

Neurologic Running Injuries

Kelly A. McKean, MSc

KEYWORDS

• Running • Jogging • Nerve entrapment

The early 1980s saw a dramatic increase in the number of people participating in running. In Canada the percent of the population running increased from 15% to 31% between 1976 to 1983.[1] The rise in running brought a focus in the sports medicine world to running-related musculoskeletal injuries, and their epidemiology and biomechanics.

Over time, training programs, footwear design, and the running demographic have evolved; however, the injury rate remains high, with 35% to 65% of runners reporting injury.[1–9] The most common location of injury is the knee, followed by the foot.[3,5,6,9–12] The recent retrospective analysis by Taunton and colleagues[13] reported patellofemoral pain syndrome, iliotibial band friction syndrome, and plantar fasciitis as the three most common diagnoses.

Of the many running injuries that are reported, few are neurological in nature. A 1983 epidemiological study reported that 5.7% of peripheral nerve injuries were sports related.[14] Furthermore, a study on peroneal nerve entrapment reported diagnosing eight athletes over 18 years of practice (seven runners and one soccer player).[15] All eight were diagnosed in the last 7 years, which the authors suggest could be secondary to increased awareness of nerve involvement or to a general increase in running activity.

Despite these reports, neurologic injuries are thought to be misdiagnosed or underdiagnosed.[16] Symptoms may present differently, depending on the degree and location of the impingement, and often require exercise to reproduce the pain. In addition, they may accompany other common running injuries, making differential diagnosis difficult. Often persistence of injury leads to implication of nerve involvement.

This article describes the etiology of nerve injuries in runners, and discusses associated musculoskeletal injuries and their differential diagnosis and treatment options.

INTERDIGITAL NERVES

The interdigital nerves arise from the medial and lateral plantar nerves, which branch from the tibial nerves. They course distally, under the transverse metatarsal ligament,

This article originally appeared in *Neurologic Clinics*, Volume 26, Issue 1.
Nike Sports Research Laboratory, One Bowerman Drive, Mia Hamm 1, Beaverton, OR 97005, USA
E-mail address: kelly.mckean@nike.com

Phys Med Rehabil Clin N Am 20 (2009) 249–262
doi:10.1016/j.pmr.2008.10.019

along the metatarsals, and terminate at the distal phalanges.[17] Morton's neuroma is an impingement of one of the interdigital nerves. Although it is referred to as Morton's neuroma, it is actually not a tumor of nerve cells as indicated by the name, but is characterized by fibrosis and demylenation of the nerve.[18] This is thought to be caused by repetitive dorsiflexion of the toes, causing microtrauma to the nerve as it is compressed either under the transverse metatarsal ligament[19] or by an inflamed intermetatarsal bursa.[20,21] It can occur between any of the metatarsals, but most commonly occurs in the third interdigital space, followed by the second interdigital space.[19,22–24]

Although the incidence in both athletes and the general population is unclear, it is considered to be a common cause of forefoot pain.[22] It is exacerbated by repetitive dorsiflexion of the toes, characteristic of the end of the stance phase in running, and by tight fitting footwear.[25] A higher incidence has been documented in females compared with males,[26–28] possibly caused by footwear differences.

Symptoms

Forefoot pain radiating to the affected interspace and numbness and tingling in the toes and interdigital space are common.[23,26,29] Pain may be relieved with gentle massage and avoiding footwear.[23,24,27] Pain is increased with weight-bearing activity and compression of the metatarsal heads.[23,24,27,29] The latter, combined with palpation of the interdigital space, may reproduce the pain and cause clicking. This is referred to as Mulder's click.[23,24,27,30]

Diagnosis

The physical examination should include a clinical history, Mulder's maneuver, and palpation of the adjacent metatarsals, phalanges, and metatarsalphalangeal joints to differentiate nerve involvement from other musculoskeletal injuries. In the case of multiple affected interspaces, more proximal nerve damage should be considered. Palpation of the proximal foot structures are indicated to determine the location of the compression.[22]

Imaging techniques can be used to aid in diagnosis; however, nonspecific interdigital masses have been found in 33% of patients who have no clinical symptoms of Morton's neuroma.[23] Therefore, weight is placed on the clinical history. Ultrasound can be used to confirm the clinical diagnosis and site of impingement. This has been shown to be more effective when done dynamically, using Mulder's maneuver.[23] It has also been successfully used to diagnose recurring injury post-surgery.[31] MRI is useful to rule out other orthopedic injuries where necessary.[24]

Treatment

Conservative treatment options include nonsteroidal anti-inflammatories and modifications to training and footwear.[26] Properly fitting footwear providing adequate width to accommodate the forefoot is essential. A metatarsal pad placed proximal to the affected interspace can be used to alleviate pressure on the affected nerve.[22] Traditional orthotics to prevent pronation or supination have been shown to have no effect on symptoms, either positive or negative.[27] If symptoms persist, corticosteroids can be injected into the interdigital space. Although the success of conservative treatment depends on the severity of the impingement, 85% reported improvement with the protocol described.[26] Twenty-one percent of patients in this study had persistent symptoms warranting surgical options.

Although nonoperative treatments should be explored first, the success of surgery for more severe cases has been positive. Using the nerve resection technique, Bennett and colleagues[26] reported a satisfactory result in 96% of patients. Some controversy exists over the surgical method. Initially, the surgical approach was to excise the impinged intermetatarsal nerve via either a plantar or dorsal approach. In 1979, Gauthier advocated transection of the intermetatarsal ligament to decompress the nerve, leaving the nerve intact.[21] Further evolution of the surgery has included a minimally invasive endoscopic technique of transecting the ligament.[32,33] Another minimally invasive technique uses an instrument for releasing carpal tunnel syndrome. Using this technique, 11 of 14 patients were symptom-free post-surgery.[34]

Failure to respond to both nonoperative and operative treatments may suggest the presence of other foot pathologies.[29]

TIBIAL NERVE

The tibial nerve arises from the sciatic nerve superior to the popliteal fossa, and courses distally through the posterior lower leg.[35] In athletes, entrapment of the tibial nerve generally only occurs at the foot and ankle region. The most common location is around the posterior edge of the medial malleolus within the tarsal tunnel, where the nerve passes to extend into the foot (**Fig. 1**).[36] The walls of the tarsal tunnel are created by the flexor retinaculum, calcaneus, talus, and medial malleolus. Several structures run through the tarsal tunnel, including the tendons of the tibialis posterior, flexor hallucis longus, flexor digitorum longus, and the posterior tibial artery and nerve.[17,19] Because of the inelasticity of the tunnel, any enlargement of the structures inside can increase pressure within the tunnel, causing nerve compression.[37]

Generally, nerve injury in this area is secondary to another pathology. For runners, this may be inflammation of the synovial sheaths lining the tendons (tenosynovitis), accessory muscles, fracture, or more rarely, ligament fibrosis from chronic ankle sprains.[19,38] Nerve compression may occur via the mechanism described above or with tension on the tibial nerve with pronation of the subtalar joint.[39] Injury to the structures of the tunnel is thought to be caused by the repetitive plantar flexion and dorsiflexion at the ankle occurring while running. Furthermore, poor mechanics, such as excessive pronation, valgus deformity, or flat feet exacerbate the problem.[38–41]

Kinoshita and colleagues[38] reported surgically treating 58 feet that had tarsal tunnel syndrome over a 16-year period; 39.1% of these were sport-related injuries. Although

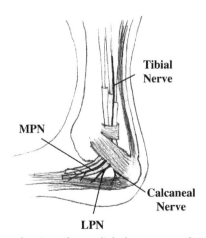

Fig. 1. The tibial nerve branches into the medial plantar nerve (MPN), lateral plantar nerve (LPN) and calcaneal nerve at the tarsal tunnel.

this injury rate appears low, tarsal tunnel syndrome is thought to be underdiagnosed because of the similarity in symptoms to plantar fasciitis, heel pad atrophy, and calcaneal fractures.[42] Plantar fasciitis is the third most commonly diagnosed injury in runners.[13] It is possible that more cases with nerve involvement present within this population, but are not differentially diagnosed.

Symptoms

Tarsal tunnel syndrome (TTS) is characterized by local tenderness behind the medial malleolus[38] and numbness, tingling, and pain over the medial heel, arch, medial sole, or sole of the foot.[37,38,43,44] Pain can be burning, sharp, shooting, or dull, and may radiate proximally up the calf or distally into the foot.[37] Pain is usually decreased with rest and increased at night, and with weight bearing, prolonged standing, running,[19,22] and the initial steps after rest. The latter is referred to as post-static dyskinesia, and is characterized by the accumulation of fluid around an injury during rest, which causes increased pressure on the nerve with subsequent weight bearing.[45] Foot weakness has also been reported.[37]

Although these are the general symptoms for TTS, symptoms vary depending on the exact location of compression of the tibial nerve or its branches (**Table 1**). Although the location of nerve branches varies among individuals, all three nerve branches originate in the region of the tarsal tunnel[46] and have been implicated in heel pain.[42] A recent review of neural heel pain differentiated symptoms according to the nerve branch

Table 1
Symptoms and diagnostics used to identify tarsal tunnel syndrome and plantar fasciitis

	TTS	PF
Symptoms	Numbness, tingling and pain in medial heel, arch, medial sole and sole	Pain in calcaneal tuberosity, origin of plantar fascia, midfoot fascia
	Sharp, shooting, dull, radiating	Localized
	Decreased with rest	
	Increased at night, running, post-static dyskinesia	Post-static dyskinesia
	Foot weakness	
	LPN—medial heel, proximal pf area, tender medial foot	
	MPN—laterally on medial arch, navicular tuberosity	
	Calcaneal nerve—medial fat pad, abductor hallucis, less over plantar fascia	
Diagnosis	History and physical	History and physical
	Tinel's	
	Sensory and motor nerve conduction of LPN, MPN	
	QST	
	Two-point discrimination	
	Modified straight leg test	

Abbreviations: LPN, lateral plantar nerve; MPN, medial plantar nerve; PF, plantar fasciitis; QST, quantitative sensory testing; TTS, tarsal tunnel syndrome.

affected.[47] Lateral plantar nerve (LPN) symptoms have been described as affecting the medial calcaneus and proximal plantar fascia area with maximum tenderness over the nerve.[48] Medial plantar nerve (MPN) symptoms occur over the medial arch and navicular tuberosity.[49] Anterior calcaneal nerve symptoms manifest in the medial fat pad and abductor hallucis, with reduced symptoms over the plantar fascia.[50]

The important differential diagnosis in this case is plantar fasciitis, in which symptoms may be slightly different, but which occurs in the same region (see **Table 1**). Plantar fasciitis is characterized by pain at the calcaneal tuberosity, or origin of the plantar fascia, continuing a few centimeters distally along the fascia over the midfoot.[43,48] The pain is more localized than tarsal tunnel syndrome, and does not include the paraesthesia or sensory deficit associated with nerve involvement. Post-static dyskinesia may also be present with plantar fasciitis.[47]

Diagnosis

Diagnosis of TTS relies on a history and physical examination. In addition to the symptoms described above, swelling over the tibial nerve may be palpable.[44] Patients experience pain on tapping the nerve (positive Tinel's sign), and may exhibit loss of two-point discrimination.[37,38] The dorsiflexion-eversion test was initially introduced as a diagnostic tool for TTS[51] that reproduces nerve pain by placing the foot in dorsiflexion and eversion with the metatarsophalangeal (MTP) joints extended. The windlass test was developed to reproduce plantar fasciitis pain by extending the MTP joints with a neutral ankle.[52] Although these diagnostic tests may aid in injury differentiation, both tests increase the strain in the tibial and plantar nerves as well as the plantar fascia.[53] Alternatively, adding a straight leg raise after dorsiflexion and eversion has been shown to further increase the strain on the tibial nerve.[54] This modified test may be useful in differential diagnosis in the future.[53]

Additional tools may be used to confirm physical examination findings, including ultrasound, radiography, quantitative sensory tests, and electrodiagnostics. Abnormal motor and sensory nerve conduction have been shown with nerve damage; however, results have been variable, and therefore the accuracy has been a topic of many studies.[36,55] In 2005, the American Association of Neuromuscular and Electrodiagnostic Medicine sponsored an effort to evaluate the existing research and determine the usefulness of these tools.[56] It was concluded that sensory nerve conduction was more sensitive than motor nerve conduction in identifying nerve injury, but less specific. Current recommendations are to use nerve conduction velocity in conjunction with physical examination and to include both motor and sensory tests of the medial and lateral plantar nerves.[56] Exposing the injured dermatome to some form of stimulus (temperature, vibration and so forth) is referred to as quantitative sensory testing. This type of test has also shown some success in identifying nerve injury, although its use for TTS has been limited thus far.[57,58]

Together, these tests, along with Tinel's sign, two-point discrimination, and potentially the modified straight leg test, will help differentiate TTS from a pure musculoskeletal injury such as plantar fasciitis (see **Table 1**).

Treatment

Initial treatment of TTS is conservative, using rest, ice, physiotherapy, nonsteroidal anti-inflammatories, corticosteroids, and footwear modifications.[38,59] Eliminating excessive pronation using varus orthotics or medially posted shoes may alleviate pain and help treat the source of the problem. This is important to correct any abnormal mechanics that may inhibit healing, especially for runners who undergo repetitive motion at the ankle.[37,38]

Initial treatment of tarsal tunnel syndrome and plantar fasciitis are similar; however, if the symptoms persist, then surgical intervention is an option and differential diagnosis becomes important. Surgical procedures involve decompressing the tibial nerve (or involved branches) while repairing the secondary pathology responsible for increased tunnel pressure. This may involve dissection of the flexor retinaculum, neurolysis of the affected nerve, tenosynovectomy, excision of bony fragments, stretching of the neurovascular bundle around foot deformities, or removal of accessory muscles.[38] Pain relief can be immediate; however, a 3-month postsurgical recovery followed by a gradual return to sport is recommended to get rid of all symptoms and avoid reinjury. Kinoshita and colleagues[38] reported a complete return to sport in 12 of 18 athletes postsurgery.

PERONEAL NERVE

The common peroneal nerve (CPN) originates from the sciatic nerve in the posterior thigh, proximal to the popliteal fossa. Distal to the popliteal fossa it winds laterally between the heads of the peroneus longus and around the neck of the fibula, where it divides into superficial peroneal nerve (SPN) and deep peroneal nerve (DPN) branches.[35]

The peroneal nerve can be entrapped in several locations along its course (**Fig. 2**). These include the fibular neck (CPN), the fascial exit above the lateral malleolus or

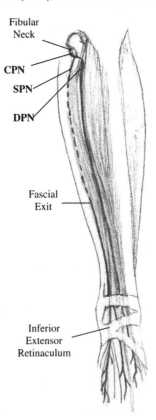

Fig. 2. Course of the common peroneal nerve (CPN) and its superficial (SPN) and deep (DPN) branches as well as locations of potential entrapment.

across the ankle joint (SPN), or the anterior tarsal tunnel (DPN). These or other locations of entrapment may occur because of chronic exercise-induced compartment syndrome (CECS), an exercise-induced increase in compartment pressure caused by a relatively greater increase in muscle size than the fascia that surrounds the compartment.[60,61] This can cause ischemia and nerve compression.[19] Although CECS is a common musculoskeletal injury in runners, it does not always lead to nerve injury; therefore a differential diagnosis becomes important and is discussed below (**Table 2**).

Common Peroneal Nerve

The most proximal location of peroneal nerve entrapment is the CPN at the fibular neck.[15,62] In runners the most likely cause is an inversion ankle sprain that stretches the peroneus longus muscle and compresses the CPN between the muscle heads.[59] This injury occurs more commonly in contact sports because of an adduction injury at the knee or blunt trauma to the area (ie, from a hockey puck).[63] It is characterized by pain, burning, and numbness in the anterolateral leg, loss of sensation on the dorsum of the foot, and motor weakness of the dorsiflexors and evertors.[15,19,59,62,63] Pain occurs with activity and decreases with rest.[15] Symptoms increase with ankle inversion and percussion of the nerve at the fibular neck.[59] Diagnosis includes a physical examination and history of the symptoms described above as well as a positive Tinel's sign at the fibular neck.[15,62] Nerve conduction velocity can also be used to confirm diagnosis.[59]

Superficial Peroneal Nerve

Distally, the SPN descends through the lateral compartment of the leg on the surface of the peroneus longus.[17] It exits the fascia 10 to 12 cm above the lateral malleolus, and gives rise to two subcutaneous branches that cross the ankle joint.[17,49] The SPN can be entrapped at the ankle joint because of inversion ankle sprains, or at the fascial exit point above the lateral malleolus.[22,64–66] The latter can also be attributed to ankle sprains that cause the edge of the fascia to compress the SPN.[49] In addition, SPN entrapments can be associated with CECS of the anterolateral compartment;[60,67] however, this has been reported in only 10% of cases.[65]

SPN symptoms include pain and cramping in the lateral leg, ankle, and dorsum of the foot, as well as numbness on the dorsum of the foot.[19,22,49,59,60,64,65] Unlike the more proximal entrapment of the CPN, there is no motor deficit.[64] Symptoms increase with activity and decrease with rest.[22,49] For entrapments at the fascial exit above the lateral malleolus local swelling may be palpable.[22,49,64] Physical examination should be done post-exercise[68] and begin at the low back, sciatic notch, and fibular neck to rule out any proximal entrapment.[16,49] Symptoms can be reproduced by any of the following three tests: (1) palpating the area of entrapment while the patient everts and dorsiflexes against resistance,[59,69] (2) percussing the nerve course while the patient passively plantarflexes and inverts the foot, and (3) the latter without percussion of the nerve.[69,70] Diagnosis includes the symptoms described above plus at least one of the three tests yielding positive results. Nerve conduction velocity tests and compartment pressure can also be used to assist with differential diagnosis.[65]

Deep Peroneal Nerve

The more medial branch of the CPN, the DPN, descends through the anterior compartment between the extensor digitorum longus and the tibialis anterior muscles.[17] It courses deep to the extensor hallucis longus and crosses the ankle joint under the extensor retinaculum.[49] The DPN can also be entrapped in more than one location. One of the most common locations is under the inferior extensor retinaculum. This is

Table 2
Symptoms and diagnosis of entrapment of the common peroneal nerve and its superficial and deep branches versus chronic exercise-induced compartment syndrome

		CPN	SPN	DPN	CECS
Symptoms		Pain and numbness in anterolateral leg	Pain and cramping lateral leg, ankle and, dorsal foot	Aching and cramping anterior leg	Aching, cramping, tightness, sharp pain in compartment
		Numbness of dorsal foot	Numbness dorsal foot	Numbness dorsal foot, first web space	
		Weak dorsiflexors, evertors (foot drop)	No motor weakness	No motor weakness	
		Increases with activity	Increases with activity	Increases with activity	Increases with activity
		Subsides with rest	Subsides with rest	Subsides with rest	Subsides with rest
		Local tenderness behind fibular head	Local swelling at fascia exit (bulge)		Diffuse swelling, tenderness over compartment
Diagnosis		Physical examination	Physical examination	Physical examination	Physical examination
		History of ankle sprains or blunt trauma	History of ankle sprains	History of ankle sprains	
		Reproduce pain with forced ankle inversion or Tinel's	Reproduce pain with one of three positive tests	Reproduce pain with dorsi flexion or plantar flexion	
		Compartment pressure	Compartment pressure	Compartment pressure	Compartment pressure
		Ncv	Ncv	Ncv	

Abbreviations: CECS, chronic exercise-induced compartment syndrome; CPN, common peroneal nerve; DPN, deep peroneal nerve; Ncv, nerve conduction velocity; SPN, superficial peroneal nerve.

referred to as anterior TTS.[71,72] It can be caused by frequent ankle sprains or trauma to the dorsum of the foot (ie, kicking). Carrying a key under the tongue of a shoe and doing sit-ups with feet hooked under a bar have also been cited as possible causative factors for runners.[49]

DPN symptoms include aching and cramping in the anterior leg and numbness in the dorsum of the foot and first web space.[19,22,49,60,71] Because this occurs in a distal branch of the CPN, no motor weakness should be present.[22] Pain occurs with activity and subsides with rest.[49] Similar to SPN entrapment, the physical examination is most revealing post-exercise, and should also begin with low back assessment to rule out proximal involvement.[49] Symptoms may be reproduced with plantar or dorsiflexion, depending on the location of entrapment.[49] Entrapment at the extensor retinaculum or anterior tarsal tunnel may be accompanied by a history of ankle sprains.[49] Entrapment elsewhere within the compartment may be related to CECS.

Part of the differential for entrapment of DPN includes CECS. Symptoms of CECS include aching and cramping of the lower leg within the involved compartment (anterior or lateral),[60,61] with pain described as tightness, squeezing, or sharp.[67] Symptoms typically occur during exercise and subside during rest.[61,67] The diffuse swelling and tenderness over the compartment differentiates this syndrome from nerve entrapment, which is characterized by localized swelling and tenderness in combination with paresthesias.[22,49]

Compartment pressure measurements may be widely used to assist in diagnosis of CECS. Intramuscular pressure is measured at rest, at 1 minute post-exercise, and at 5 minutes post-exercise. Both elevated pressure and increased time to recovery to rest pressure can be indicative of pathology.[61] Resting pressure equal to or greater than 15 mmHg, equal to or greater than 30mmHg at 1 minute post-exercise, or equal to or greater than 20 mmHg at 5 minutes post-exercise combined with clinical symptoms are considered diagnostic.[73]

Treatment

CPN contusion caused by blunt trauma can have functional recovery within days to weeks, and minimal treatment intervention is required.[63] Conversely, nontraumatic entrapments of the peroneal nerve and its branches do not respond well to conservative treatment.[15,19,49] Surgical decompression of the nerve is often recommended.[22,59]

For cases related to CECS, fasciotomy of the involved compartment is done for decompression of the nerve; however, it is not uncommon for symptoms to persist post-fasciotomy. Schepsis and colleagues[69] studied a group of 18 patients having revision surgery for anterior CECS, and found that 44% had symptoms and surgical findings consistent with SPN entrapment. At 2 years post-surgery, patients who had concurrent SPN entrapment had 100% recovery, whereas the patients who did not have the SPN entrapment had only 50% recovery. The authors hypothesized that the original surgery may have stimulated scar tissue formation and subsequent compression of the nerve.[69] Slimmon and colleagues[74] studied the effects of partial fasciectomy with the goal of decreasing scar tissue formation, but recurrent symptoms persisted long term.

OTHER INJURIES

The following injuries occur less frequently in the lower extremity of runners.

Sural nerve entrapment has been documented in a few runners.[49,75] The sural nerve branches from the tibial nerve in the popliteal fossa and descends between the heads of the gastrocnemius.[17] In the distal calf the nerve exits the deep aponeurosis and descends adjacent to the Achilles tendon.[17] In all patients reported by Fabre and colleagues[75] entrapment occurred as the nerve exits the fascia in a fibrotic aponeurosis. Sural nerve entrapment is characterized by calf pain (sometimes radiating), and tenderness along the Achilles tendon.[49,75] Symptoms may be exacerbated by exercise, pressure over the entrapment site, and plantar flexion.[75] It can be misdiagnosed as Achilles tendinopathy;[59] however, nerve conduction velocity and Tinel's may help differentiate the conditions.[49,75] In cases where the nerve is compressed in fibrotic scar tissue, surgical excision is indicated.[49,75]

Joplin's neuroma is described as compression of the medial plantar (digital) nerve over the first MTP/medial aspect of the foot,[76] with common symptoms including pain and paresthesia over the medial side of the great toe. There is a controversial relationship with wearing of tight footwear.[59,76] Abnormal forefoot biomechanics may be a predisposing factor.[59] Treatments include footwear modification or surgical neurolysis in some cases.

Transient forefoot numbness during exercise has been rarely documented in the literature, and has been reported anecdotally in both orthopedic clinics and the footwear industry. This phenomenon, also referred to as transient parasthetica or digitalgia parasthetica, has been reported in military marchers, long-distance backpackers, individuals wearing cowboy boots, and those using stair climbing machines.[77–81]

This phenomenon may be caused by decreased neural perfusion in the forefoot. In compressive footwear or on exercise equipment in which the foot remains in contact with the machine and is pressure loaded, the muscle pump effect is lost, and arterial/venous stasis ensues. This perfusion loss may progress to neural ischemia and the symptoms of dysesthesia or anesthesia in the affected nerve's dermatomal region (Neil A. Manson, MD, FRCSC, personal communication, 2007). This hypothesis has also been corroborated by Vereschagin and colleagues.[77] Although the numbness is generally transient, a review by Schon[22] suggests the symptoms may be indicative of initial injury that could develop into a chronic neuropathy of the interdigital nerves, or potentially the plantar or tibial nerves. Further research is required to determine the etiology of this phenomenon and identify methods of prevention.

SUMMARY

Nerve injuries caused by running account for a small percentage of running injuries. These include injury to the interdigital, tibial, peroneal, and sural nerves. Awareness of the differences in symptoms between these and musculoskeletal injuries is important for good diagnostic specificity. Ultimately, early differential diagnosis will aid in appropriate treatment and rapid return to running.

REFERENCES

1. Government of Canada. Fitness and lifestyle in Canada. Fitness & Amateur Sport; 1983. Ottawa, Canada.
2. Lysholm J, Wiklander J. Injuries in runners. Am J Sports Med 1987;15(2):168–71.
3. McKean KA, Manson NA, Stanish WD. Musculoskeletal injury in the masters runners. Clin J Sport Med 2006;16(2):149–54.
4. Macera C, Pate R, Powell K, et al. Predicting lower extremity injuries among habitual runners. Arch Intern Med 1989;149:2565–8.
5. Koplan JP, Rothenberg RB, Jones EL. The natural history of exercise: a 10-yr follow-up of a cohort of runners. Med Sci Sports Exerc 1995;27(8):1180–4.
6. Koplan JP, Powell KE, Sikes RK, et al. An epidemiologic study of the benefits and risks of running. JAMA 1982;248(23):3118–21.

7. Taunton JE, Ryan MB, Clement DB, et al. A prospective study of running injuries: the Vancouver Sun Run "In Training" clinics. Br J Sports Med 2003;37(3):239–44.

8. Jacobs S, Berson B. Injuries to runners: astudy of entrants to a 10,000 meter race. Am J Sports Med 1986;14(2):151–5.

9. Walter SD, Hart LE, McIntosh JM, et al. The Ontario Cohort Study of Running-Related Injuries. Arch Intern Med 1989;149:2561–8.

10. Macintyre JG, Taunton JE, Clement DB, et al. Running injuries: a clinical ttudy of 4173 cases. Clin J Sport Med 1991;1:81–7.

11. Brunet ME, Cook SD, Brinker MR, et al. A survey of running injuries in 1505 competitive and recreational runners. J Sports Med Phys Fitness 1990;30(3):307–15.

12. Clement DB, Taunton JE, Smart GW, et al. A survey of overuse running injuries. Phys Sportsmed 1981;9(5):47–58.

13. Taunton JE, Ryan MB, Clement DB, et al. A retrospective case-control analysis of 2002 running injuries. Br J Sports Med 2002;36(2):95–101.

14. Hirasawa Y, Sakakida K. Sports and peripheral nerve injury. Am J Sports Med 1983;11(6):420–6.

15. Leach RE, Purnell MB, Saito A. Peroneal nerve entrapment in runners. Am J Sports Med 1989;17(2):287–91.

16. Rosenow DE. Superficial peroneal nerve. J Neurosurg 2007;106(3):520–2.

17. Sarrafian SK. Anatomy of the foot and ankle: descriptive topographic function. 2nd edition. Philadelphia: J.B. Lippincott; 1993.

18. Graham CE, Graham DM. Morton's neuroma: a microscopic evaluation. Foot Ankle 1984;5(3):150–3.

19. Lorei MP, Hershman EB. Peripheral nerve injuries in athletes. Treatment and prevention. Sports Med 1993;16(2):130–47.

20. Bossley CJ, Cairney PC. The intermetatarsophalangeal bursa—its significance in Morton's metatarsalgia. J Bone Joint Surg Br 1980;62-B(2):184–7.

21. Gauthier G. Thomas Morton's disease: a nerve entrapment syndrome. A new surgical technique. Clin Orthop Relat Res 1979;142:90–2.

22. Schon LC. Nerve entrapment, neuropathy, and nerve dysfunction in athletes. Orthop Clin North Am 1994;25(1):47–59.

23. Bencardino J, Rosenberg ZS, Beltran J, et al. Morton's neuroma: is it always symptomatic? AJR Am J Roentgenol 2000;175(3):649–53.

24. Perini L, Del BM, Cipriano R, et al. Dynamic sonography of the forefoot in Morton's syndrome: correlation with magnetic resonance and surgery. Radiol Med (Torino) 2006;111(7):897–905.

25. Hockenbury RT. Forefoot problems in athletes. Med Sci Sports Exerc 1999; 31(Suppl 7):S448–58.

26. Bennett GL, Graham CE, Mauldin DM. Morton's interdigital neuroma: a comprehensive treatment protocol. Foot Ankle Int 1995;16(12):760–3.

27. Kilmartin TE, Wallace WA. Effect of pronation and supination orthosis on Morton's neuroma and lower extremity function. Foot Ankle Int 1994;15(5):256–62.

28. Greenfield J, Rea J Jr, Ilfeld FW. Morton's interdigital neuroma. Indications for treatment by local injections versus surgery. Clin Orthop Relat Res 1984;185: 142–4.

29. Okafor B, Shergill G, Angel J. Treatment of Morton's neuroma by neurolysis. Foot Ankle Int 1997;18(5):284–7.

30. Mulder JD. The causative mechanism in morton's metatarsalgia. J Bone Joint Surg Br 1951;33-B(1):94–5.

31. Levine SE, Myerson MS, Shapiro PP, et al. Ultrasonographic diagnosis of recurrence after excision of an interdigital neuroma. Foot Ankle Int 1998;19(2):79–84.

32. Barrett SL, Pignetti TT. Endoscopic decompression for intermetatarsal nerve entrapment—the EDIN technique: preliminary study with cadaveric specimens; early clinical results. J Foot Ankle Surg 1994;33(5):503–8.
33. Shapiro SL. Endoscopic decompression of the intermetatarsal nerve for Morton's neuroma. Foot Ankle Clin 2004;9(2):297–304.
34. Zelent ME, Kane RM, Neese DJ, et al. Minimally invasive Morton's intermetatarsal neuroma decompression. Foot Ankle Int 2007;28(2):263–5.
35. Romanes GJ. Cunninghams manual of practical anatomy. New York: Oxford Medical Publications; 1989.
36. Fu R, DeLisa JA, Kraft GH. Motor nerve latencies through the tarsal tunnel in normal adult subjects: standard determinations corrected for temperature and distance. Arch Phys Med Rehabil 1980;61(6):243–8.
37. Jackson DL, Haglund BL. Tarsal tunnel syndrome in runners. Sports Med 1992; 13(2):146–9.
38. Kinoshita M, Okuda R, Yasuda T, et al. Tarsal tunnel syndrome in athletes. Am J Sports Med 2006;34(8):1307–12.
39. Daniels TR, Lau JT, Hearn TC. The effects of foot position and load on tibial nerve tension. Foot Ankle Int 1998;19(2):73–8.
40. Bracilovic A, Nihal A, Houston VL, et al. Effect of foot and ankle position on tarsal tunnel compartment volume. Foot Ankle Int 2006;27(6):431–7.
41. Trepman E, Kadel NJ, Chisholm K, et al. Effect of foot and ankle position on tarsal tunnel compartment pressure. Foot Ankle Int 1999;20(11):721–6.
42. Schon LC, Glennon TP, Baxter DE. Heel pain syndrome: electrodiagnostic support for nerve entrapment. Foot Ankle 1993;14(3):129–35.
43. Jackson DL, Haglund B. Tarsal tunnel syndrome in athletes. Case reports and literature review. Am J Sports Med 1991;19(1):61–5.
44. Lam SJ. Tarsal tunnel syndrome. J Bone Joint Surg Br 1967;49(1):87–92.
45. Davidson MR, Copoloff JA. Neuromas of the heel. Clin Podiatr Med Surg 1990; 7(2):271–88.
46. Dellon AL, Mackinnon SE. Tibial nerve branching in the tarsal tunnel. Arch Neurol 1984;41(6):645–6.
47. Alshami AM, Souvlis T, Coppieters MW. A review of plantar heel pain of neural origin: differential diagnosis and management. Man Ther 2007, epub ahead of print.
48. Baxter DE, Pfeffer GB. Treatment of chronic heel pain by surgical release of the first branch of the lateral plantar nerve. Clin Orthop Relat Res 1992;(279):229–36.
49. Schon LC, Baxter DE. Neuropathies of the foot and ankle in athletes. Clin Sports Med 1990;9(2):489–509.
50. Henricson AS, Westlin NE. Chronic calcaneal pain in athletes: entrapment of the calcaneal nerve? Am J Sports Med 1984;12(2):152–4.
51. Kinoshita M, Okuda R, Morikawa J, et al. The dorsiflexion-eversion test for diagnosis of tarsal tunnel syndrome. J Bone Joint Surg Am 2001;83-A(12):1835–9.
52. De GD, Dean D, Requejo SM, et al. The association between diagnosis of plantar fasciitis and windlass test results. Foot Ankle Int 2003;24(3):251–5.
53. Alshami AM, Babri AS, Souvlis T, et al. Biomechanical evaluation of two clinical tests for plantar heel pain: the dorsiflexion-eversion test for tarsal tunnel syndrome and the windlass test for plantar fasciitis. Foot Ankle Int 2007;28(4): 499–505.
54. Coppieters MW, Alshami AM, Babri AS, et al. Strain and excursion of the sciatic, tibial, and plantar nerves during a modified straight leg raising test. J Orthop Res 2006;24(9):1883–9.

55. Galardi G, Amadio S, Maderna L, et al. Electrophysiologic studies in tarsal tunnel syndrome. Diagnostic reliability of motor distal latency, mixed nerve and sensory nerve conduction studies. Am J Phys Med Rehabil 1994;73(3):193–8.
56. Patel AT, Gaines K, Malamut R, et al. Usefulness of electrodiagnostic techniques in the evaluation of suspected tarsal tunnel syndrome: an evidence-based review. Muscle Nerve 2005;32(2):236–40.
57. Dellon AL. Management of peripheral nerve problems in the upper and lower extremity using quantitative sensory testing. Hand Clin 1999;15(4):697–715, x.
58. Tassler PL, Dellon AL. Pressure perception in the normal lower extremity and in the tarsal tunnel syndrome. Muscle Nerve 1996;19(3):285–9.
59. McCrory P, Bell S, Bradshaw C. Nerve entrapments of the lower leg, ankle and foot in sport. Sports Med 2002;32(6):371–91.
60. Black KP, Schultz TK, Cheung NL. Compartment syndromes in athletes. Clin Sports Med 1990;9(2):471–87.
61. Martens MA, Backaert M, Vermaut G, et al. Chronic leg pain in athletes due to a recurrent compartment syndrome. Am J Sports Med 1984;12(2):148–51.
62. Moller BN, Kadin S. Entrapment of the common peroneal nerve. Am J Sports Med 1987;15(1):90–1.
63. Kopell H, Thompson W. Peripheral entrapment neuropathies of the lower extremity. N Engl J Med 1960;262:56–60.
64. Yang LJ, Gala VC, McGillicuddy JE. Superficial peroneal nerve syndrome: an unusual nerve entrapment. Case report. J Neurosurg 2006;104(5):820–3.
65. Styf J. Entrapment of the superficial peroneal nerve. Diagnosis and results of decompression. J Bone Joint Surg Br 1989;71(1):131–5.
66. Acus RW III, Flanagan JP. Perineural fibrosis of superficial peroneal nerve complicating ankle sprain: a case report. Foot Ankle 1991;11(4):233–5.
67. Detmer DE, Sharpe K, Sufit RL, et al. Chronic compartment syndrome: diagnosis, management, and outcomes. Am J Sports Med 1985;13(3):162–70.
68. Styf J. Chronic exercise-induced pain in the anterior aspect of the lower leg. An overview of diagnosis. Sports Med 1989;7(5):331–9.
69. Schepsis AA, Fitzgerald M, Nicoletta R. Revision surgery for exertional anterior compartment syndrome of the lower leg: technique, findings, and results. Am J Sports Med 2005;33(7):1040–7.
70. Styf J. Diagnosis of exercise-induced pain in the anterior aspect of the lower leg. Am J Sports Med 1988;16(2):165–9.
71. Barr KP, Harrast MA. Evidence-based treatment of foot and ankle injuries in runners. Phys Med Rehabil Clin N Am 2005;16(3):779–99.
72. Borges LF, Hallett M, Selkoe DJ, et al. The anterior tarsal tunnel syndrome. Report of two cases. J Neurosurg 1981;54(1):89–92.
73. Pedowitz RA, Hargens AR, Mubarak SJ, et al. Modified criteria for the objective diagnosis of chronic compartment syndrome of the leg. Am J Sports Med 1990;18(1):35–40.
74. Slimmon D, Bennell K, Brukner P, et al. Long-term outcome of fasciotomy with partial fasciectomy for chronic exertional compartment syndrome of the lower leg. Am J Sports Med 2002;30(4):581–8.
75. Fabre T, Montero C, Gaujard E, et al. Chronic calf pain in athletes due to sural nerve entrapment. A report of 18 cases. Am J Sports Med 2000;28(5):679–82.
76. Still GP, Fowler MB. Jopliin's neuroma or compression neuropathy of the plantar proper digital nerve to the hallux: clinicopathologic study of three cases. J Foot Ankle Surg 1998;37(6):524–30.

77. Vereschagin KS, Firtch WL, Caputo LJ, et al. Transient paresthesia in stair-climbers' feet. Phys Sportsmed 1993;21(2):63–9.
78. Meharg JG. Cowbot boot neuropathy. JAMA 1984;251:2659–60.
79. Stein M, Shlamkovitch N, Finestone A, et al. Marcher's digitalgia paresthetica among recruit. Foot Ankle 1989;9(6):312–3.
80. Boulware DR. Backpacking-induced paresthesias. Wilderness Environ Med 2003;14(3):161–6.
81. Massey EW. Digitalgia parethetica in the foot. JAMA 1978;239(14):1393–4.

Neurologic Injuries from Scuba Diving

Jodi Hawes, MD, PT, E. Wayne Massey, MD, FAAN, FACP*

KEYWORDS

- Scuba diving • Decompression
- Arterial gas embolism • Decompression illness

Interest in scuba (self-contained underwater breathing apparatus) diving increased in the 1970s, and undersea diving continues to be a popular sport early in the 21st century, with approximately 3 million certified divers in the United States.[1] The Divers Alert Network (DAN), an institution created in 1981 by the Commerce Department, National Oceanic and Atmospheric Administration, has collected diving injury data for US and Canadian divers since 1987 that can be studied to suggest the epidemiologic characteristics of diving.

The 2006 annual DAN Diving Report on Diving Injuries and Diving Fatalities[2] is based on data collected during 2004. This diving report presents information on Project Dive Exploration (PDE), which is a prospective observational study of recreational diving yearly data since 1995. PDE divers are volunteers from the general recreational diving population, but they are not necessarily representative of this population. Most PDE divers are 30 to 50 years of age; 22% are over the age of 50, and 4% are under 20 years of age. Thirty percent of the divers are female. Sixty-six percent of the female divers hold open water, advanced open water, or specialty certification, verses 46% of the males.

The annual number of injury cases reported has increased from 1987 to 2004, with about 600 cases in 1987 and 1100 cases in 2002 (**Fig. 1**).[2] The dramatic dip noted in 2003 represents decreased data collection because of the Health Insurance Portability and Accountability Act (HIPAA). The mean age of divers in the DAN injury population was 39 years (**Fig. 2**).[2] Interestingly, divers with advanced certification had the highest percentage of injuries, but this may be due to unknown diving frequency and may differ between the varying certification categories (**Fig. 3**).

The annual record of US and Canadian diving fatalities, began in 1971 by John McAniff of the University of Rhode Island, was transitioned to DAN in 1989.[2] The number of fatalities reported from 1970 to 2004 ranges from 80 to 120 annually, with a stable number of fatalities (**Fig. 4**).[2] The general diving population seems to be aging, as a larger percentage of divers have been diving for more than a decade

This article originally appeared in *Neurologic Clinics*, volume 26, issue 1.
Duke University Medical Center, Box 3909, Durham, NC 27710, USA
* Corresponding author.
E-mail address: masse010@mc.duke.edu (E.W. Massey).

Phys Med Rehabil Clin N Am 20 (2009) 263–272
doi:10.1016/j.pmr.2008.10.018
1047-9651/08/$ – see front matter © 2009 Elsevier Inc. All rights reserved.

pmr.theclinics.com

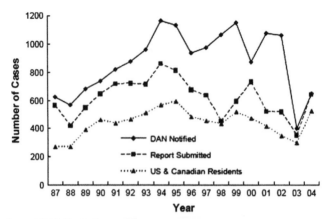

Fig. 1. Annual record of dive injury cases.

since certification. This aging of the diving population may account for the increase in the mean age of diving fatalities from 1989 to 2002. The mean age of divers experiencing injuries also increased from 33 to 39 years during this time.[2]

Medical history (limited) was available in 40% of the fatality cases, and the most frequently reported medical conditions were heart disease and high blood pressure. Most of the fatalities in the DAN Report had open water or advanced certification, and 25% had been certified 10 years or greater, whereas 45% had 1 year or less.[2] This report does not specify the dive frequency among the fatalities. The most common cause of death in the judgment of the DAN pathologist reviewing each case was drowning, whereas the next most common causes were an acute heart condition or an arterial gas embolism. The cause of death was not determined in 10% of the cases, either because the body was not found or the cause was not identified by the local medical examiner.

DECOMPRESSION SICKNESS

Decompression sickness occurs when inert gas comes out of solution, forming bubbles following the reduction of surrounding pressure (decompression). This commonly occurs with breathing compressed air while diving. As the diver descends and is exposed to elevated environmental pressure, increased amounts of inert gas dissolve in the tissues. This is in accordance with Henry's law, which states that the

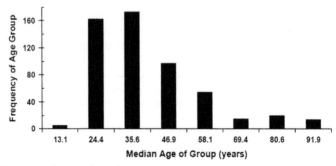

Fig. 2. Median age of group (years).

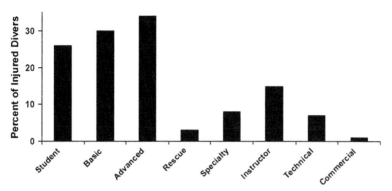

Fig. 3. Certification level of injured divers.

amount of gas dissolved in a fluid is directly proportional to the partial pressure of that gas. The amount of inert gas dissolved depends on the depth and the duration of the dive. If the diver ascends too quickly, the inert gas taken up during the dive exceeds solubility at the reduced pressure, and leads to bubble formation in tissues and in venous blood. The extent of bubble formation depends on the depth and duration of the dive and the rate of the ascent.

The likelihood of decompression sickness is related to the extent of bubble formation. A few bubbles coming out of solution may cause only minor symptoms; however, a large bubble load may result in multisystem failure and death. There are two general types of decompression sickness, Type I and Type II. Small gas loads typically cause Type I decompression sickness, which is characterized by pain in the joints and limbs and itching in the skin (niggles). Decompression sickness Type II is serious, and is characterized by neurologic problems such as weakness or paralysis, limb paresthesias, disturbance of vision, bowel and bladder dysfunction, and vertigo. Most often, the target organ is the spinal cord, usually the thoracic level. The thoracic level is probably targeted because of the vascular anatomy of the spinal cord. The

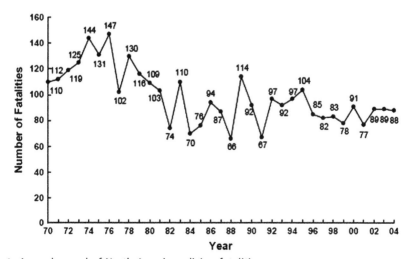

Fig. 4. Annual record of North American diving fatalities.

paravertebral veins (Batson's plexus) allows for bubbles to collect because of stagnant flow resulting in venous infarction in the spinal cord. Cerebral involvement occurs in 30% of the cases of Type II decompression sickness. Divers who have cerebral involvement may complain of confusion, lethargy, mental cloudiness, difficulty with concentration, visual disturbances and dysphagia. Symptoms typically begin within an hour of surfacing, but may be delayed for several hours. An earlier symptom onset may indicate a greater bubble load and a worse prognosis.

The diagnosis of decompression illness is based on the clinical examination, including the neurologic examination, and the dive history. Laboratory and imaging studies sometimes add to the diagnosis. In 2004 Freiberger[3] identified important diagnostic factors using simulated diving injury cases. The top five diagnostic factors in order of importance were: (1) a neurologic symptom as the primary presenting symptom, (2) onset time to symptoms, (3) joint pain as a presenting symptom, (4) any relief after recompression treatment, and (5) maximum depth of the last dive.[3] Age, gender, or physical characteristics were not statistically important.[3]

DECOMPRESSION SICKNESS: CASE ONE

A 32-year-old sport diver with several years experience was in the fifth day of a diving vacation trip to the South Pacific. On each of the previous days, he had made two or three dives, and at least one dive each day had exceeded 100 feet. He was using a decompression computer and was quite sure that he had stayed within the parameters required by the computer throughout his trip. On the fifth day, he made one dive to 150 feet and three dives to 90 feet, each separated by surface intervals that met the requirements of his computer. About 5 minutes after surfacing from his third 90-foot dive, as he was sitting on the bench, he had an aching, pressurelike pain around his flanks and into his groin. The right side was somewhat worse than the left, but as the pain became more intense, both sides were equally affected. A few minutes later, he got to his feet and was unable to walk without assistance. His companions and the boat captain helped him to the bench, where he lay down and was treated with oxygen. Symptoms did not improve. Arrangements were made to evacuate him to a recompression chamber on an island several hundred miles distant. The flight was delayed by darkness. When he arrived at the chamber the next day, about 10 hours after onset, he had moderate weakness in both thighs and virtually no strength in his left foot and lower leg, with his right foot less affected. He had altered sensation and patchy loss of sensation from the umbilicus downward, although he could feel pressure in his feet. He was unable to void without pressing on his abdomen. On urinary catheterization, he had 1500 mL residual urine. Reflexes were hyperactive.

He was treated according to US Navy Table 6. He made some improvement during the first 2 hours and treatment was extended to a full 10 hours. At the conclusion of treatment, his quadriceps and thigh strength had largely returned; his left foot was still nearly flaccid, but his right was only slightly weak. Sensation was improved, and pain resolved. The indwelling catheter was removed on the second day, and he was able to void with a Crede maneuver.

He was retreated on Table 5 (shorter oxygen table) for each of the following 3 days. He made no further improvement after the first treatment.

A week after completion of treatment, he returned to the United States by commercial aircraft. There was no change in his symptoms. In the ensuing year, he reported slow improvement in his mobility and in bladder control. One year after the event, he had persistent spastic paraparesis. He was able to ambulate without a cane or crutches, but with moderate discernable weakness and bilateral hyperreflexia. Sensation about the perineum was decreased and was nearly normal in the feet.

This case typifies serious decompression sickness with delayed treatment and with partial response. Although this patient was diving "within the rules," he had accumulated a large gas load.[4]

DECOMPRESSION SICKNESS: CASE TWO

A 46-year-old woman, an experienced diver, surfaced after an uneventful dive to 110 feet for 27 minutes, conservatively decompressing for 13 minutes at 10 feet (only 7 minutes normally required). On climbing into the boat, about 10 minutes after the dive, her right foot felt hot, then tingly (as if it were going to sleep); the limb became progressively numb from foot to thigh over 20 minutes while the left leg also became warm and tingly, and she had low back pain. Reaching the shore after 30 minutes, she could not walk. She recovered sensation and strength while breathing pure oxygen for 60 minutes. For several days, her left leg felt strange, and there was some loss of feeling in the left foot, but she felt normal after 1 week. This is a representation of a typical case of mild decompression sickness.[5]

ARTERIAL GAS EMBOLISM

Arterial gas embolism occurs when a diver breathing compressed air at depth ascends without exhaling air from the lungs. This occurs as a consequence of Boyle's law, which states that the product of pressure times volume is constant, or as pressure decreases, volume increases and the alveoli rupture as a consequence of pulmonary overinflation.

When aveoli rupture, air escapes or dissects into the surrounding spaces. Air entering the pleural cavity results in pneumothorax; air escaping into the mediastinum causes subcutaneous or mediastinal emphysema or air dissecting into the pericardium causes pneumopericardium. More dangerous yet, air may enter the pulmonary capillaries, reaching the pulmonary vein in the left heart, and be pumped into the arterial circulation. Emboli that enter the cerebral vessels cause strokelike events that typically occur within minutes of surfacing.

Patients experiencing arterial gas embolism or pulmonary over-inflation will experience pain and respiratory distress, coughing, hemoptysis, headache, unconsciousness, seizures, hemiparesis, quadriparesis, and cortical blindness. The mortality rate is high and immediate treatment is essential.

Pulmonary overpressure accidents occur most commonly in inexperienced divers. Inexperienced divers may simply forget to exhale during ascent. More commonly, this may occur during an emergency ascent, perhaps from an out-of-air situation or equipment failure.

Similar to making the diagnosis of decompression sickness, the diagnosis of arterial gas embolism is entirely based on clinical findings. The top five diagnostic factors for arterial gas embolism cited by Freiberger and colleagues[3] are: (1) the onset time of symptoms, (2) altered consciousness, (3) any neurologic symptoms as a presenting symptom, (4) motor weakness, and (5) seizure as the primary presenting symptom.[3] The National Institute of Health Stroke Scale (NIHSS), when applied to cerebral neurologic diving injuries, is a tool for severity stratification and has adequate predictive ability while providing a more standardized scale.[6]

ARTERIAL GAS EMBOLISM: CASE STUDY

A 28-year-old man made a certification dive in a fresh water lake as part of a primary scuba course. The students were performing an emergency drill in which they made a free ascent from 30 feet, simulating an out-of-air situation. They were instructed to take a full breath and then swim to the surface while exhaling constantly.

He reached the surface, had a generalized convulsion, and lost consciousness. He was towed to shore by his companions and carried to the truck. Oxygen was not available and the patient was transported about 60 miles in the back of a pick-up truck to an emergency medical facility. During this transit, he was conscious, but stuporous and uncommunicative. The emergency department physician found that he had a right hemiparesis and was aphasic, and recommended the likelihood of arterial gas embolism. The patient was treated with oxygen and transported by helicopter to a recompression chamber 200 miles away. Dysphagia and hemiparesis persisted. He was treated in a monoplace oxygen chamber for 90 minutes, at a depth equivalent to 50 feet of sea water. Directly after he was removed from the chamber, he had a generalized and largely right-sided seizure. Oxygen treatment was continued and he was not recompressed. Over the next several hours, the hemiparesis improved and he began to utter simple words. Oxygen was continued. The next morning, he had a minimal persisting hemiparesis and a moderate aphagia. He was discharged after 3 days, substantially improved, but with minimum persisting findings. Two months after the event, his hemiparesis was no longer apparent, his speech had improved to normal, and he was functioning at near his normal level.

This case typifies the sudden onset of a cerebral event in arterial gas embolism. It also illustrates the usually good prognosis in patients who survive the initial insult.[4]

PREVENTION OF DYSBARIC ILLNESS

Divers attempt to protect themselves from decompression sickness by adherence to diving tables. Diving tables were designed by the US Navy and other agencies based on theoretical and empirical data. The tables were created from the theoretical picture of the body consisting of different tissues that accept and relieve gas at different rates, and the decompression tables are designed to allow the diver to surface at a rate compatible with the slowest tissue for the depth and duration of the dive.[7] The tables are not perfect. The US Navy reports incidence of "the bends" of approximately 0.5% with strict adherence to the tables.[7] Adherence to the diving tables can be challenging because the diver has no communication with the surface and must keep track of depth and time at the bottom. Decompression computers are used by many divers and provide real-time simulation of body uptake of inert gas.

Several medical illnesses increase the risk of decompression sickness and arterial gas embolism in the diver. The most common is pulmonary dysfunction, including obstructive pulmonary disease, particularly asthma, which is a relatively absolute contraindication to diving.[8] Individuals who have pulmonary dysfunction should be evaluated by a physician. Several neurologic diseases such as migraine, in particular complicated migraine, epilepsy, muscle dystrophy, multiple sclerosis, and spinal disease can increase the risk of dysbaric illness. These should be discussed with a physician knowledgeable with the challenges of diving to assess the risk.

It is generally accepted that inert gas bubbles in the tissue and venous system cause decompression sickness, and the greater the bubble load, the higher the risk of developing decompression sickness. Research has attempted to identify ways to decrease the bubble formation in diving. Duplessis and colleagues evaluated prophylactic Atorvastatin in 16 trained military divers, but this failed to reduce the number of intravascular bubbles observed following a dry chamber dive.[9] Exercise, both pre- and post-dive, has been studied as a possible means of decreasing inert gas load and bubble formation. Dujic and colleagues studied strenuous exercise after an open sea dive in seven male military divers, and their results suggest that post-dive strenuous exercise reduces post-dive gas bubble formation in well-trained military divers.[10] The current practice is to avoid strenuous exercise after diving because its effect on bubble formation remains controversial. Pre-dive exercise was found to significantly reduce the number of bubbles in the right heart and to protect divers from decompression sickness.[11] In another study, short-acting exogenous nitric oxide before a dive was found to reduce bubble formation.[12] The use of alcohol increases the risk of dysbaric illness in divers because it adversely effects judgment, making adherence to diving tables more difficult.

TREATMENT OF DYSBARIC ILLNESS

Scuba divers breathing from a compressed air source are subject to trauma, hypothermia, asphyxiation, and water aspiration, but may also have decompression sickness or arterial gas embolism. The neurologic outcome of dysbaric illness is greatly influenced by effective early management. Typically, the diagnosis must be suspected and made in the field by a companion or dive supervisor.

Prompt recognition within the diving party is essential to begin on-site treatment. Development of pulmonary or cerebral symptoms on reaching the surface or immediately after leaving the water suggests pulmonary over-pressure injury. If cerebral symptoms such as convulsion, cortical blindness, hemiplegia, or aphasia are present, air embolism must be assumed. Symptoms delayed minutes to hours after surfacing and localizing to the spinal cord implicate decompression sickness. Prompt recompression treatment is necessary in all cases.

Once the presumptive diagnosis of dysbaric illness is established, the most important on-site treatment is administration of 100% oxygen. Most sport dive boats do carry oxygen, and ideally a close-fitting mask and reservoir that will provide high fraction of inspired oxygen and a large oxygen supply to allow for treatment until the patient is delivered to a recompression chamber.

The purpose of oxygen is to increase the rate of nitrogen removal. The damaging lesion is nitrogen bubbles within the tissue; it interrupts blood flow and damages neural structures. The basis of oxygen treatment for dysbaric illness was termed "the oxygen window" by Behnke and Shaw, which describes the changing pressure of nitrogen in the alveoli.[7] The administration of 100% oxygen creates a nitrogen gradient that tends to eliminate nitrogen bubbles from tissue. At the surface, the nitrogen bubbles have a calculated pressure of 633 torr and the alveoli air has a pressure of approximately 573 torr, making the off-gassing gradient 60 torr.[7] When the patient breathes pure oxygen, the alveolar nitrogen pressure becomes 0 torr and the gradient is then 633 torr, creating a tremendous treatment advantage, "the oxygen window." This is the critical part of treatment of both decompression sickness and arterial gas embolism. An even greater advantage is achieved by breathing oxygen under pressure.

In the field, the next crucial step is timely transportation to a recompression chamber. This can be exceedingly difficult because diving injuries occur off-shore, frequently at significant distances from emergency medical treatment and recompression facilities. An evacuation plan and communication are essential for a successful emergency evacuation. Air evacuation, when possible, must be done at low altitude, because ascent from sea level further complicates dysbaric illness.

Nitrogen bubbles within tissues and occluding vessels cause ischemia and space-occupying lesions. Bubble volume decreases as absolute pressure increases in accordance with Boyle's law. If pressure is doubled, bubble volume is reduced by half and allows bubbles in vessels to pass downstream, thus reducing the area of ischemia and in other tissues decreasing the space-occupying lesions. The ambient pressure is increased by recompression in a chamber, but there are limits to the use of pressure. Enormous pressures are required to redissolve the nitrogen bubble; however, greater pressure increases allow further absorption of nitrogen, thus 6 atmospheres (165 feet) is the maximum conventional treatment depth.[7,8]

Decompression commonly follows the treatment schedules established by the US Navy in the late 1960s.[7,8,13] The diver is recompressed to 60 feet and breathes pure oxygen, interrupted with air breaks, for 90 minutes. Air breaks are necessary to prevent oxygen toxicity, which can cause pulmonary irritation and loss of compliance. After 90 minutes, the pressure is decreased to 30 feet over a period of 30 minutes, and the diver continues oxygen breathing for 2 additional hours. Finally, the diver ascends to the surface at one foot a minute while still breathing oxygen. The total treatment time is 4 hours and 45 minutes. Treatment schedules may be extended if diver improvement is less than complete. Treatment can be extended to 12 to 13 hours if necessary.

Cianci and Slade[13] present an alternative treatment table more suitable for monoplace chambers that was found to be effective in the treatment of decompression sickness. The use of short oxygen treatment tables, as originally described by Hart and Kindwall, were effective in the treatment of decompression sickness even with long delays to definitive recompression.[13] Bennett and colleagues[14] showed that the addition of an NSAID or the use of heliox (helium and oxygen) was found to reduce the number of recompressions required, but neither improved the odds of recovery.

DIAGNOSTIC STUDIES

The diagnosis of decompression illness is entirely based on clinical findings, because there is no objective "gold standard." The history, especially the details of the dive, assists in understanding the injury; however, in many cases the dive history is innocent. No laboratory test exists that can confirm or reject the diagnosis of decompression illness, and tests rarely assist in guiding treatment.

Divers do develop dysbaric illness in spite of diving responsibly.[6] One possible etiology in these individuals is a patent foramen ovale (PFO) resulting in bubble passage from the right to left side of the heart.[15] When this occurs the bubbles can be arterialized. Divers who have PFO have an increased risk of paradoxical brain embolization. Honek and colleagues[16] examined 28 scuba divers, 15 of whom had decompression sickness associated with the ascent. PFO was diagnosed in 53% of the 15 divers by transesophageal echocardiogram. Among asymptomatic divers, PFO was found in only 8%. The authors concluded that PFO detection is clinically useful after repeated decompression sickness and in all frequent divers and instructors.[16] Transesophageal echocardiogram is the gold standard.

Neuropsychological testing has been studied in commercial and recreational divers with conflicting results, but generally adds little to the clinical examination.[8] Neuroimaging such as CT scanning is not always sensitive enough to detect structural abnormalities associated with cerebral decompression sickness or arterial gas embolism. MRI may be helpful in the diagnosis of decompression sickness in the spinal cord. In a small series, 4 out of 5 patients who had clinical spinal cord decompression sickness had high-intensity lesions in the spinal cord on MRI.[17] In the same series, there were 15 patients who had clinical cerebral decompression sickness, but MRI failed to identify cerebral lesions in any of the patients,[17] even though it can demonstrate cerebral events in some cases. Cerebral profusion studies (SPECT-HMPAO) have not been found to be helpful in the diagnosis of dysbaric illness.[8]

In the setting of dysbaric illness, electroencephalogram (EEG) demonstrates nonspecific abnormalities in some divers.[17] EEG demonstrated nonspecific abnormalities in only one third of the cases.[17] The value of electronystagmography and evoked potential studies is limited.

LONG-TERM NEUROLOGIC CONSEQUENCES OF DYSBARIC ILLNESS

Fortunately, most deep sea divers are young and healthy, and if treated promptly, ideally in the field, achieve a complete recovery from dysbaric illness. In contrast, when there are long delays to treatment or negligent diving profiles, outcomes may not be as good, as supported by the 2005 Divers Alert Network Report, in which only 70% of the divers obtained complete relief at discharge and 29.7% had residual symptoms.[18]

The residual symptoms and signs may be obvious and debilitating, such as spasticity, urinary incontinence, or weakness, or may be mild, such as peripheral paresthesias.

Similarly, divers who survive arterial gas embolism typically make a full recovery. The youth of the divers and the presence of a healthy circulatory and neurologic symptom likely contribute to their favorable prognosis. The most common residual symptoms reported by divers after arterial gas embolism are difficulties in short-term memory and concentration.[8]

The question of cumulative neurologic damage from asymptomatic diving is less clear. A multivariant analysis demonstrated that divers had significantly more neurologic symptoms and signs than non-divers,[19] with the divers more likely to complain of difficulties with concentration and long- and short-term memory. The most prominent abnormal finding was distal spinal cord and nerve root dysfunction.[19] The occurence of symptoms and abnormal findings was higher in divers who have had a previous recognized decompression sickness episode.

REFERENCES

1. Denoble PJ, Uguccioni D, Forbes R, et al. The incidence of decompression illness in recreational divers is not homogenous. Undersea Hyperb Med 2003;30(3):208.
2. Vann R, Denoble P, Uguccioni D, et al. DAN report on decompression illness, diving fatalities and project dive exploration. 2006 edition. Durham (NC): Divers Alert Network; 2006.
3. Freiberger JJ, Lyman SJ, Denoble PJ, et al. Consensus factors used by experts in the diagnosis of decompression illness. Aviat Space Environ Med 2004;75(12): 1023–8.
4. Greer HD, Massey EW. Neurological injury from undersea diving. In: Evans RW, editor. Neurology and trauma. Philadelphia: W.B. Saunders Company; 1996. p. 529–39.
5. Dick APK, Massey EW. Neurologic presentation of decompression sickness and air embolism in sport divers. Neurology 1985;35(5):667–71.
6. Holck P, Hunter RW. NIHSS applied to cerebral neurological dive injuries as a tool for dive injuries severity stratification. Undersea Hyperb Med 2006;33(4):271–80.
7. Greer HD. Neurologic complications of scuba diving and water sports. In: Jordan BD, Tsairis P, Warren RF, editors. Sports neurology. Rockville (MD): Aspen Publishes, Inc; 1989. p. 279–90.

8. Massey EW. Neurological injury from undersea diving. In: Evans RW, editor. Neurology and trauma. 2nd edition. Oxford (NY): Oxford University Press; 2006. p. 549–58.

9. Duplessis CA, Fothergill D, Schwuller D, et al. Prophylactic statins as a possible method to decrease bubble formation in diving. Aviat Space Environ Med 2007; 78(4):430–4.

10. Dujic Z, Obad A, Palada I, et al. Venous bubble count declines during strenuous exercise after an open sea dive to 30 meters. Aviat Space Environ Med 2006; 77(6):592–6.

11. Blatteau JE, Boussuges A, Gempp E, et al. Hemodynamic changes induced by submaximal exercise before a dive and its consequences on bubble formation. Br J Sports Med 2007;41:375–9.

12. Dujic Z, Palada I, Valic Z, et al. Exogenous nitric oxide and bubble formation in divers. Med Sci Sports Exerc 2006;38(8):1432–5.

13. Cianci P, Slade JB Jr. Delayed treatment of decompression sickness with shunt, no-air-break tables: review of 140 cases. Aviat Space Environ Med 2006;77(10): 1003–8.

14. Bennett MH, Lehm JP, Mitchell SJ, et al. Recompression and adjunctive therapy for decompression illness. Cochrane Database of Systemic Reviews 2007;(2). Art. No.:CD005277.

15. Moon RE, Camporesi EM, Kisslo JA. Patent foramen ovale and decompression illness in divers. Lancet 1989;1:513–4.

16. Honek T, Veselka J, Tomek A, et al. Paradoxical embolization and patent foramen ovale in scuba divers: screening possibilities. Vnitr Lek 2007;53(2):143–6.

17. Gronning M, Risberg J, Skeidsvoll H, et al. Electroencephalography and magnetic resonance imaging in neurological decompression illness. Undersea Hyperb Med 2005;32(6):397–402.

18. Vann R, Denoble P, Uguccioni D, et al. DAN report on decompression illness, diving fatalities and project dive exploration. 2005 edition. Durham (NC): Divers Alert Network; 2005. p. 63–5.

19. Todnem K, Nyland H, Kambeetad BK, et al. Influence of occupational diving upon the nervous system: epidemiological study. Br J Ind Med 1990;47(10):708–14.

Neurologic Disorders Associated with Weight Lifting and Bodybuilding

Kevin Busche, BSc, MD, FRCPC Neurology[a,b]

KEYWORDS

- Weightlifting • Bodybuilding • Nerve entrapment

Weight lifting and other forms of strength training are becoming more universal because of an increased awareness of the need to maintain individual physical fitness. Emergency room data indicate that injuries caused by weight training have become more common over time, likely because of increased participation rates.[1] Neurological injuries can result from lifting and related practices. Although predominantly peripheral nervous system (PNS) injuries have been described, central nervous system (CNS) disease may also occur. This article illustrates the type of neurologic disorders associated with weight lifting.

WEIGHT TRAINING

Training completed by overcoming resistance is called "resistance training." Weight training is a method of resistance training in which a load (in the form of free weights or a weight stack on a machine) is pushed or pulled as a form of resistance.[2] Weight training can be used as a component of a general fitness program or as part of overall training in order to improve an individual's capability for sports performance or to satisfy overall fitness goals.

Power lifting is a specific sport in which three lifts are executed: the squat, bench press, and deadlift. Weight lifting (also known as Olympic lifting) is a separate sport in which the lifts performed include the snatch and the clean and jerk.[2] Bodybuilding is a performance competition emphasizing an appearance of extreme muscular

---

This article originally appeared in *Neurologic Clinics*, Volume 26, Issue 1.

Division of Neurology, Department of Clinical Neurosciences, Faculty of Medicine, University of Calgary Health Sciences Center, 3330 Hospital Drive NW, Calgary, Alberta, Canada T2N 4N1.

[a] Division of Neurology, Department of Clinical Neurosciences, Faculty of Medicine, University of Calgary Health Sciences Center, 3330 Hospital Drive NW, Calgary, Alberta, Canada T2N 4N1

[b] Division of Neurology, Calgary Health Region, Rockyview General Hospital, 7007 14th Street SW, Calgary, Alberta, Canada T2V 1P9

E-mail address: kdbusche@ucalgary.ca

Phys Med Rehabil Clin N Am 20 (2009) 273–286

doi:10.1016/j.pmr.2008.10.017

1047-9651/08/$ – see front matter © 2009 Elsevier Inc. All rights reserved.

hypertrophy achieved by weight training. In the vernacular, "weight lifting" is often used interchangeably with "weight training," and will be used as such in this article.

Nervous system injury can occur in relation to the process of weight lifting or through drugs such as anabolic steroids or growth hormone used to enhance the effectiveness of training. Nervous system injury can result from the injection, the physiologic effects of the substances used, or the resultant muscular hypertrophy as a contributor to injury. The use of these drugs and other supplements, both legal and illegal, is reported to be common and increasing.[3–5]

PERIPHERAL NERVOUS SYSTEM

An excellent, recent review of peripheral nerve injury in weight lifters and bodybuilders incorporating all aspects of diagnosis, pathophysiology and treatment has recently been published.[6]

Peripheral nerve injuries are relatively uncommon in cohort studies that examine types of injury associated with sporting activities, with an estimate that peripheral nerve injuries account for perhaps 0.5% of all injuries associated with athletic endeavors.[7] When specifically related to injuries caused by weight training, the percentages of injuries in studies of 71 power lifters and 354 high-school football players that involved nerve injury were 3.1% and 3.7%, respectively.[8]

Chronic damage to the PNS caused by weight training may occur secondary to prolonged compression or traction of nerves, caused either by the positions and movements required while weight lifting or by the resultant muscular hypertrophy or soft tissue injury. Chronic PNS injury of this type is more common than acute injury, which appears to be rare. Chronic or acute compressive injury often produces a combination of focal segmental demyelination and focal axonal injury.[6,9]

In two case series examining nerve injury in athletes in a single EMG laboratory, the percentages of confirmed PNS injuries caused by weight lifting were only 16% and 15%, respectively.[10,11] Several other nerve injuries in athletes from other sports, however, were felt to be related to weight training undertaken for these sports, suggesting that this may be an underestimation.

Distinguishing nerve injuries from more common soft tissue injuries is important in considering the need for investigations, determining prognosis, and assessing the need for aggressive or operative management. Clinical diagnosis can be supplemented by nerve conduction studies and electromyography. In the vast majority of cases cited in the literature, avoidance of the provoking activity (thereby removing the injurious stimulus) and rest usually achieve significant if not complete recovery. This speaks to the nature of the injury, which is usually caused by chronic compression, without nerve laceration or transection.

MEDIAN NERVE

Median nerve entrapment at the wrist, referred to as carpal tunnel syndrome (CTS), is the most common entrapment neuropathy seen in the general population.[12,13] Typical symptoms include numbness, tingling, and pain in a median nerve distribution. A nocturnal predominance to episodic symptoms is characteristic. Weakness and wasting in median innervated hand muscles can be seen in more severe cases.

The nerve injury occurs as a consequence of chronic, repeated mechanical compression that results from a combination of positioning with wrist flexion and external factors, including local soft tissue edema and hypertrophy.[12–14] Repetitive, forceful, muscular activity of the hand and wrist is also seen as a contributing factor to the development of CTS.[13,14] As such, weight training involving the upper extremities can be considered a risk factor for the development of CTS.[15]

In one study of athletes who had peripheral nerve injuries on EMG, the majority of cases of CTS were seen in weight lifters.[16] In a series of athletes assessed with electrodiagnostic studies, median nerve injuries were seen in 28 of 190 sports-related nerve injuries.[10] Of these, 24 were cases of CTS, 6 symptomatic and 18 asymptomatic. Three of the symptomatic cases occurred in athletes identified as weight lifters; in the others, identified as wrestlers or football players, weight training was included as regular part of their training regimen.

A case series of pediatric patients who had CTS was reported that included 13 male patients who frequently participated in weight training,[17] suggesting that this may have been associated with the development of the condition, because the rate of CTS is generally low in children.

Case reports have described competitive bodybuilders who developed bilateral carpal tunnel syndrome while using recombinant human growth hormone to enhance muscular hypertrophy achieved by weight training, a not uncommon practice among competitive bodybuilders.[18,19] In one case, the bilateral CTS was accompanied by bilateral ulnar neuropathies.[19] It is thought that this is similar to the pathophysiology seen in acromegalics, with soft tissue hypertrophy secondary to elevated systemic levels of growth hormone.

Acute, self-limiting CTS was also described in a bodybuilder who underwent a "body sculpting" procedure with tumescent liposuction, where fluid is injected into the subcutaneous fat to aid in fat removal. It is felt that fluid redistribution may have occurred, leading to swelling within the carpal tunnel to produce this acute, temporary nerve compression.[20]

Treatment modalities for CTS include splinting, local steroid injections, and carpal tunnel release surgery.[12–14]

More proximal median neuropathies, pronator syndrome (PS) and anterior interosseous neuropathy (AIN), can be seen in the elbow and forearm region. Although most athletic median nerve injuries are found at the elbow,[9] few are specifically described in association with weight lifting. PS, with proximal median nerve compression at the elbow, generally presents with activity-provoked, deep, proximal, volar, forearm pain. This may be associated with parathesiae in a median nerve distribution. AIN classically presents with proximal, volar forearm pain worsened by exercise involving the affected limb. Weakness of the flexor digitorum profundus and flexor pollicis longus muscles lead to the inability to completely flex the distal phalanges of the index finger and thumb. Both PS[21] and AIN[9,22] are reported to be associated with weight lifting, in which repetitive forceful gripping and pronation are required. Muscular hypertrophy in the forearm is considered a risk factor for these conditions. There is a single reported case of AIN that initiated during weight training,[23] although no details were provided as to the presence or absence of muscular hypertrophy in this particular patient.

ULNAR NERVE

The ulnar nerve is most commonly injured at the cubital tunnel or ulnar groove at the elbow and within Guyon's canal at the wrist. Both sites of injury are seen in weight lifters and bodybuilders.[5]

Ulnar neuropathy at the elbow is a common condition in the general population. The injury occurs secondary to a combination of direct compression of the ulnar nerve (caused by resting the elbow on hard surfaces) and tension of the ulnar nerve around the elbow caused by prolonged flexion of the elbow joint.[13] This is also true in athletes.[24] Symptoms of ulnar neuropathy typically include numbness and tingling in the medial aspect of the hand—potentially involving both the volar and dorsal surfaces—as well as in the medial one-and-a-half digits. Symptoms often have a nocturnal predominance. Weakness and wasting of ulnar innervated hand muscles can develop in more severe entrapment of the ulnar nerve.

Weight lifting occasionally be causative for at the elbow,[9] because many exercises completed in the gym may involve resting the elbow on a firm or partially padded surface to minimize use of other muscles, such as when doing bicep exercises.[11] It is also noted that muscular hypertrophy of the medial head of the triceps or the flexor carpi ulnaris can lead to acquired compressive ulnar neuropathy.[11,25] Such hypertrophy is not uncommon in weight lifters and bodybuilders. A surgically treated case of ulnar neuropathy at the elbow in a competitive weight lifter allowed for direct visualization of compression of the ulnar nerve between the heads of the flexor carpi ulnaris.[26]

Specific case reports or case series of ulnar neuropathy at the elbow directly related to bodybuilding and weight lifting are few in the medical literature, perhaps because this is a common condition in the general population, and although cases may be related to activities of weight training, the underlying problem is one of tension and compression of the ulnar nerve at the elbow, and therefore is considered unremarkable.

Bilateral ulnar neuropathies at the elbows were described as part of a multi-entrapment syndrome in a bodybuilder using growth hormone to supplement his strength training.[19] The pathophysiology was proposed to be increased soft tissue swelling caused by the growth hormone combined with the repetitive activities while lifting weights.

Snapping of the medial head of the triceps over the medial epicondyle at the elbow is not uncommon, and can occur in susceptible individuals with either extension or flexion of the elbow. This is associated with displacement of the ulnar nerve, potentially causing nerve injury. A case series of 17 patients who had recurrent displacement of the medial head of the triceps included a description of 9 patients who had symptoms (one bilateral) attributable to ulnar neuropathy.[27] It was noted by the study authors that weight lifting activities, particularly those with resisted flexion at the elbow past 90° or resisted extension, may produce triceps snapping. It was further noted that several of the symptomatic patients had first noted symptoms only after beginning extensive weight training, suggesting that relative hypertrophy of the triceps may also be a contributor to this condition. A further 2 patients were subsequently described by the same author with a similar presentation after initiating weight lifting.[28]

There is a single case report that described rupture of the tendon of the triceps in a power lifter, with subsequent hematoma formation causing acute compression of the ulnar nerve.[29] Although other cases of triceps tendon rupture have been published, no other reports describe such secondary ulnar nerve injury.

Ulnar nerve injury at the wrist is less common than ulnar neuropathy at the elbow. With a distal ulnar neuropathy, various combinations of injury to the distal motor and sensory branches can occur, depending on the exact site of the nerve injury in Guyon's canal.

Ulnar neuropathy at the wrist can be provoked by strength training exercises that involve lifting weights with the hands, because direct compression on Guyon's canal can result. Several patients have been diagnosed with such, thought to be related to gripping barbells in an improper fashion, thereby increasing the pressure applied over Guyon's canal to produce nerve injury.[30] This is also reported as having been seen in one of 180 nerve injuries demonstrated on EMG in a case series looking at nerve injuries sustained in various athletic endeavors.[11] In a patient who underwent serial electrodiagnostic testing,[31] multiple repetitions of exercises with weights held across the lower to mid palm induced direction compression of Guyon's canal, leading to conduction block in the ulnar nerve at the wrist that improved with cessation of exercise.

Similar ulnar nerve entrapment has also been described in a patient undertaking a regimen of push-ups on a hard surface;[32] EMG demonstrated isolated injury to the first dorsal interosseous muscle of the affected hand. Symptoms resolved over 3 months with cessation of the excessive push-ups.

RADIAL NERVE

Proximal radial neuropathy can occur because of weight lifting,[9] although actual reports are rare.[7] Patients who have proximal radial nerve injury typically present with weakness of wrist and finger extension and sensory alteration over the lateral dorsal aspect of the hand. Proximal radial neuropathy may also cause weakness in supination and elbow. More proximal injury of the radial nerve may lead to weakness of the triceps and altered sensation of the posterior upper arm.

A 45-year-old elite bodybuilder presented with a gradual-onset wrist drop over 2 weeks,[33] without provoking trauma. Clinical and electrophysiologic evaluation showed a severe, axonal radial nerve lesion at the level of the spiral groove, and surgical exploration revealed compression by a markedly hypertrophied teres major. It was felt that the nerve injury was as a direct result of the patient's bodybuilding and subsequent muscular hypertrophy.

More distal involvement of the radial nerve, posterior interosseous nerve (PIN), may also be associated with weight training. Radial tunnel syndrome (RTS) has occurred in a power lifter who used anabolic steroids to boost performance.[34] Pain developed in the region of the right brachioradialis during specific exercises, and this pain could be reproduced with deep palpation over the same location. There were no motor or sensory deficits on history or examination; electrophysiologic studies were not completed. Transient relief occurred with injection, and the symptoms subsequently resolved with cessation of the excessive weight lifting. It was hypothesized that the extreme muscular hypertrophy of the supinator muscle predisposed the patient to PIN entrapment.

Radial nerve injury has also been reported as a complication of steroid injection. A recreational bodybuilder presented with sensory alteration in the territory of the left distal radial nerve and mild wrist extensor weakness following the self-injection of steroids into the left triceps, producing trauma to the radial nerve.[35]

MUSCULOCUTANEOUS NERVE

The musculotaneous nerve (MCN), an uncommon site of injury in the general population, can be injured in weight lifters. MCN injury presents as painless weakness of elbow flexion, which can be accompanied by sensory alteration in the territory of the lateral antebrachial cutaneous nerve. In two male weight lifters using anabolic steroids presenting with weakness and atrophy of the biceps, electromyograph (EMG) identified denervation in the biceps muscle.[36] This nerve injury may have resulted from either direct compression of a terminal motor branch of the MCN (related to muscular hypertrophy) or from stretching of the MCN nerve during weight training. In another small case series, two of three patients reported to have MCN injuries with EMG confirmation had a history of habitual weight lifting.[37]

Injury to the MCN has been reported in a patient who did excessive, frequent push-ups, leading to onset of progressive atrophy of the left upper arm and decrease in elbow flexion strength, with electrophysiologic studies demonstrating neurogenic changes within the biceps and brachialis consistent with injury to the MCN.[38]

SUPRASCAPULAR NERVE

The suprascapular nerve (SSN) is typically injured in volleyball players and baseball pitchers, in whom repetitive overhead motions occur, but SSN injury is also reported as a consequence of weight training.[9] The nerve can be injured at the suprascapular notch (thus affecting both the supra- and infraspinatus muscles) or at the spinoglenoid notch (affecting the infraspinatus in isolation). The latter of the two sites is more commonly seen in injury caused by weight lifting or bodybuilding.[7] In some cases, anatomic abnormalities such as ganglia are present at the suprascapular or spinoglenoid notch,[39] and the neuropathy may be related more to this than the muscular hypertrophy common to other weight lifting and bodybuilding entrapment neuropathies.

In a series of 28 patients who had EMG-documented SSN injury, 16 had symptoms related to athletic activities.[40] Of these, one was identified as a bodybuilder and another as a weight lifter. Two separate case series of peripheral nerve injuries in weight lifters each include a case of SSN.[36,41] One case occurred in a female bodybuilder who was using anabolic steroids, whereas the other was in a recreational weight lifter not taking steroids. Both presented with mild pain with SSN injury present at the level of the spinoglenoid notch, with isolated denervation in the infraspinatus muscle found during EMG.

Other weight lifting-induced injuries at the level of the suprascapular notch[39,42] have also occurred soon after an aggressive weight training program was initiated. In both cases, a suprascapular localization for SSN injury was documented by both EMG and MRI, and in one patient, surgical release of the nerve at the suprascapular notch led to a full recovery.

LONG THORACIC NERVE

Long thoracic nerve (LTN) injury leads to isolated weakness of the serratus anterior muscle and to scapular winging. This has been reported in association with weight training activities in a very small number of cases.[6] Bilateral LTN palsies have been described in a single patient undertaking a weight training program without other obvious contributing causes.[43]

MEDIAL PECTORAL NERVE

One nerve injury that appears quite specific to weight lifters and bodybuilders is medial pectoral nerve (MPN) injury. Patients present with painless weakness and significant atrophy of pectoral muscles. Electrodiagnostic studies confirm the neuropathic changes within pectoralis major. In most cases, cessation of the provoking activity (weight training) leads to either partial or complete recovery. Again, MPN injury may be caused by direct compression secondary to muscular hypertrophy.

In two reported cases there was unilateral MPN palsy with isolated clinical and EMG changes in the sternocostal head of the pectoralis major.[36,41] Both of these patients were using anabolic steroids to supplement weight training. Another case of unilateral MPN injury also included evidence of an associated thoracodorsal neuropathy, with changes seen on EMG in both the pectoralis major and the latissimus dorsi.[36]

Rossi and colleagues[44] describe a case of bilateral MPN palsy, with severe pectoral wasting beginning during intensive weight training, presumably caused by intramuscular nerve entrapment. In this case the patient denied anabolic steroid use. Also unique to this case, the patient presented approximately 2 years after the beginning of symptoms, and even with cessation of his intensive weight lifting regimen, no recovery occurred.

Finally, MPN injury may also occur secondary to a pectoralis muscle tear and hematoma sustained while bench pressing.[45]

OTHER NERVES

Case series in the literature describe other unusual mononeuropathies specifically in bodybuilders, often in association with steroid use. These cases include a single report describing injury to the dorsoscapular nerve with denervation in the rhomboids, and a case of isolated thoracodorsal nerve injury with denervation in the latissimus dorsi without medial pectoral involvement.[41]

BRACHIAL PLEXUS AND CERVICAL NERVE ROOTS

Although brachial plexus injuries are the most common nerve injury in sports such as football or wrestling[11] (so called "burners" or "stingers" possibly caused by acute traction of nerve roots or plexus, causing transient pain, parathesiae and numbness), they are quite rare in weight lifting and bodybuilding. Burners have been reported after lifting heavy weights up from the floor.[46] Krivickas and Wilbourn[10] document cervical radiculopathies and brachial plexus lesions in weight lifters, with five of the former and one of the latter in 27 patients who had documented nerve injuries on EMG. More chronic brachial plexus injury in a bodybuilder documented with careful MRI imaging[47] followed 3 years of weight training leading to excessive muscularity. The muscular hypertrophy combined with degenerative changes of the acromioclavicular joint decreased the size of the thoracic inlet leading to compression of the brachial plexus.

LOWER EXTREMITY NERVES

Lower extremity nerve injuries caused by weight lifting are less common than those of the upper extremity. Between 0% and 14% of all sport-related nerve injuries have occurred in the leg, and none of these were specifically reported to be related to weight lifting.[10,11] Data are therefore largely derived from case reports.

Femoral nerve injury has been reported in bodybuilders. In one reported case, there was unilateral involvement of a distal portion of the vastus lateralis muscle,[48] while in another, denervation changes were restricted to the vastus medialis,[36] suggesting in both cases an entrapment of a terminal branch of the femoral nerve within the muscle itself. In these cases, painless weakness and atrophy developed subacutely in bodybuilders who had considerable quadriceps hypertrophy. Direct compression and tension of the nerve was proposed, related to muscle hypertrophy and shear forces during muscle movement.

Localized femoral nerve injury has also occurred secondary to nerve trauma following steroid injection in the anterior thigh.[49] Proposed mechanisms for the nerve injury were direct compression due to the liquid or a toxic effect of the testosterone preparation.

Meralgia paresthetica, entrapment of the lateral femoral cutaneous nerve of the thigh at the level of the inguinal ligament, is often produced by low-slung belts (eg, tool belts), but can also occur with weight lifting belts.[46] These wide belts are tightly cinched around the waist by some weight lifters to increase intra-abdominal pressure, ostensibly to support the lower back during heavy lifting.

Saphenous nerve entrapment neuropathy has been reported in a single case of a competitive female bodybuilder.[50] Progressive, unilateral medial knee pain developed subacutely, and examination showed sensory impairment over the territory of the saphenous nerve. Somatosensory-evoked potentials documented saphenous nerve injury, with injury localized to the subsartorial canal. Repetitive trauma caused by aggressive weight training was hypothesized to produce the nerve injury.

Focal, unilateral lateral plantar nerve entrapment developed in a power lifter secondary to loading forces during heavy weight lifting,[51] with improvement in symptoms was occurring following the use of foot orthotics during heavy lifts. Nerve conduction studies pre- and post-orthotic use demonstrated recovery of nerve injury.

CENTRAL NERVOUS SYSTEM

The vast majority of neurological conditions associated with weight lifting and bodybuilding are injuries within the PNS. There are, however, a few recognized CNS disorders that may present in the weight lifter. These are thought to be rare, although no estimation of prevalence has been attempted.

BENIGN HEADACHE

A survey found that 35% of university athletes experienced headache associated with sports activities; weight training was the second most frequent headache-related sport after running.[52] Of those who had headache, 60% described effort-related headaches.

Three different types of benign headaches are thought to occur with relative frequency in weight lifters: benign exertional headache (BEH), cervicogenic headache, and exercise-induced migraine.[53]

BEH is recognized by the International Headache Society as a primary headache condition.[54] The headache begins during exercise, is typically bilateral, and is described as explosive or throbbing from onset. The headache may last anywhere from 5 minutes to 24 hours, and can be reliably prevented with avoidance of excessive exertion.

The pathophysiology of BEH may be related to either acute venous or arterial distention secondary to breath holding and Valsalva maneuver during exertion, particularly weight lifting. Marked elevations in both systolic and diastolic blood pressure occur during times of maximal effort in weight lifters. This may translate to the intracranial vessels.[55] Increased intrathoracic and intra-abdominal pressure during exertion may also be transmitted through the vascular system, increasing intracranial arterial and venous pressures.[56]

Several authors have described the use of indomethacin, either as acute treatment or before exercise, to be effective for BEH. Ergotamine tartrate, methysergide,[57] intravenous dihydroergotamine, and propranolol[55] have also been attempted as treatments. Other authors have suggested that a warm-up period before exercise may prevent BEH.[58]

A recognized variant of exertional headache is "weight lifter's headache".[57] It has been suggested that the pathophysiology of this headache is related to cervical ligamentous strain or stretch,[59] but, other authors feel it is more likely vascular in origin and thus a type of benign exertional headache.[57] Supporting the vascular hypothesis is a case report of a weight lifter's headache that was only brought on by doing heavy leg presses on a weight machine.[60] In this exercise there would be relatively little activation of pain sensitive cervical structures but great increases in blood pressure, making a vascular process more likely. Similarly, in a series of four patients presenting to an emergency department with benign exertional headache during weight lifting,[61] two had the onset of headache while doing leg presses or leg extensions, both unlikely to produce significant cervical stretch.

Cervicogenic headache is recognized by the International Headache Society as one of the descriptors for "headaches associated with disorders of the cervical spine".[54] Many different pain sensitive structures in the neck have been postulated as the pain generator in this condition, including joints, ligaments, periosteum, annulus fibrosis, cervical muscles, cervical nerve roots and the vertebral and carotid arteries. As noted above, Paulson[59] proposed that weight lifters headache was a cervicogenic headache, but little further support for this has emerged.

Effort-induced migraine is not always clearly differentiated from BEH in the literature.[53,55] Effort-induced migraine is more common in patients who experience episodic migraine without exercise. These headaches tend to be provoked by maximal or submaximal aerobic exercise and are therefore relatively uncommon in weight lifters. Often, the provoking factor is unclear, as weight lifters also may undertake aerobic exercise as well. These headaches, like other migraines, are often unilateral, as opposed to BEH, which are typically bilateral. There may be other migrainous features, particularly an aura.[53] Treatment is similar to that for typical migraine.

Another uncommon cause for headache in the weight lifter is low cerebrospinal fluid (CSF) pressure. This headache is typically postural (worsens when upright). This condition occurs because of a CSF leak, with a dural tear most often occurring in dural sleeves surrounding spinal nerve roots at the thoracic level.[62] In many cases minor trauma can precipitate this condition, and it has been reported in one case to have begun 2 hours following an informal weight-lifting competition.[63] Complete recovery can occur with several days of forced recumbency, permitting healing of the tiny dural tear, although in recalcitrant cases blood patches can be used therapeutically.

CENTRAL NERVOUS SYSTEM LESIONS

More sinister intracranial conditions have been associated with weight lifting. Many of these are thought to be associated with marked increases in intra-abdominal,[64] intrathoracic,[65] and intra-arterial[66] pressure during Valsalva maneuver in the midst of moving heavy weights. Intra-arterial pressure can be transmitted directly to intracranial vessels, with the increased intrathoracic pressure also increasing central venous pressure, thereby impeding venous outflow and leading to increased intracranial pressure.[67]

Subarachnoid hemorrhage (SAH) in association with weight training may be caused by increase in the aneurysmal transmural pressure secondary to increased mean arterial pressure.[67] Reported cases of intracranial aneurysmal rupture have occurred during bilateral bicep curl exercises or during bilateral leg press exercises.

SAH caused by ruptured ateriovenous malformations (AVM) is less common. A single patient has been reported as suffered spinal AVM rupture during weight lifting.[68] Vascular pressure changes during Valsalva maneuvers again appeared to increase the risk of AVM rupture.

Nontraumatic subdural hematomas (SDH) are distinctly uncommon in young patients. Two young (24- and 32-year-old) male patients were described as having developed non-traumatic SDH;[69] both had been weight lifters for several years using combinations of anabolic steroids and growth hormone. It was felt by the authors that excessive muscular hypertrophy may produce even greater pressure changes systemically during the Valsalva maneuver, predisposing weight lifters (particularly those using steroids) to the development of SDH. Other authors feel that the period of sudden relative intracranial hypotension following Valsalva cause cerebral retraction and subsequent tearing of bridging veins leading to SDH.[70]

Spinal epidural hematoma (EDH), a neurologic emergency, has occurred causing acute partial quadriplegia in a patient doing sit-up exercises while performing a Valsalva maneuver.[71] Although no underlying vascular abnormality was found, it was felt that the transmission of elevated intrathoracic and intra-abdominal pressures to the spinal epidural venous plexus led directly to the rupture.

Intracranial hemorrhage (ICH) in young, healthy individuals who have no underlying structural, vascular lesion or coagulopathy is uncommon, but may occur in the weight lifter.[72,73] In one case[72] the patient was in the midst of lifting at submaximal capacity, suggesting that the changes in systemic and intracranial pressures would be less than those seen during maximal effort and therfore the ICH may be unrelated to the weight-lifting. A second case is reported,[73] but, in this case, the 27-year-old patient had been using anabolic steroids for several years to augment weight training as a bodybuilder. He sustained a fatal right cerebellar hemorrage with subarachnoid and intraventricular extension. No underlying vascular abnormality or coagulation disorder was found to explain this unusual occurrence, and it was felt to be related to the steroid use, although the mechanism was unclear.

Hemorrhage into an acoustic neuroma during heavy weight training has also been reported.[74] Although acoustic neuromas are not uncommon (representing approximately 8% of all brain tumors), hemorrhage into these tumors is rare, with only a few cases in the literature. The thin-walled vessels in these hypervascular tumors may be susceptible to rupture when subjected to the markedly increased arterial pressures seen in weight lifting.

A middle cerebral artery territory stroke has been described with no stroke risk factors.[75] In the 6 weeks prior to his stroke, he had been consuming compounds containing the equivalent of 40 to 60 mg of ephedra alkaloids, 400 to 600 mg of caffeine, and 6000 mg of creatine monohydrate daily. Ephedrine is recognized as a sympathomimetic and vasoconstrictor, and has been associated with stroke and intracranial hemorrhage, and may have precipitated stroke, either alone or in association with the other supplements used in this case.

Stroke has also occurred in a bodybuilder who had a 4-year history of anabolic steroid use.[76] In this case, steroid use may have promoted platelet aggregation and hypercoagulability,[77,78] as no other cause for the stroke was found.

Ischemic stroke in the left posterior cerebral artery (PCA) territory has occurred in a healthy 37-year-old man while performing sit ups with Valsalva maneuver.[71] This was proposed to be due to an intracranial vascular dissection of the PCA, although no such pathology was conclusively demonstrated.

A single case of ischemic stroke occurring during weight training was attributed to Valsalva maneuver causing reversal of flow through a patent foramen ovale.[79] While the mechanism is theoretically plausible, during echocardiography the patient completed a Valsalva maneuver and yet no alteration in the degree of right to left shunt was observed.

Dural sinus thrombosis has been attributed to the use of androgens by bodybuilders.[77,78] A healthy 37-year-old man who had a 5-year history of using multiple steroids developed an acute onset of headache during a weight training session, with unilateral facial weakness and papilledema identified on later examination.[77] A second case has occurred with a healthy 22-year-old man who used anabolic steroids developing progressive headache, nausea, and vomiting. Examination showed evidence of bilateral papilledema. In both cases, neuroimaging demonstrated the presence of sagittal and transverse sinus thrombosis without another identifiable cause for hypercoagulability. Androgens can increase platelet aggregation and increase coagulation, possibly leading to dural sinus thrombosis in these cases.

SUMMARY

Both benign and sinister complications of weight training and associated practices may affect the central and peripheral nervous systems. Most of the information in the literature describing these disorders is in the form of case reports and case series, making it difficult to estimate the frequency with which they will be seen. Weight lifting is becoming more prevalent in the general population which may presage an increase in incidence of these conditions.

REFERENCES

1. Jones C, Christensen C, Young M. Weight training injury trends: a 20-year survey. Phys SportsMed 2000;28(7):61–72.
2. Stone M, Pierce K, Sands W, et al. Weight lifting: a brief overview. Strength and Conditioning Journal 2006;28(1):50–66.
3. Frankle M, Cicero C, Payne J. Use of androgenic anabolic steroids by athletes. JAMA 1984;252:484.
4. McCabe S, Brower K, West B, et al. Trends in non-medical use of anabolic steroids by U.S. college students: results from four national surveys. Drug Alcohol Depend 2007; epub ahead of print.
5. VandenBerg P, Neumark-Sztainer D, Cafri G, et al. Steroid use among adolescents: longitudinal findings from Project EAT. Pediatrics 2007;119(3):476–86.
6. Lodhia K, Brahma B, McGillicuddy J. Peripheral nerve injuries in weight training: sites, pathophysiology, diagnosis and treatment. Phys Sportsmed 2005;33(7): 24–37.
7. Lorei M, Hershman E. Peripheral nerve injuries in athletes: treatment and prevention. Sports Med 1993;16(2):130–47.
8. Mazur L, Yetman J, Risser W. Weight-training injuries: common injuries and preventative methods. Sports Med 1993;16(1):57–63.
9. Elman L, McCluskey L. Occupational and sport related traumatic neuropathy. The Neurologist 2004;10(2):82–96.
10. Krivickas L, Wilbourn A. Sports and peripheral nerve injuries: report of 190 injuries evaluated in a single electromyography laboratory. Muscle Nerve 1998; 21:1092–4.
11. Krivickas L, Wilbourn A. Peripheral nerve injuries in athletes: a case series of over 200 injuries. Semin Neurol 2000;20(2):225–32.
12. Bayromoglu M. Entrapment neuropathies of the upper extremity. Neuroanatomy 2004;3:18–24.
13. Dawson D. Entrapment neuropathies of the upper extremity. N Engl J Med 1993; 329(27):2013–8.
14. Katz J, Simmons B. Carpal tunnel syndrome. N Engl J Med 2002;346(23): 1807–12.
15. Izzi J, Dennison D, Noerdlinger M, et al. Nerve injuries of the elbow, wrist and hand in athletes. Clin Sports Med 2001;20(1):203–17.
16. Wilbourn A. Electrodiagnostic testing of neurologic injuries in athletes. Clin Sports Med 1990;9(2):229–45.
17. Berenson F, Wilbourn A. Carpal tunnel syndrome in pediatrics: frequency and etiologies. Neurology 1995;45:A348.

18. Dickerman R. Bilateral median neuropathy and growth hormone use: a case report. Arch Phys Med Rehabil 2000;81:1594–5.

19. Caliandro P, Padua L, Aprile I, et al. Adverse effects of GH self administration on peripheral nerve. J Sports Med Phys Fitness 2004;44:41–3.

20. Lombardi A, Quirke T, Rauscher G. Acute median nerve compression associated with tumescent fluid administration. Plastic Reconstr Surg 1998;102(1):235–7.

21. Behr C, Altchek D. The elbow. Clin Sports Med 1997;16(4):681–704.

22. Kim D, Murovic J, Kim Y-Y, et al. Surgical treatment and outcomes in 15 patients with anterior interosseous nerve entrapments and injuries. J Neurosurg 2006; 104(5):757–65.

23. Goulding P, Schady W. Favourable outcome in non-traumatic anterior interosseous nerve palsy. J Neurol 1993;240:83–6.

24. Glousman R. Ulnar nerve problems in the athlete's elbow. Clin Sports Med 1990; 9(2):365–77.

25. Aldrige J, Bruno R, Strauch R, et al. Nerve entrapment in athletes. Clin Sports Med 2001;20(1):95–122.

26. Dangles C, Bilos Z. Ulnar nerve neuritis in a world champion weightlifter. Am J Sports Med 1980;8(6):443–5.

27. Spinner R, Goldner R. Snapping of the medial head of the triceps and recurrent dislocation of the ulnar nerve: anatomical and dynamic factors. J Bone Joint Surg Am 1998;80:239–47.

28. Spinner R, Wenger D, Barry C, et al. Episodic snapping of the medial head of the triceps due to weight lifting. J South Orthop Assoc 1999;8(4):288–92.

29. Duchow J, Kelm J, Kohn D. Acute ulnar nerve compression syndrome in a power-lifter with triceps tendon rupture—a case report. Int J Sports Med 2000;21:308–10.

30. Haupt H. Upper extremity injuries associated with strength training. Clin Sports Med 2001;20(3):481–90.

31. Montoya L, Felice K. Recovery from distal ulnar motor conduction block injury: serial EMG studies. Muscle Nerve 2002;26:145–9.

32. Walker O, Troost BT. Push-up palmar palsy. JAMA 1988;259(1):45–6.

33. Ng A, Borhan J, Ashton H, et al. Radial nerve palsy in an elite bodybuilder. Br J Sports Med 2003;37(2):185–6.

34. Dickerman R, Stevens Q, Cohen A, et al. Radial tunnel syndrome in an elite power athlete: a case of direct compressive neuropathy. J Peripher Nerv Syst 2002;7(4): 229–32.

35. Evans N. Local complications of self administered anabolic steroid injections. Br J Sports Med 1997;31:349–50.

36. Bird S, Brown M. Acute focal neuropathy in male weight lifters. Muscle Nerve 1996;19:897–9.

37. Braddom R, Wolfe C. Musculocutaneous nerve injury after heavy exercise. Arch Phys Med Rehab 1978;59:290–3.

38. Pecina M, Bojanic I. Musculocutaneous nerve entrapment in the upper arm. Int Orthop 1993;17:232–4.

39. Zeiss J, Woldenberg L, Saddemi S, et al. MRI of suprascapular neuropathy in a weight lifter. J Comput Assist Tomogr 1993;17(2):303–8.

40. Antonadis G, Richter H, Rath S, et al. Suprascapular nerve entrapment: experience with 28 cases. J Neurosurg 1996;85(6):1020–5.

41. Mondelli M, Cioni R, Federico A. Rare mononeuropathies of the upper limb in bodybuilders. Muscle Nerve 1998;21:809–12.

42. Agre J, Ash N, Cameron M, et al. Suprascapular neuropathy after intensive progressive exercise: case report. Arch Phys Med Rehabil 1987;68(4):236–8.

43. Ebata A, Kokubun N, Miyamoto T, et al. The bilateral long thoracic nerve palsy presenting with "scapula alata" as a result of weight training. A case report. Rinsho Shinkeigaku 2005;45(4):308–11 [in Japanese].
44. Rossi F, Triggs W, Gonzalez R, et al. Bilateral medial pectoral neuropathy in a weight lifter. Muscle Nerve 1999;22:1597–9.
45. Borg-Stein J, Mostoufi S, Hirschberg R. Chronic pectoral pain following medial pectoral nerve injury: a case report. J Back Musculoskeletal Rehabil 2006; 19(1):7–11.
46. Feinberg J, Nadler S, Krivickas L. Peripheral nerve injuries in the athlete. Sports Med 1997;24(6):385–408.
47. Collins J, Shaver M, Disher A, et al. Compromising abnormalities of the brachial plexus as displayed by magnetic resonance imaging. Clin Anat 1995;8:1–16.
48. Padua L, D'Aloya E, LoMonaco M, et al. Mononeuropathy of a distal branch of the femoral nerve in a bodybuilding champion. J Neurol Neurosurg Psychiatry 1997; 63:669–71.
49. Dickerman R, Kramer E, Pertusi R, et al. Peripheral neuropathy and testosterone. Neurotoxicology 1997;18(2):587–8.
50. Dumitru D, Windsor R. Subsartorial entrapment of the saphenous nerve in a competitive bodybuilder. Phys Sportsmed 1989;17(1):116–25.
51. Johnson E, Kirby K, Leiberman J. Lateral plantar nerve entrapment: foot pain in a power lifter. Am J Sports Med 1992;20(5):619–20.
52. Williams S, Nakuda J. Sport and exercise headache: part 1. Prevalence among university students. Br J Sports Med 1994;28:90–5.
53. Rifat S, Moeller J. Diagnosis and management of headache in the weight lifting athlete. Curr Sports Med Rep 2003;2:272–5.
54. Headache Classification Committee of the International Headache Society. The international classification of headache disorders. 2nd edition. Cephalalgia 2004;24(Suppl 1):9–160.
55. McRory P. Headaches and exercise. Sports Med 2000;30(3):221–9.
56. Haykowsky M, Eves N, Warburton D, et al. Resistance exercise, the Valsalva maneuver and cerebrovascular transmural pressure. Med Sci Sports Exerc 2003;35:65–8.
57. Lance J, Goadsby P. Miscellaneous headaches unassociated with a structural lesion. In: Tfelt-Hansen P, Welch K, Olesen J, editors. The headaches. 2nd edition. Philadelphia: Lippincott Williams and Wilkins; 2000. p. 751–62.
58. Lambert R, Burnet D. Prevention of exercise induced migraine by quantitative warm up. Headache 1985;25:317–9.
59. Paulson G. Weightlifter's headache. Headache 1983;23:193–4.
60. Powell B. Weight lifter's cephalgia. Ann Emerg Med 1982;11(8):449–51.
61. Imperato J, Burstein J, Edlow J. Benign exertional headache. Ann Emerg Med 2003;42(1):98–103.
62. Vilming S, Campbell J. Low cerebrospinal fluid pressure. In: Olesen J, Tfelt-Hansen P, Welch K, editors. The headaches. 2nd edition. Philadelphia: Lippincott Williams and Wilkins; 2000. p. 831–9.
63. Knutson G. Intracranial hypotension causing headache and neck pain: a case study. J Manipulative Physiol Ther 2006;29(8):682–4.
64. McGill S, Norman R, Sharrall M. The effect of an abdominal belt on trunk muscle activity and intra-abdominal pressure during squat lifts. Ergonomics 1990;33: 147–60.
65. Lentini A, McKelvie R, McCartney N, et al. Left ventricular response in healthy young men during heavy-intensity weight-lifting exercise. J Appl Physiol 1992; 75:2703–10.

66. Compton D, Hill P, Sinclair J. Weight lifter's blackout. Lancet 1973;2:1234–7.
67. Haykowsky M, Findlay J, Ignaszewski A. Aneurysmal subarachnoid hemorrhage associated with weight training: three case reports. Clin J Sport Med 1996;6: 52–5.
68. Rosenow J, Rawanduzy A, Weitzner I, et al. Type IV spinal arteriovenous malformation. I. Association with familial pulmonary vascular malformations: case report. Neurosurgery 2000;46(5):1240–5.
69. Alaraj A, Chamoun R, Dahdaleh N, et al. Spontaneous sudural hematoma in anabolic steroids dependent weight lifters: reports of two cases and review of the literature. Acta Neurochir (Wien) 2005;147:85–8.
70. Dickerman R, Morgan J. Pathogenesis of subdural hematoma in healthy athletes: postexertional intracranial hypotension? Acta Neurochir (Wien) 2005;147:349–50.
71. Uber-Zak L, Venkatesh S. Neurologic complications of sit-ups associated with the Valsalva maneuver: 2 case reports. Arch Phys Med Rehabil 2002;83:278–82.
72. Cayen B, Cullen N. Intracerebral hemorrhage in previously healthy adults following aerobic and anaerobic exercise. Brain Inj 2002;16(5):397–405.
73. Kennedy M, Corrigan A, Pilbeam S. Myocardial infarction and cerebral hemorrhage in a young bodybuilder taking anabolic steroids. Aust NZ J Med 1993; 23:713.
74. Goetting M, Swanson S. Massive hemorrhage into intracranial neurinomas. Surg Neurol 1987;27:168–72.
75. Vahedi K, Domigo V, Amarenco P, et al. Ischaemic stroke in a sportsman who consumed MaHuang extract and creatine monohydrate for body building. J Neurol Neurosurg Psychiatry 2000;68:112–3.
76. Frankle M, Eichberg R, Zachariah S. Anabolic steroids and a stroke in an athlete: case report. Arch Phys Med Rehabil 1988;69:632–3.
77. Sahraian M, Mottamedi M, Azimi A, et al. Androgen-induced cerebral venous sinus thrombosis in a young body builder: case report. BMC Neurol;4:22.
78. Jaillard A, Hommel M, Mallaret M. Venous sinus thrombosis associated with androgens in a healthy young man. Stroke 1994;25:212–3.
79. Sweeney B, Rossor M. Medial medullary syndrome associated with patent foramen ovale in a weightlifter. Eur Neurol 1996;36:391.

Head Injuries in Winter Sports: Downhill Skiing, Snowboarding, Sledding, Snowmobiling, Ice Skating and Ice Hockey

Brian Chaze, BA[a], Patrick McDonald, MD, MHSc, FRCSC[a,b,*]

KEYWORDS

- Skiing • Snowboarding • Sledding
- Snowmobiling • Skating • Hockey • Head injury

Popular winter sports and recreational activities often combine high rates of speed with the potential for collision with other participants or large, stationary objects. Head injuries in winter sports range from seemingly inconsequential minor trauma to life-threatening intracranial pathology. Factors that appear to influence head injury incidence and severity include mechanism of injury, participant skill level, age, terrain and venue conditions, helmet use, risky behaviors, and sport-specific regulations. Prevention strategies include education and helmet use programs, legislation, and sport-specific rules. Despite efforts to increase helmet use and head injury awareness, sports such as skiing and snowboarding have not yet shown wide acceptance of helmet use. Conversely, in ice hockey, where helmet use is ubiquitous, concussion remains a common diagnosis among injured players. It is important for physicians to be aware of risk factors and types of head injuries specific to particular sports in order to anticipate, help prevent, and treat these injuries.

Injuries as a result of winter sporting activities can also bring a unique set of challenges to the treating physician, including hypothermia and difficulties related to remote and often difficult-to-access locations.

This article originally appeared in *Neurologic Clinics*, Volume 26, Issue 1.
[a] Section of Neurosurgery, University of Manitoba, GB126-820 Sherbrook Street, Winnipeg, Manitoba, Canada R3A 1R9
[b] Pediatric Neurosurgery, Winnipeg Children's Hospital, GB 126 820 Sherbrook Street, Winnipeg, Manitoba, Canada R3A 1R9
* Corresponding author. Section of Neurosurgery, University of Manitoba, GB126-820 Sherbrook Street, Winnipeg, Manitoba, Canada R3A 1R9.
E-mail address: pmcdonald@hsc.mb.ca (P. McDonald).

Phys Med Rehabil Clin N Am 20 (2009) 287–293
doi:10.1016/j.pmr.2008.10.016
1047-9651/08/$ – see front matter © 2009 Elsevier Inc. All rights reserved.

This article provides an overview of the epidemiology and treatment of injuries seen in some of the more commonly enjoyed winter sports, with a focus on the unique aspects of injuries as they relate to specific sports.

DOWNHILL SKIING

Downhill skiing is enjoyed by more than 200 million people worldwide.[1] Downhill skiers are at risk of serious head injury through falls or collisions, sometimes at high speeds, which can lead to long-term disability or death.[2,3] Head injury incidence is estimated to be in the range of 0.77 to 3.8/100,000 ski visits, with most cases involving beginner or intermediate-level enthusiasts.[2,6] Head injuries are the leading cause of death in downhill skiing accidents, with an the average age of head-injured skiers of approximately 30 years,[1,4] but traumatic brain injury is also the leading cause of downhill skiing injury fatalities in children.[5] Head injury is also the most common diagnosis among child and adolescent skiers requiring admission to hospital.[7,8] In s study of skiing related fatalities in Colorado from 1980 to2001, 42.5% of 174 deaths in that era resulted from head injury.[9]

Approximately 50% of head injuries result from falls on the slopes, whereas 42% to 47% result from collisions.[1,2] Collisions with other skiers and snowboarders account for 58% and 34% of collision-related head injuries respectively, whereas collisions with trees and lift towers account for only 4% and 3% respectively.[2] Jumping accounts for only 2.5% of head injuries among skiers.[2] The pattern of injury by head region is: occipital (31%), frontal (29%), diffuse (23%), temporal (14%), and parietal (3%).[2] Most head injuries in skiing are mild, with concussion as the most frequent diagnosis.[1] The most common organic head injury among skiers is skull fracture. Wearing a helmet has been shown to reduce the risk of head injuries in downhill skiers, even when other potential risk factors are considered.[10,11] It was once assumed that helmet use would increase the incidence of cervical spine injuries in downhill skiers, but this controversial assumption has been shown to be unlikely.[12]

Despite clear evidence that helmet use prevents or reduces the severity of injuries, use remains less than widely accepted.[13] In one study examining helmet use in child enthusiasts, only 30% of injured skiers and snowboarders wore helmets.[12] It has also been suggested that no suitable helmet exists to protect all skiers, and that helmet development should be based on injury data analysis and strict standards.[14]

There are very few published data on the risk and nature of head injury among Nordic or cross-country skiers.

SNOWBOARDING

Snowboarding is a downhill alpine sport that was initially assumed to have injury patterns similar to those of skiing, but recent studies have shown that the incidence of head and spinal injuries in snowboarding is higher than previously documented.[15] Injuries to the head and face represent 25% of all snowboarding injuries, and the rate of head and neck injury among snowboarders is one and a half to three that of skiers.[1,2,16,17] The incidence of head injury for snowboarders is estimated to be 6.5/100,000 visits, compared with 3.8/100,000 visits for skiers.[18] Head-injured snowboarders tend to be an average of 3.6 to 6.3 years younger than their skiing counterparts, and are more likely to be male.[2,4] It is speculated that higher risk-taking behavior in younger males may be responsible for higher incidences of head injury. Most head injuries occur as a result of falls on mild to moderate slopes among beginner to intermediate-level participants.[2] Jumping accounts for 30% of head injury cases among snowboarders, compared with only 2.5% of cases in skiers,[2] reflecting the differences between the two activities. Most severe head injuries have occurred on gentle or moderate slopes resulting from the "opposite edge" phenomenon, in which the edge of the snowboard facing upslope catches a ridge of snow during a turn at low speeds, causing the rider to lose balance and fall.[18] The occipital region of the head is the area most frequently affected in snowboarding head injuries, with a pattern of injury by head region being: occipital (48%), diffuse (23%), frontal (19%), temporal (9%), and parietal (1%).[2] Snowboarders suffer intracranial hemorrhage more than twice as often as skiers, and require a craniotomy nearly three times as often.[19] The reason for the difference in injury patterns in snowboarders compared with those in skiers is unclear, but may be related to the rails and jumps commonly found in snowboard parks.

The most common organic head injury among snowboarders is subdural hematoma, as opposed to skiers, who exhibit a higher frequency of skull fractures.[2] Acute subdural hematomas are related to falls on the slope, falling backward, and occipital impact, whereas subcortical hemorrhagic contusions are thought to be related to falling during a jump, temporal impact, and falling on a jump platform.[18] Mild snowboarding head injuries may rarely lead to chronic subdural hematoma, even in the absence of other predisposing factors.[20,21] Snowboarders suffering head injuries more frequently require longer terms of rehabilitation and ongoing care compared with skiers who have head injuries,[19] suggesting that the injuries themselves are more severe. Helmet use in snowboarders has shown similar efficacy as in skiers, leading to a reduction in head injury even after other risk factors have been considered.[10,11] As with downhill skiing, helmet use does not significantly increase the risk of cervical spine injuries in snowboarders.[12]

SLEDDING/TOBOGGANING

Injuries in sledding affect a larger and younger contingent of winter sport participants than injuries in skiing or snowboarding, likely owing to its easy accessibility, high speeds of descent, limited control and stability, and dangerous venues fraught with hazards such as trees, rocks, and roadways.[4,7] Sledding is the winter activity most commonly associated with admission to hospital for children under 16 years of age, with head injury being the most common diagnosis.[7] The average age of a severely injured sledder is 18.8 plus or minus 11.9 years; 12 years younger than the average skier, and more than 5 years younger than the average snowboarder.[4] More than half (59%) of injured children sledders are male. Injured children sledders are almost three times as likely to require hospital admission compared with children injured in other sports.[22,23] Although head injuries represent 13% of all sledding injuries in general, they account for 55% of severe sledding injuries.[4,22] In most pediatric studies examining sledding injuries requiring emergency department assessment, head/neck injuries are the most frequent type of injury.[24–26] Among childhood sledding injuries, younger children (≤6 yrs) are more likely to experience head/neck trauma compared with older children, with a relative risk of 2.60 ($P<.001$).[24] The most serious sledding injuries were incurred after the rider struck a tree or another stationary object in 60% and 76% of injuries.[25,26] Although the incidence of collisions with motor vehicles is low, these often have catastrophic consequences,[26,27] with head injury much more common.[28] Although many studies advocate helmet use for sledders, the efficacy of helmet use in sledding is uncertain, and there are no specific helmets designed for sledding.. Helmet use among sledders is significantly lower than for downhill skiing or snowboarding, with only about 3% of sledders wearing some form of head protection.[24] In addition to helmet use, familiarity with the terrain, proper lighting conditions, and proper supervision in children may also lower the risk of injury.

SNOWMOBILING

Snowmobiles are an increasingly popular form of winter recreation in Canada and the northern United States. Snowmobiles can weigh over 600 pounds, and reach speeds in excess of 90 mph.[29] Each year in North America more than 200 people die from injuries sustained while snowmobiling, and more than 14,000 people present to hospitals with snowmobile-related injuries.[29] Only 15% of snowmobile accidents take place on groomed trails, where 80% of riding occurs, whereas 31% occur on roadways.[29,30] Head injuries represent 13% to 34% of all snowmobiling injuries, and are the leading cause of snowmobile injury fatalities in both adult and pediatric populations.[30–34] Snowmobile fatalities have a strong male predominance.[29] Collision is the most common mechanism of injury in adult population snowmobilers, and is also the most common mechanism for fatality in the pediatric population.[30,33] In a study of severe snowmobile injuries presenting to a level 1 trauma care center in Manitoba over 10 years, 27.6% of patients died of their injuries.[30] Risk factors included excessive speed (54%), suboptimal lighting conditions (86%), and blood alcohol level greater than 0.08 (70%).[30] Fifty-four percent of accidents in the adult population involve excessive speed, compared with 33% in the pediatric population,[30,35] whereas alcohol is implicated in 40% to 70% of snowmobile-related fatalities.[29,30] Among cases with fatality, only 35% of riders were wearing a helmet in one study;[36] lack of helmet use should be considered a major risk factor for snowmobile injury death. For pediatric patients who had snowmobile injuries requiring admission to a trauma center, only 68% of children were wearing a helmet at the time of injury.[34] Moreover, whereas older children are more likely to suffer serious snowmobile related injuries, younger children are less likely to wear a helmet while snowmobiling.[34,35] A review of snowmobile legislation in states where pediatric deaths have occurred revealed that few helmet laws or age restrictions exist, and children as young as 8 years may legally operate a snowmobile in some jurisdictions.[33] Snowmobile injuries, including head injuries, may be reduced through initiatives such as trail development and improvement, driver education about intoxication and riding, innovative helmet use programs, and mandatory snowmobile registration and driver licensure.[36] In Sudbury, Ontario, a significant decrease in snowmobile related injuries and fatalities was noted after the institution of a community-based snowmobile policing program.[29]

ICE SKATING

Under the age of 18, head injuries compose 13.3% of ice skating injuries, compared with only 5.0% of in-line skating injuries and 4.4% of roller skating injuries. Ice skaters suffer five times as many concussions as in-line skaters, and seven times as many concussions as roller skaters.[37] Children injured while skating have a mean age of 10.9 years, with a male-to-female ratio of 1:1.[37] Most pediatric ice skating head injuries result from falls, which take place when the child is not wearing a helmet or other protective equipment.[37,38] Ice skating falls causing head injury are predominantly from falling forward, and involve head contact with the ice surface.[39] Helmet use is widely recommended as a means to reduce the risk of head injury in ice skating.[38,39] The observation that, during forward falls, the ice skater often attempts to brace against the ice with outstretched hands, has also led to the recommendation of a wrist-guard with a non-slip palm to protect the skater against head and wrist injury.[39] Although ice skating fatalities are rare, the authors recently were involved in a case of a helmetless 4-year-old female who died from a severe head injury after she fell while skating, following which she had another skater land on her.

There is a paucity of data regarding head injury in completive speed skaters.

ICE HOCKEY

Hockey-related injuries are covered in a separate article in this issue, but are covered briefly below.

With the exception of rare cases of intracranial hemorrhage, concussions compose the majority of head injury cases in ice hockey.[40] Moreover, concussion is the most common injury diagnosis overall in minor league, collegiate men's, and university women's ice hockey.[41–43] Because of a lack of appropriate studies and a noted trend of under-reporting of concussion throughout youth ice hockey organizations, the overall incidence of head injury in ice hockey is difficult to gauge.[40,44] Contact with an opposing player through body checking is the most common mechanism of concussion in hockey, followed by collision with the ice surface, or with the goal post or boards.[41,45,46] Smaller ice surfaces increase the risk of concussion among high level hockey players.[47] Ice hockey players experience 65% of their injuries during games, even though games account for only 23% of total exposures.[42] In addition to mandatory helmet use in organized hockey, other methods of injury prevention have been considered. In a large study examining head injuries presenting to American emergency departments,[48] it was noted that the rate of concussion for ice hockey players dropped significantly the same year that USA Hockey implemented stricter rules surrounding body checking. The one-time showing of a hockey-specific injury prevention video to 11- to 12-year-old Canadian minor hockey players resulted in fewer body checking related penalties, as well as an increase in the ability of players to name common mechanisms of head and spinal cord injuries in hockey.[49] Although controversial, some critics have advocated for the delay of the introduction of body contact in minor hockey until the age of 16 as a means of reducing the incidence of concussion in ice hockey. When the authors began playing minor hockey in the early 1970s and 1980s, full body contact was prior to 6 years of age, whereas Hockey Canada has since instituted rules that disallow body contact in hockey leagues until the age of 11.

SUMMARY

The most common theme among head injuries related to winter sports is speed, because skiing, snowboarding, snowmobiling, sledding, ice skating and ice hockey can all be associated with high speeds. Not surprisingly, the pairing of speed with a slippery surface, be it snow or ice, commonly results in a loss of control and subsequent injury. For virtually every winter-related sporting activity in which head injury can occur, the use of a protective helmet, usually activity or sport specific, has been shown to reduce both the incidence and severity of head injury. The authors are strong advocates for legislated helmet use in high-risk activities, especially among children, who should also participate in public awareness programs demonstrating the importance of helmet use.

REFERENCES

1. Levy AS, Hawkes AP, Hemminger LM, et al. An analysis of head injuries among skiers and snowboarders. J Trauma 2002;53(4):695–704.
2. Fukuda O, Takaba M, Saito T, et al. Head injuries in snowboarders compared with head injuries in skiers. A prospective analysis of 1076 patients from 1994 to 1999 in Niigata, Japan. Am J Sports Med 2001;29(4):437–40.
3. Hagel BE, Pless IB, Platt RW. Trends in emergency department reported head and neck injuries among skiers and snowboarders. Can J Public Health 2003; 94(6):458–62.
4. Federiuk CS, Schlueter JL, Adams AL. Skiing, snowboarding, and sledding injuries in a northwestern state. Wilderness Environ Med 2002;13(4):245–9.
5. Xiang H, Stallones L, Smith GA. Downhill skiing injury fatalities among children. Inj Prev 2004;10:99–102.

6. Diamond PT, Gale SD, Denkhaus HK. Head injuries in skiers: an analysis of injury severity and outcome. Brain Inj 2001;15(5):429–34.

7. Hackam DJ, Kreller M, Pearl RH. Snow-related recreational injuries in children: assessment of morbidity and management strategies. J Pediatr Surg 1999;34(1): 65–8 [discussion: 69].

8. Skokan EG, Junkins EP Jr, Kadish H. Serious winter sport injuries in children and adolescents requiring hospitalization. Am J Emerg Med 2003;21(2):95–9.

9. Xiang H, Stallones L. Deaths associated with snow skiing in Colorado 1980–1981 to 2000–2001 ski seasons. Injury 2003;34(12):892–6.

10. Sulheim S, Holme I, Ekeland A, et al. Helmet use and risk of head injuries in alpine skiers and snowboarders. JAMA 2006;295(8):919–24.

11. Hagel BE, Pless IB, Goulet C, et al. Effectiveness of helmets in skiers and snowboarders: case-control and case crossover study. BMJ 2005;330(7486):281–5.

12. Macnab AJ, Smith T, Gagnon FA, et al. Effect of helmet wear on the incidence of head/face and cervical spine injuries in young skiers and snowboarders. Inj Prev 2002;8(4):324–7.

13. Hennessey T, Morgan SJ, Elliot JP, et al. Helmet availability at skiing and snowboarding rental shops. a survey of Colorado ski resort rental practices. Am J Prev Med 2002;22(2):110–2.

14. McCrory P. The role of helmets in skiing and snowboarding. Br J Sports Med 2002;36(5):314.

15. Ferrera PC, McKenna DP, Gilman EA. Injury patterns with snowboarding. Am J Emerg Med 1999;17(6):575–7.

16. Yamagami T, Ishihara H, Kimura T. Clinical features of snowboarding injuries. J Orthop Sci 2004;9(3):225–9.

17. Hagel BE, Goulet C, Platt RW, et al. Injuries among skiers and snowboarders in Quebec. Epidemiology 2004;15(3):279–86.

18. Nakaguchi H, Fujimaki T, Ueki K, et al. Snowboard head injury: prospective study in Chino, Nagano, for two seasons from 1995 to 1997. J Trauma 1999;46(6): 1066–9.

19. Hentschel S, Hader W, Boyd M. Head injuries in skiers and snowboarders in British Columbia. Can J Neurol Sci 2001;28(1):42–6.

20. Uzura M, Taguchi Y, Matsuzawa M, et al. Chronic subdural haematoma after snowboard head injury. Br J Sports Med 2003;37(1):82–3.

21. Rajan GP, Zellweger R. Half pipe snowboarding: an (un)forgettable experience or an increasing risk of head injury? Br J Sports Med 2004;38(6):e35.

22. Voaklander DC, Kelly KD, Sukrani N, et al. Sledding injuries in patients presenting to the emergency department in a northern city. Acad Emerg Med 2001;8(6): 629–35.

23. Wynne AD, Bota GW, Rowe BH. Sledding trauma in a northeastern Ontario community. J Trauma 1994;37(5):820–5.

24. Ortega HW, Shields BJ, Smith GA. Sledding-related injuries among children requiring emergency treatment. Pediatr Emerg Care 2005;21(12):839–43.

25. Shorter NA, Mooney DP, Harmon BJ. Childhood sledding injuries. Am J Emerg Med 1999;17(1):32–4.

26. Kim PC, Haddock G, Bohn D, et al. Tobogganing injuries in children. J Pediatr Surg 1995;30(8):1135–7.

27. Lee F, Osmond MH, Vaidyanathan CP, et al. Descriptive study of sledding injuries in Canadian children. Inj Prev 1999;5(3):198–202.

28. Rowe BH, Bota GW. Sledding deaths in Ontario. Can Fam Physician 1994;40: 68–71.

29. Pierz JJ. Snowmobile injuries in North America. Clin Orthop 2003;409:29–36.
30. Stewart RL, Black GB. Snowmobile trauma: 10 years' experience at Manitoba's tertiary trauma centre. Can J Surg 2004;47(2):90–4.
31. Beilman GJ, Brasel KJ, Dittrich K, et al. Risk factors and patterns of injury in snowmobile crashes. Wilderness Environ Med 1999;10(4):226–32.
32. Sy ML, Corden TE. The perils of snowmobiling. WMJ 2005;104(2):32–4.
33. Rice MR, Avanos L, Kenney B. Snowmobile injuries and deaths in children: a review of national injury data and legislation. Pediatrics 2000;105(3 Pt 1):615–9.
34. Decou JM, Fagerman LE, Riopele D, et al. Snowmobile injuries and fatalities in children. J Pediatr Surg 2003;38(5):784–7.
35. Nayci A, Stavlo PL, Zarroug AE, et al. Snowmobile injuries in children and adolescents. Mayo Clin Proc 2006;81(1):39–44.
36. Landen MG, Middaugh J, Dannenberg AL. Injuries associated with snowmobiles, Alaska, 1993–1994. Public Health Rep 1999;114(1):48–52.
37. Knox CL, Comstock RD, McGeehan J, et al. Differences in the risk associated with head injury for pediatric ice skaters, roller skaters, and in-line skaters. Pediatrics 2006;118(2):549–54.
38. McGeehan J, Shields BJ, Smith GA. Children should wear helmets while ice-skating: a comparison of skating-related injuries. Pediatrics 2004;114(1):124–8.
39. Knox CL, Comstock RD. Video analysis of falls experienced by paediatric ice skaters and roller/inline skaters. Br J Sports Med 2006;40(3):268–71.
40. Toth C, McNeil S, Feasby T. Central nervous system injuries in sport and recreation: a systematic review. Sports Med 2005;35(8):685–715.
41. Emery CA, Meeuwisse WH. Injury rates, risk factors, and mechanisms of injury in hockey. Am J Sports Med 2006;34(12):1960–9.
42. Filk K, Lyman S, Marx RG. American collegiate men's ice hockey: an analysis of injuries. Am J Sports Med 2005;33(2):183–7.
43. Schick DM, Meeuwisse WH. Injury rates and profiles in female ice hockey players. Am J Sports Med 2003;31(1):47–52.
44. Williamson IJS, Goodman D. Converging evidence for the under-reporting of concussions in youth ice hockey. Br J Sports Med 2006;40(2):128–32.
45. Goodman D, Gaetz M, Meichenbaum D. Concussions in hockey: there is cause for concern. Med Sci Sports Exerc 2001;33(12):2004–9.
46. Delaney JS, Puni V, Rouah F. Mechanisms of injury for concussions in university football, ice hockey, and soccer: a pilot study. Clin J Sport Med 2006;16(2):162–5.
47. Wennberg R. Effect of ice surface size on collision rates and head impacts at the world junior hockey championships, 2002 to 2004. Clin J Sport Med 2005;15(2):67–72.
48. Delaney JS. Head injuries presenting to emergency departments in the united states from 1990 to 1999 for ice hockey, soccer, and football. Clin J Sport Med 2004;14(2):80–7.
49. Cook DJ, Cusimano MD, Tator CH, et al. Evaluation of the *ThinkFirst Canada, Smart Hockey Brain and Spinal Cord Injury Prevention* video. Inj Prev 2003;9(4):361–6.

Index

Note: Page numbers of article titles are in **boldface** type.

A

AAN. See *American Academy of Neurology (AAN).*
Acidosis, in peripheral fatigue, 166
Age, as factor in return-to-play decision, 47–48
ß-Agonists, adverse effects of, 142
All-terrain vehicle riding, peripheral nerve injuries related to, 94
All-terrain-vehicle riding, nervous system injuries related to, epidemiology of, 15–16
American Academy of Neurology (AAN), 40
American Orthopedic Society for Sports Medicine (AOSSM), 45
Amino acid oxidation, during endurance exercise, 105
Anabolic agents, adverse effects of, 140
AOSSM. See *American Orthopedic Society for Sports Medicine (AOSSM).*
Appetite suppressants, adverse effects of, 144
Archery, peripheral nerve injuries related to, 77, 86
Arm wrestling, peripheral nerve injuries related to, 79
Aromatase inhibitors, adverse effects of, 142
Arterial gas embolism, scuba diving and, 267–268
Athlete(s), PEDs and, **133–148.** See also *Performance-enhancement drugs (PEDs).*
Athlete morningness/eveningness scale, in pilot study of sleep quality and circadian sleep phase in competitive athletes, 154–155
Australian rules football
    head injuries related to, biomechanical aspects of, 34
    nervous system injuries related to, epidemiology of, 14
    peripheral nerve injuries related to, 93
Auto racing
    nervous system injuries related to, epidemiology of, 2
    peripheral nerve injuries related to, 79
Axillary neuropathy, in baseball players, 182–185
    anatomy related to, 182
    causes of, 182–183
    clinical evaluation of, 183
    treatment of, 184–185

B

Ballet dancing, peripheral nerve injuries related to, 79
Baseball
    biomechanics in, 175–177
    catastrophic spine injuries related to, considerations for, 66
    described, 175
    nervous system injuries related to, epidemiology of, 2–3
    peripheral nerve injuries related to, 79, 80, 84–85

Phys Med Rehabil Clin N Am 20 (2009) 295–311
doi:10.1016/S1047-9651(08)00106-X
1047-9651/08/$ – see front matter © 2009 Elsevier Inc. All rights reserved.

pmr.theclinics.com

Moving?

Make sure your subscription moves with you!

To notify us of your new address, find your **Clinics Account Number** (located on your mailing label above your name), and contact customer service at:

E-mail: elspcs@elsevier.com

800-654-2452 (subscribers in the U.S. & Canada)
314-453-7041 (subscribers outside of the U.S. & Canada)

Fax number: 314-523-5170

Elsevier Periodicals Customer Service
11830 Westline Industrial Drive
St. Louis, MO 63146

*To ensure uninterrupted delivery of your subscription, please notify us at least 4 weeks in advance of move.

Printed and bound by CPI Group (UK) Ltd, Croydon, CR0 4YY

03/10/2024

01040462-0010